Respiratory Endoscopy

Takehiro Izumo • Shinji Sasada
Tomohiko Aso • Kazuko Nasu • Yasuaki Arai
Editors

Respiratory Endoscopy

With contributions by Christine Chavez

Springer

Editors
Takehiro Izumo
Department of Respiratory Medicine
Japanese Red Cross Medical Center
Tokyo, Japan

Tomohiko Aso
Department of Radiological Techonology
National Cancer Center Hospital
Tokyo, Japan

Yasuaki Arai
Department of Diagnostic Radiology
National Cancer Center Hospital
Tokyo, Japan

Shinji Sasada
Department of Respiratory Medicine
Tokyo Saiseikai Central Hospital
Tokyo, Japan

Kazuko Nasu
Nursing Service Department
National Cancer Center Hospital
Tokyo, Japan

Original Japanese edition published by Iryo Kagakusha, INC., Tokyo, 2015

This English translation is based on; Kokyuki Naishikyou Jissen Manual by Takehiro Izumo

ISBN 978-981-13-5726-8 ISBN 978-981-287-916-5 (eBook)
DOI 10.1007/978-981-287-916-5

Softcover re-print of the Hardcover 1st edition 2017

Printed on acid-free paper

This Springer imprint is published by Springer Nature
The registered company is Springer Nature Singapore Pte Ltd.
The registered company address is: 152 Beach Road, #22-06/08 Gateway East, Singapore 189721, Singapore

Preface

Respiratory endoscopy is an essential tool in cases of both malignant diseases, such as lung cancer, and non-malignant diseases, such as interstitial pneumonia. In 1966, flexible bronchoscopy was developed and first introduced at the National Cancer Center, Japan, by Dr. Shigeto Ikeda. Fifty years later, the basic procedure has dramatically evolved to include a myriad of techniques for both diagnosis and treatment.

In Japan, the current clinical practice of respiratory endoscopy, such as transbronchial biopsy for peripheral lung lesions, frequently employs X-ray fluoroscopy guidance. In this book, we describe in detail the applications of respiratory endoscopy procedures combined with X-ray fluoroscopy. At our institution, improvements in the techniques have been possible through close collaboration with radiologic technologists, who work with us in ensuring procedural quality and safety, including radiation exposure management.

The topics in this book are descriptions of the actual work that we do, with emphasis on respiratory endoscopy, a field that is deep-rooted in this hospital. All authors are current or former doctors, nurses, and radiologic technologists who were engaged in practice at the National Cancer Center, Japan. We thank all the contributing authors who shared their expertise in this book.

In recent years, medical care has realized the value of a team approach, with contributions from all healthcare workers. In this book, we discuss the components of a concerted effort among doctors, nurses, and radiologic technicians in delivering quality service, particularly for a minimally invasive procedure such as respiratory endoscopy. After all, developing an efficient and safe medical system cannot be accomplished single-handedly, even by the most skilled individual. Lastly, we hope that this book will help aspiring respiratory endoscopists in learning and, potentially, further improving this craft.

Tokyo, Japan

Takehiro Izumo
Shinji Sasada
Tomohiko Aso
Kazuko Nasu
Yasuaki Arai

Pasig, Philippines

Christine Chavez

May 2016

Contents

Part I Edition for Radiological Technicians

1 **The Role of X-Ray Fluoroscopy in Bronchoscopy** 3
Yuichi Nagai and Yuzuru Kouno

2 **Development of X-Ray Fluoroscopy Devices** 9
Mayumi Kitagawa and Yuzuru Kouno

3 **Characteristics of X-ray Fluoroscopy** 13
Yuichi Nagai and Yuzuru Kouno

4 **Image Processing in X-Ray Fluoroscopy and Digital Tomography** 17
Jun Torii and Yuzuru Kouno

5 **Quality Control in X-Ray Fluoroscopy and Digital Tomography** 27
Takumi Iwase and Yuzuru Kouno

6 **Computed Tomography Imaging to Bronchoscopic Navigation** 33
Hirobumi Nagasawa and Yuzuru Kouno

Part II Edition for Doctors

7 **Fluorographic and Radiographic Conditions in Bronchoscopy Using X-Ray Fluoroscopy** 41
Yuichi Nagai, Takehiro Izumo, and Yuzuru Kouno

8 **Identification of the Involved Bronchus to Peripheral Pulmonary Lesions on Computed Tomography** 47
Takaaki Tsuchida

9 **Anesthesia for Bronchoscopy** 53
Masahiro Katsurada and Takehiro Izumo

10 **Processing Samples** ... 59
Takaaki Tsuchida and Takehiro Izumo

11 **Rapid On-Site Cytology Evaluation** ... 67
Takaaki Tsuchida and Takehiro Izumo

12 **Type and Selection of Flexible Bronchoscope** ... 75
Shinji Sasada

13 **Latest in Bronchoscopy (High-Vision Scope with Rotation Function)** ... 85
Takehiro Izumo

14 **Basic Flexible Bronchoscopy** ... 91
Shinji Sasada

15 **Tomography-Guided Transbronchial Biopsy for Peripheral Pulmonary Lesions** ... 103
Takehiro Izumo

16 **Radial Endobronchial Ultrasound Findings** ... 109
Takehiro Izumo

17 **Radial EBUS Findings for Ground Glass Opacity: Comparison of Radiologic and Pathologic Findings** ... 117
Takehiro Izumo

18 **Endobronchial Ultrasound with a Guide Sheath for Peripheral Pulmonary Lesions** ... 125
Yuji Matsumoto and Takehiro Izumo

19 **Transbronchial Needle Aspiration Through a Guide Sheath for Peripheral Pulmonary Lesions** ... 137
Moto Takai and Takehiro Izumo

20 **Virtual Bronchoscopic Navigation for Peripheral Pulmonary Lesions** ... 143
Yuji Matsumoto and Takehiro Izumo

21 **Virtual Bronchoscopic Simulation by CT Workstation** ... 151
Yuji Matsumoto, Takehiro Izumo, and Yasuyuki Mizumori

22 **The Dose and Risk Factors for Radiation Exposure from X-Ray Fluoroscopy During EBUS-GS for Peripheral Pulmonary Lesions** ... 159
Masahiro Katsurada and Takehiro Izumo

23 **Endobronchial Ultrasound-Guided Transbronchial Needle Aspiration** ... 163
Hibiki Udagawa and Takehiro Izumo

24 Endobronchial Ultrasound Elastography 177
Takehiro Izumo

25 Flex-Rigid Pleuroscopy Under Local Anesthesia 183
Yukio Watanabe and Shinji Sasada

26 Stent Placement Under X-Ray Fluoroscopy 205
Shinji Sasada

27 Therapeutic Bronchoscopy for Central Airway Obstruction (Balloon, Argon Plasma Coagulation, High Frequency) 213
Yukio Watanabe and Shinji Sasada

28 Endoscopic Bronchial Occlusion with Silicone Spigots 219
Yasuyuki Mizumori and Shinji Sasada

29 Photodynamic Therapy for Lung Cancer 229
Takaaki Tsuchida and Takehiro Izumo

Part III Edition for Nurses

30 Actual Nursing in Respiratory Endoscopy 245
Akiko Kobayashi, Sugako Hirata, Mayumi Ohga, Akemi Sakatsume, Kaori Shimada, and Junko Kaneko

Part I
Edition for Radiological Technicians

Chapter 1
The Role of X-Ray Fluoroscopy in Bronchoscopy

Yuichi Nagai and Yuzuru Kouno

Abstract X-ray fluoroscopy is one of the ways to make real-time observations of the internal anatomic structures of a patient. This technique has been applied in the field of interventional radiology and during bronchoscopy, myelography, and digestive tract contrast inspection. With the use of barium sulfate and iodine-based or oily contrast media, radiography may be enhanced for better imaging. For bronchoscopy, high-quality fluoroscopy and multidirectional radiography are needed while maintaining the lowest possible radiation exposure dose to the staff and patients. To ensure efficient and safe imaging procedures, domestic regulation limits should be applied.

Keywords X-ray fluoroscopy • Radiation control of medical staff • Bronchoscopy

1.1 Introduction

X-ray fluoroscopy is one of the ways to visualize the internal structures of a subject in real time. This technique has been constantly applied in interventional radiology, bronchoscopy, myelography, and digestive tract contrast inspection. With the use of barium sulfate and iodine-based or oily contrast media, radiography may be enhanced for better imaging. Table 1.1 indicates the components of X-ray fluoroscopy equipment.

There has been an ongoing discussion on the increased radiation dose absorbed from medical imaging [1]. In 1980, medical imaging accounted for 15% of the average annual radiation exposure of the US population (0.54 out of 3.6 mSv/year);

Y. Nagai
Department of Radiology, National Hospital Organization East Saitama National Hospital, 4147, Kurohama, Hasuda, Saitama 349-0196, Japan

Y. Kouno (✉)
Department of Radiological Technology, National Cancer Center Hospital, 5-1-1, Tsukiji Chuo-ku, Tokyo 104-0045, Japan
e-mail: ykouno@ncc.go.jp

T. Izumo et al. (eds.), *Respiratory Endoscopy*,
DOI 10.1007/978-981-287-916-5_1

Table 1.1 Components of X-ray fluoroscopy

No	Components
1.	Power supply
2.	X-ray tube bulb
3.	Fluoroscopy and radiography
4.	Imaging by DR or FPD[a]
5.	Image display

[a]*DR* digital radiography, *FPD* flat panel detector

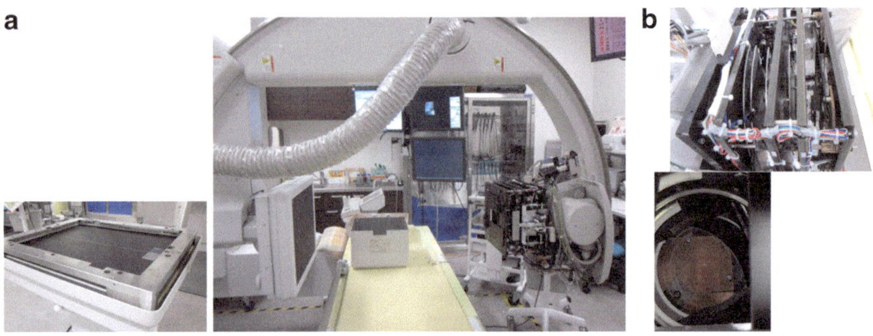

Fig. 1.1 The ideal setup of an X-ray fluoroscopy equipment. (**a**) An X-ray grid is installed in front of an X-ray detector. (**b**) Metal filters are installed close to the X-ray tube bulb

in 2006, this proportion has grown to 50% (3.0 out of 6.0 mSv/year) [2]. Although this increasing trend of radiation exposure was due to the more frequent use of computed tomography (CT) and nuclear cardiology, new techniques that reduce radiation dose to patients and staff are strongly desired.

Figure 1.1 shows an ideal setup of an X-ray fluoroscopy. We underscore that the quality and measurement of the metal filter greatly affect both the amount of radiation exposure and image quality. Providing a comfortable procedure to patients is also important to ensure long-lasting clinical examination and treatment. Figure 1.2 is a good example showing sponge mat.

1.2 X-Ray Fluoroscopy Equipment for Bronchoscopy

Multidirectional fluorography and high-quality radiography images are needed for bronchoscopy. Figure 1.3 illustrates an example setup that is equipped with C-arm and over tube. Information about the clinical demands, space of the room, etc. is necessary in order to select a suitable device. Multipurpose X-ray fluoroscopy may be recommended when the purpose is for use during diagnostic and therapeutic endoscopy procedures, both respiratory and gastrointestinal. Some ancillary and peripheral devices would be needed for fluoroscopy during bronchoscopy (Fig. 1.4). These are enumerated below:

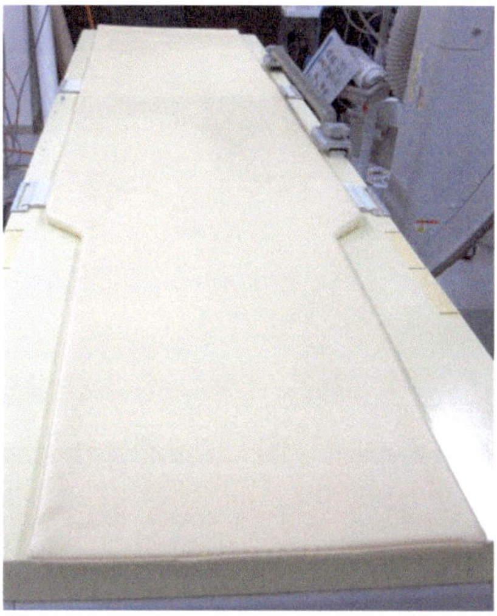

Fig. 1.2 An example of X-ray fluoroscopy accessory, such as a mattress, that is especially designed to ensure patient comfort during procedures

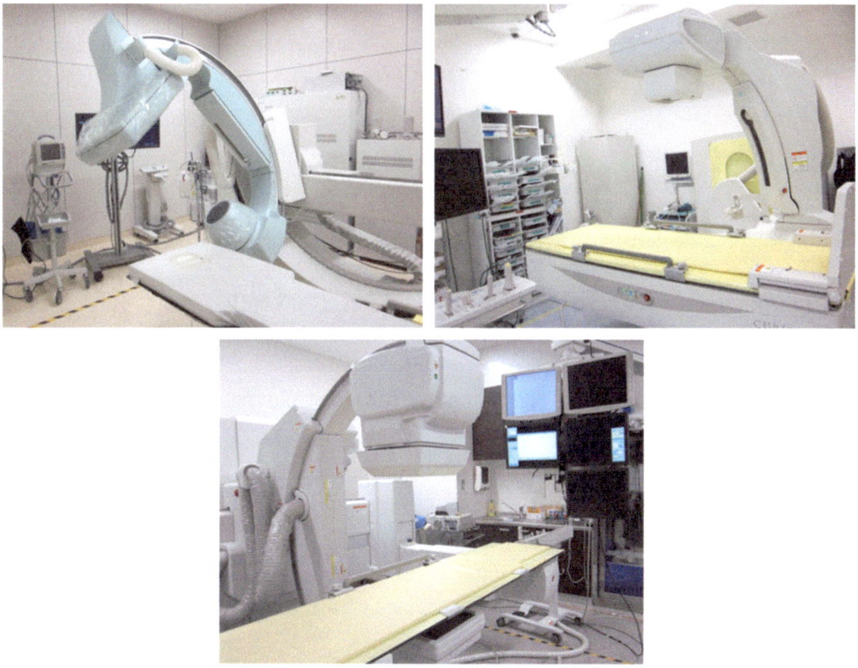

Fig. 1.3 The X-ray fluoroscopy system includes a C-arm-type under tube, an over tube, and a C-arm-type over tube

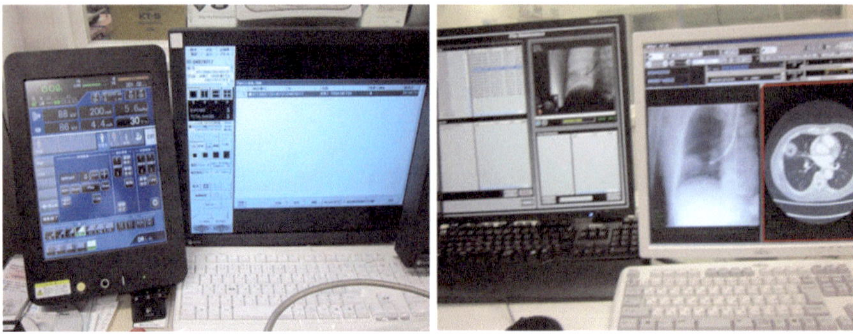

Fig. 1.4 Ancillary devices for the X-ray fluoroscopy equipment

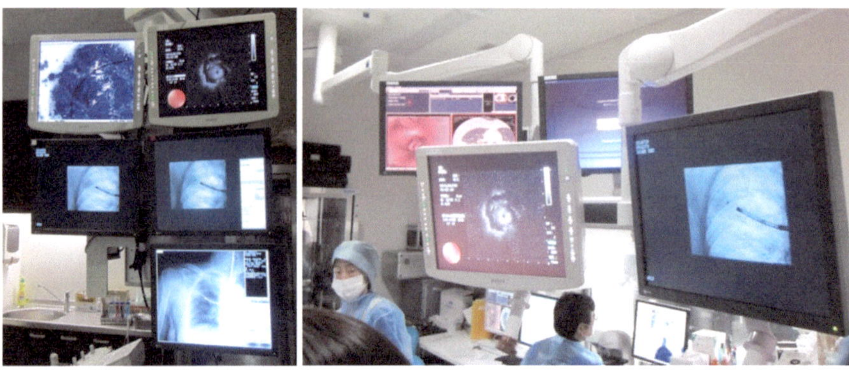

Fig. 1.5 Monitors in the examination room

1. Control panel to regulate acquisition parameters
2. Image display monitor for data processing, as well as for reference of past data
3. Image display monitor for the radiography image
4. Video recording apparatus and computer for video playback and display
5. Electronic medical record

Two monitors for radiography and fluorography are essential for the doctor who will perform the clinical procedure. Some manufacturers provide monitors that can simultaneously display the medical records of patients and reconstructed bronchoscopy navigation images from CT data. Each institution should choose a system to fulfill their particular clinical purpose and needs (Fig. 1.5).

1.3 Dose Control for Staff During Bronchoscopy

Radiation dose to the staff must be recorded and reported to their employer, who is responsible for radiation protection. The European Atomic Energy Community published the Directive 96/29 Euratom – ionizing radiation to establish uniform basic

Table 1.2 Dose limits according to the Euratom Council Directive 96–29 [3]

	Effective dose	Equivalent dose		
	Whole body	Eye lens	Skin	Extremities
Exposed workers	20 mSv per year[a]	150 mSv	500 mSv/cm^2	500 mSv
	Max. 50 mSv in 1 year			

[a]Average value over a 5-year period

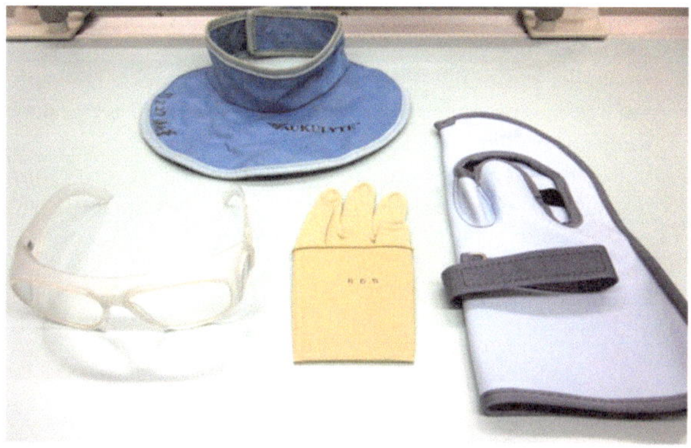

Fig. 1.6 Apparatus for radiation exposure protection

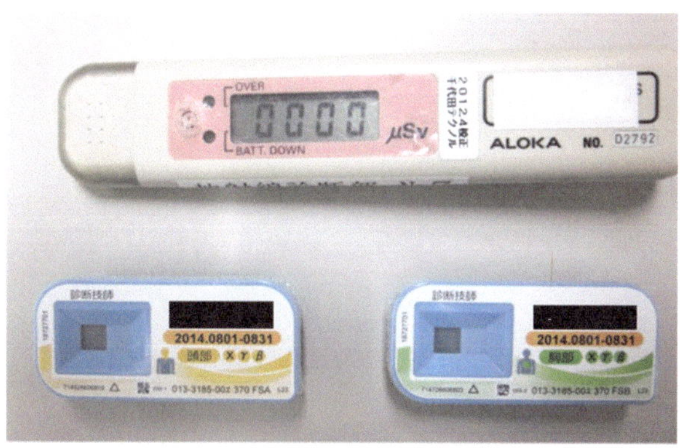

Fig. 1.7 Wearable radiation dosimetry

safety standards to protect the health of workers (Table 1.2) [3]. Each staff working in the bronchoscopy unit must wear a personal dosimeter (glass badge or electric dosimeter) (Fig. 1.6) and an apparatus for radiation exposure protection, such as a lead gown, during the procedure (Fig. 1.7). Dosimeters should be worn at an appropriate position and working practices should be evaluated [4]. If an individual is to be exposed at a high radiation level that is close to the limit, special attention and instruction should be given to optimize administered radiation dose [5].

Dealing with staff exposure is an everyday challenge. Appropriate shielding devices and robust safety regulation programs are required for each institution. Staff radiation dose must be maintained as low as possible and at reasonably achievable levels without compromising best patient care.

References

1. Amis ES, Butler PF, Applegate KE, et al. American college of radiology white paper on radiation dose in medicine. J Am Coll Radiol. 4:272–84.
2. National Council on Radiation Protection and Measurement. Ionizing radiation exposure of the population of the United States, Report NCRP 93. Washington, DC: National Council on Radiation Protection and Measurement; 1987.
3. Council Directive 96/29 Euratom of 13 May 1996 laying down the basic safety standards for the protection of the health of workers and the general public against the dangers arising from ionizing radiation.
4. Donadille L, Carinou E, Ginjaume M, Jankowski J, Rimpler A, Sans Merce M, et al. An overview of the use of extremity dosimeters in some European countries for medical applications. Radiant Prot Dosim. 2008;131:62–6.
5. ICRP (International Commission on Radiological Protection). 1990 recommendations of the international commission on radiological protection 60. Oxford: Program Press; 1991.

Chapter 2
Development of X-Ray Fluoroscopy Devices

Mayumi Kitagawa and Yuzuru Kouno

Abstract Radiology has evolved over the past 120 years since it was introduced by Wilhelm Röentgen. Photomultipliers, which enable visualization of weak photons to improve diagnostic radiology, were invented in 1955. Since 1961, remotely operated X-ray fluoroscopy has been developed; this was followed by widespread clinical application of the image intensifier (I.I.) system for analog fluoroscopy in the 1980s. Ten years after, fluoroscopy was further enhanced by image intensifier digital radiography (IIDR), which began to be utilized in the clinics in the 1990s.

Keywords Photomultiplier • Image intensifier • Image intensifier digital radiography

2.1 Photomultiplier

Wilhelm Röentgen produced and detected X-rays on November 8, 1895; soon after in October 1896, the use of radiography was started in Japan. However, a diagnostic system was not established then because of some technical difficulties with fluorescent screens. In the 1950s, the invention of an image intensifier (I.I.) system drastically improved diagnostic radiology (Fig. 2.1) by allowing low-intensity X-rays to be converted to bright light outputs that may be visible even in lighted rooms. The addition of a camera enabled separate and remote visualization of the images to reduce the risk of radiation exposure. With these innovations, it was possible to view images on screen under normal lighting conditions; subsequent improvements included coupling of video cameras to enable recording of cine images and electronic storage of still images.

M. Kitagawa • Y. Kouno (✉)
Department of Radiological Technology, National Cancer Center Hospital,
5-1-1, Tsukiji, Chuo-ku, Tokyo 104-0045, Japan
e-mail: ykouno@ncc.go.jp

T. Izumo et al. (eds.), *Respiratory Endoscopy*,
DOI 10.1007/978-981-287-916-5_2

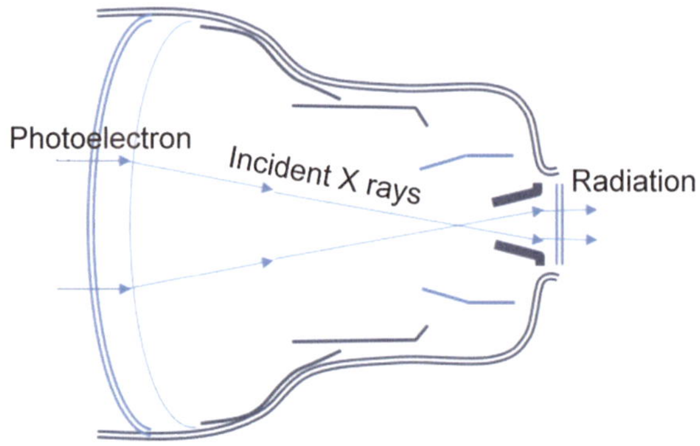

Fig. 2.1 An example of an image intensifier system

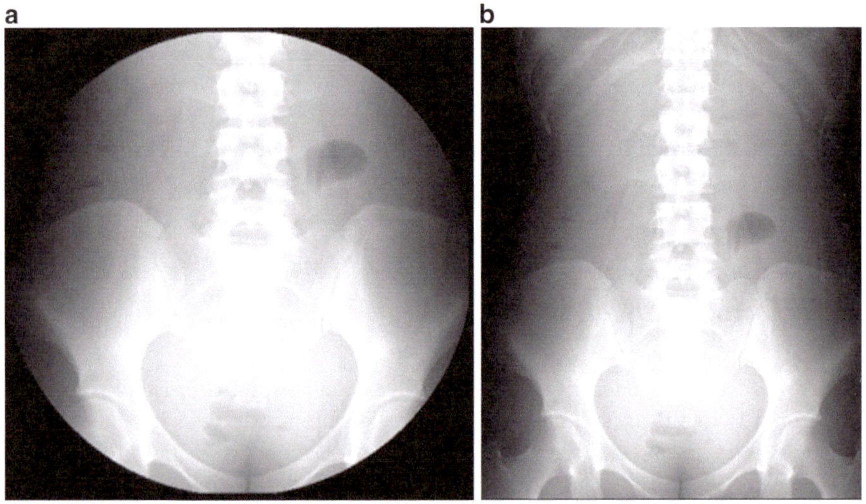

Fig. 2.2 Further improvements in diagnostic radiology. (**a**) An example image in image intensifier and digital radiography (*IIDR*) system. (**b**) An example image in flat panel detector (*FPD*) system

2.2 Analog and Digital X-Rays

Originally, all X-ray images were recorded on film and real-time visualization was not possible. In 1988, a system that utilizes C-arm type of X-ray fluoroscopy was developed and has become an essential technique during bronchoscopy. The factors for analog and digital imaging are basically the same. A sensor converts X-rays into a medium, followed by conversion of the image signal from analog to digital (a–d) format and transfer into a computer.

Imaging plates (IPs) enable efficient imaging recording. In the 1990s, image intensifier digital radiography (IIDR) system and flat panel detector (FPD) system, in which a conventionally produced image is digitalized (Figs. 2.2 and 2.3), were

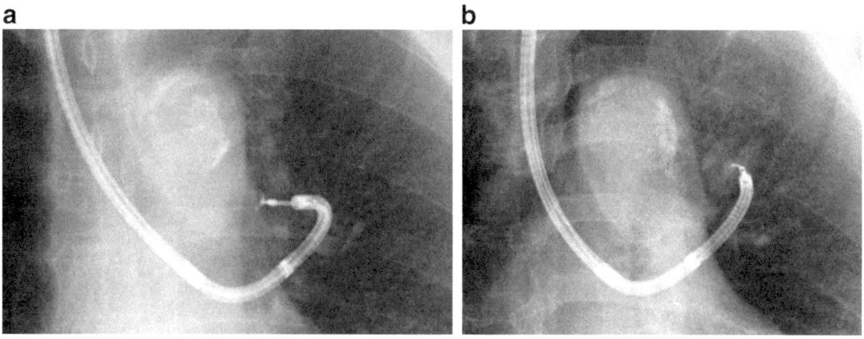

Fig. 2.3 Examples of X-ray fluoroscopic imaging in bronchoscopy. (**a**) Anterior-posterior projection. (**b**) Left anterior projection of 20°

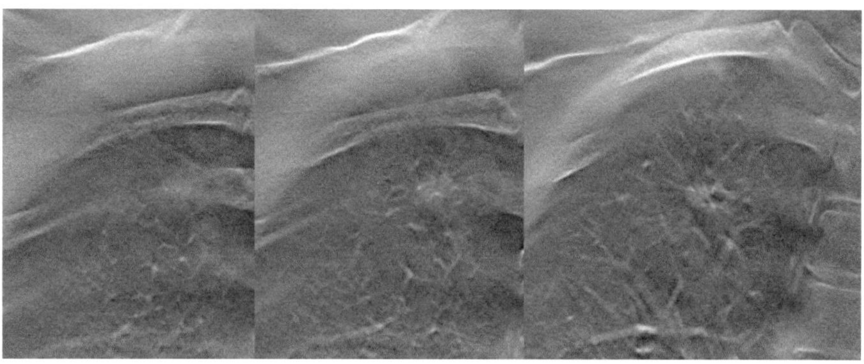

Fig. 2.4 An example of tomosynthesis

invented for fluoroscopy and fluorography. However, questions on the substantial advantages of digital processing still remain.

2.3 Latest Technology

A new technique, tomosynthesis (Fig. 2.4), enables acquisition of information on depth of a subject. Advanced computed tomography (CT) imaging techniques and work stations produce three-dimensional (3D) images to help operators navigate and capture images of microscopic abnormalities (Fig. 2.5). A 3D CT scan allows fast and high-quality imaging of organs, blood vessels, bones, etc. (Fig. 2.6a). Each CT image is layered on top of another to form a virtual model (Fig. 2.6b); this enables more precise depiction of anatomical structures, as well as structural defects, tumors, and lesions, compared with conventional radiology techniques.

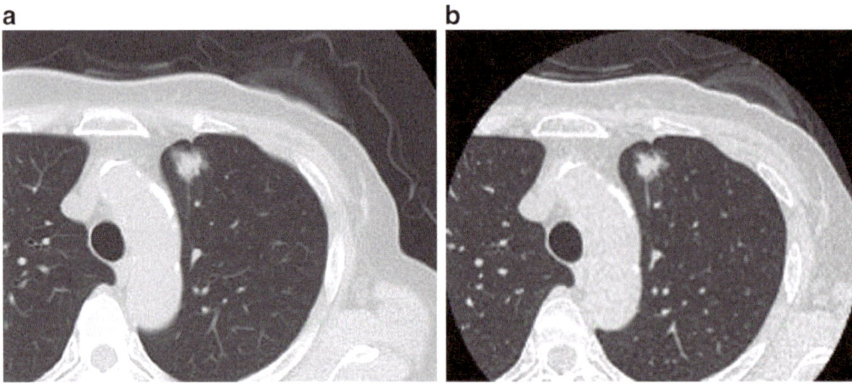

Fig. 2.5 Computed tomography imaging. (**a**) Slice thickness of 5 mm. (**b**) Slice thickness 1 mm

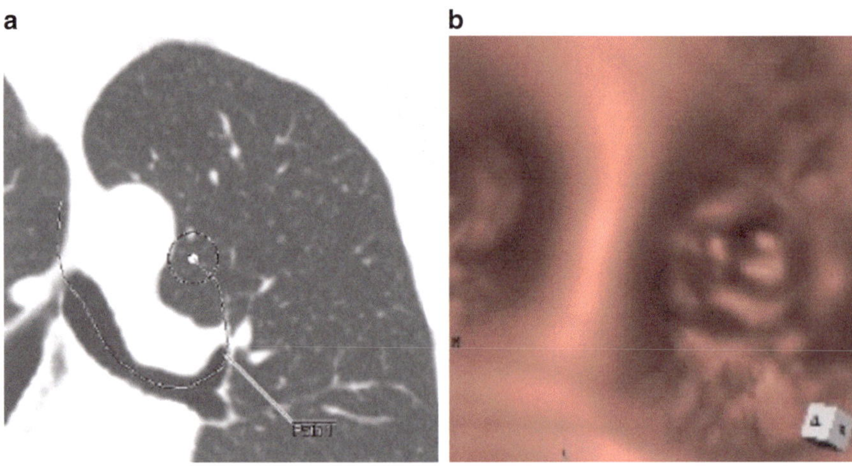

Fig. 2.6 Reconstructed computed tomography imaging. (**a**) Multiplanar reconstruction (*MPR*). (**b**) Volume-rendered 3D CT imaging

Bibliography

1. Hirano H. Digital de Yomigaeru Tomosynthesis no Sekai. Innervision. 2011;26(7):2–3.
2. Houshasen Gijutsushi Hensan Tokubetsu Iinkai. X-Ray Souchi・X-Ray Kan Oyobi Fuzokuhin. In: Nihon Houshasen Gijutsushi Vol. 1, 2000. http://www.jsrt.or.jp/data/about/outline-02/. Accessed 29 June 2016.
3. Kansai-chiku CR Kenkyukai. FCR Cho-kiso Kouza. Tokyo: Iryo Kagakusha; 2013.
4. Makino S. Nihon no Houshasen-kiki Sengo Hattenshi (Zempen). Nihon Houshasen Gijutsu Gakkai Zasshi. 2000;56(10):1181–93.

Chapter 3
Characteristics of X-ray Fluoroscopy

Yuichi Nagai and Yuzuru Kouno

Abstract The quality of x-ray fluoroscopy images relates with radiation exposure. The appropriate parameters for image acquisition and reconstruction should be established by balancing image quality and radiation exposure to the patient. X-ray fluoroscopy is equipped with either over or under x-ray tube, each of which has its own characteristics and should be chosen according to the clinical need.

Keywords Under x-ray tube • Over x-ray tube

3.1 Characteristics of X-ray Fluoroscopy Device

Figure 3.1 shows three commercially available x-ray fluoroscopy devices, which are equipped with a flat panel detector (FPD) that converts x-rays into signals and pictures. There are two types of FPDs: one directly converts x-rays into pictures, whereas the other converts x-rays into pictures after improvement. Each manufacturer has its unique parameter for radiography and fluorography acquisition. Figure 3.2 shows the correlation among tube voltage, acrylic plate depth, and fluoroscopic dosage rate for each device. Each device has its unique characteristics, which is the result of additional filter and pulse x-rays. The initial settings of radiography machines vary among devices, and users should optimize the parameters for image acquisition and reconstruction (Fig. 3.3).

Y. Nagai
Department of Radiology, National Hospital Organization, East Saitama National Hospital, 4147, Kurohama, Hasuda, Saitama 349-0196, Japan

Y. Kouno (✉)
Department of Radiological Technology, National Cancer Center Hospital, 5-1-1, Tsukiji Chuo-ku, Tokyo 104-0045, Japan
e-mail: ykouno@ncc.go.jp

T. Izumo et al. (eds.), *Respiratory Endoscopy*,
DOI 10.1007/978-981-287-916-5_3

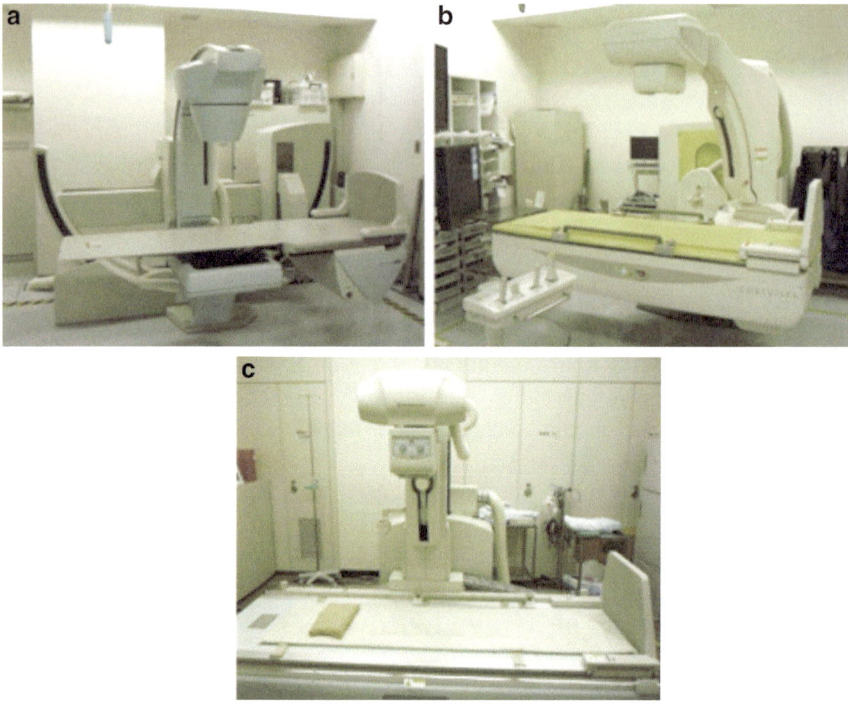

Fig. 3.1 Examples of x-ray fluoroscopy devices with a flat panel detector. (**a**) Cvision safire 17 (Shimadzu Ltd., Japan). (**b**) CUREVISTA (Hitachi Medical Systems Ltd., Japan). (**c**) SONIALVISION Safire 17 (Shimadzu Ltd., Japan)

3.2 Characteristics of Under and Over X-ray Tubes

Some C-arm x-ray equipment can operate both as under and over x-ray tubes, according to the purpose of its use; VersiFlex VISTA (Hitachi Medical Systems Ltd., Japan) is an example. We compared and estimated the radiation dose to the operator in each mode (Figs. 3.4 and 3.5). Our results showed that the under x-ray tube mode led to reduced scatter radiation dose and absorption by the couch, but field of view was smaller (Table 3.1). Therefore, an over x-ray tube mode should be recommended during bronchoscopy with fluoroscopy guidance.

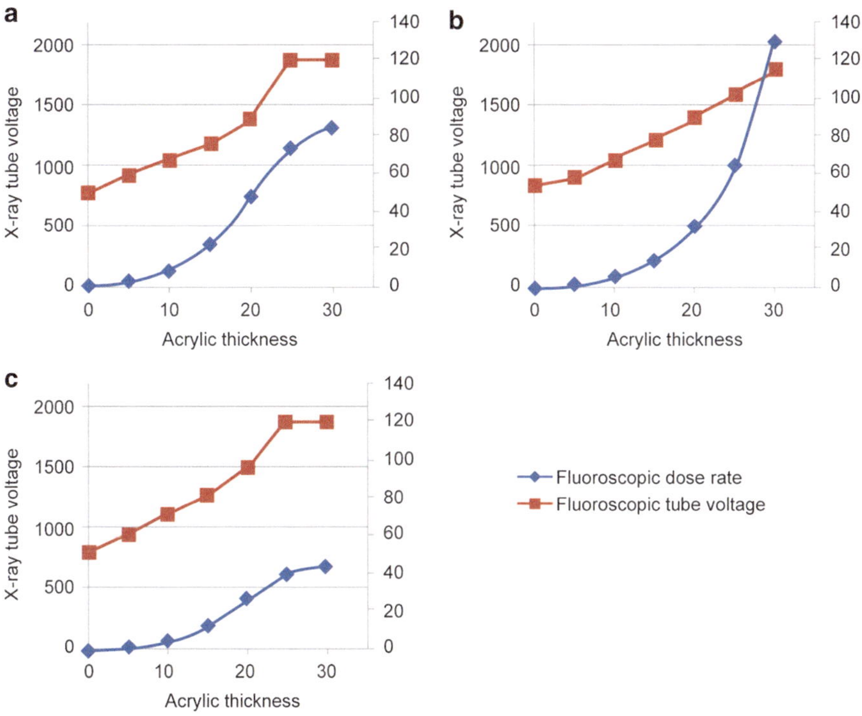

Fig. 3.2 Characteristics of three x-ray fluoroscopy devices: (**a**) Cvision safire 17, (**b**) CUREVISTA, (**c**) SONIALVISION Safire 17. All data were acquired in an autoexposure control (*AEC*) mode

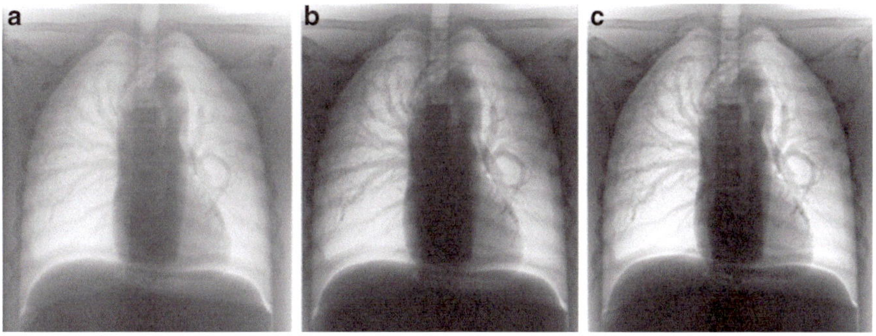

Fig. 3.3 Body phantom radiography taken by (**a**) Cvision safire 17, (**b**) CUREVISTA, and (**c**) SONIALVISION Safire 17. All radiographies were acquired in the autoexposure control (*AEC*) mode and reconstructed in an initial mode

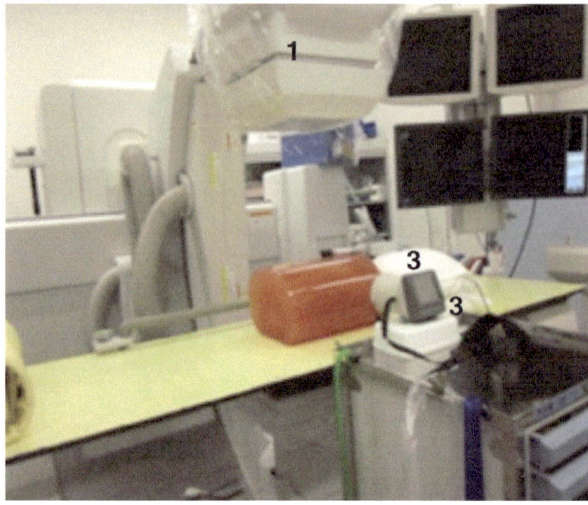

Fig. 3.4 Measurement of scatter radiation on a body phantom during fluoroscopy using VersiFlex VISTA in over x-ray tube mode; the over x-ray tube (1) and ionization chamber model 9015 (3) (Radical Corporation) are shown

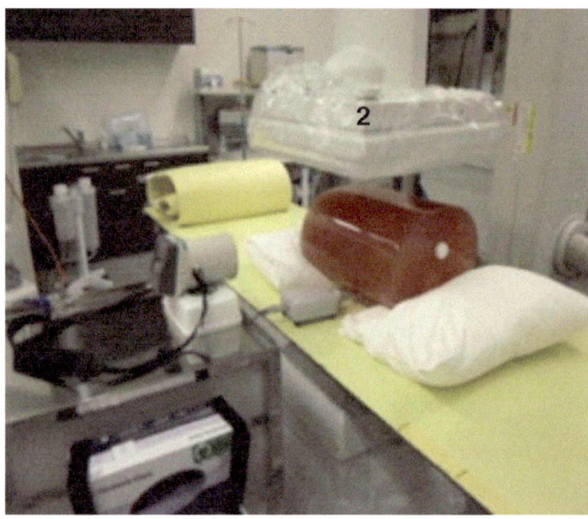

Fig. 3.5 Measurement of scatter radiation on a body phantom during fluoroscopy using VersiFlex VISTA in under x-ray tube mode; the flat panel detector (2) is shown

Table 3.1 Measurement of scatter radiation in each x-ray tube mode

Acquisition mode	Over x-ray tube	Under x-ray tube
Scatter radiation (mSv/h)	3.53	2.78

Bibliography

1. Nihon Houshasen Gijutsu Gakkai. Rinsho Kenkyu no Tame no Digital Gazou Shori no Kiso to Pasokon-sofuto Katsuyo-jutsu. Tokyo: Medical Tribune; 2013.
2. Ogawa W. Houshasen Gazoukei no Gazou Hhyoka. Tokyo: Iryo Kagakusha; 2007.
3. Shinryo Houshasen Gishi Kokuritsu Byoin Seisaku Iryo-han. Shinryo Housyasen Gishi no Tame no Step UP Q & A. Tokyo: Iryo Kagakusha; 2010.

Chapter 4
Image Processing in X-Ray Fluoroscopy and Digital Tomography

Jun Torii and Yuzuru Kouno

Abstract It is well known that optimal image processing is important to enhance the diagnostic quality and value of radiography and fluorography. The new technique of tomosynthesis provides more detailed information and depiction of abnormalities, compared with traditional x-ray radiography and fluorography. Furthermore, it may improve outcomes and diagnostic accuracy of imaging examinations.

Keywords Image processing • Tomosynthesis • Digital tomography

4.1 Image Processing in X-Ray Fluoroscopy

X-ray fluoroscopy is utilized for many clinical purposes, ranging from barium enema (Fig. 4.1) to postoperative treatment (Fig. 4.2). Each fluorography is to be optimized according to the type and purpose of the examination. The factors affecting image quality are sharpness, graininess, after-image phenomenon, and so on. Compared with a combination of optimal factors, sharpness, and graininess, for example, application of the best value of a single factor during radiography would be less effective. Another rational option would be to select a few factors to optimize, depending on the anatomical region and clinical procedure. Owing to technological development, there is now a wide variety of image processing methods available. In this chapter, we will introduce three of these new modalities that are usually applied for the mediastinum during diagnostic and therapeutic bronchoscopy procedures.

J. Torii • Y. Kouno (✉)
Department of Radiological Technology, National Cancer Center Hospital,
5-1-1, Tsukiji Chuo-ku, Tokyo 104-0045, Japan
e-mail: ykouno@ncc.go.jp

T. Izumo et al. (eds.), *Respiratory Endoscopy*,
DOI 10.1007/978-981-287-916-5_4

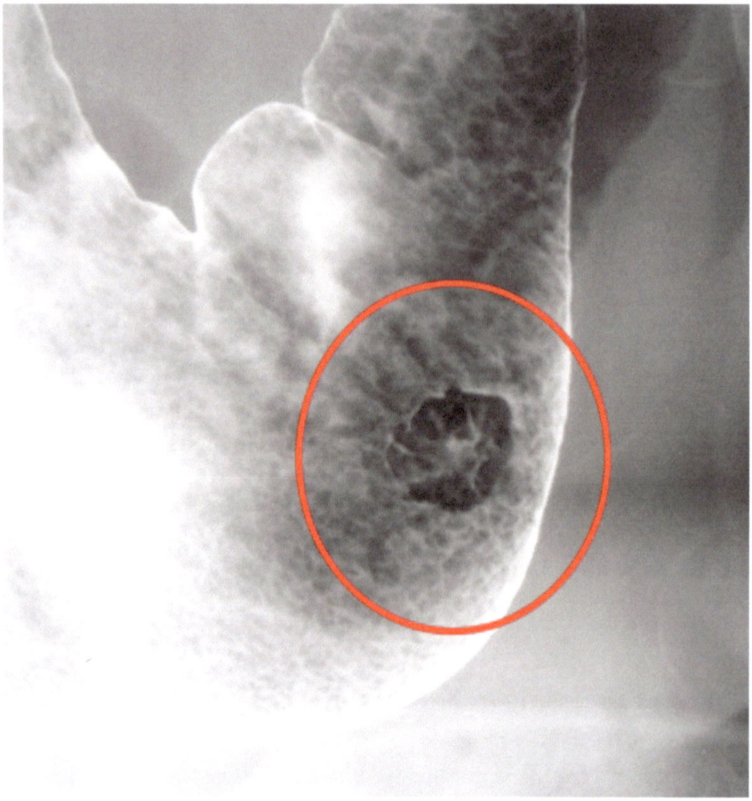

Fig. 4.1 An example of radiography use during barium enema to evaluate the mucosa and microscopic folds of the stomach

4.1.1 Dynamic Range Compression

Chest radiographs should be displayed on a large dynamic range because the thorax is composed of a large variety of anatomical tissues. Dynamic range compression (DRC) is a technique that can successfully preserve a detailed high contrast and reduce the dynamic range viewing systems. This technique makes it possible to change black-mashed areas to areas that are visible enough for adequate diagnosis (Fig. 4.3). Blurred images from the high-frequency component are removed from the original images to render the final contour-enhanced images. This final image shows an improved "black-mashed" image while maintaining the contour-enhanced area.

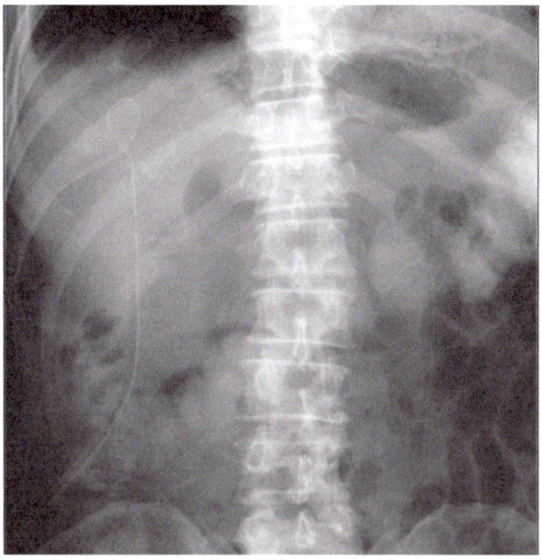

Fig. 4.2 An example of radiography use during postoperative treatment to observe the entire abdomen and to confirm the position of a catheter tip

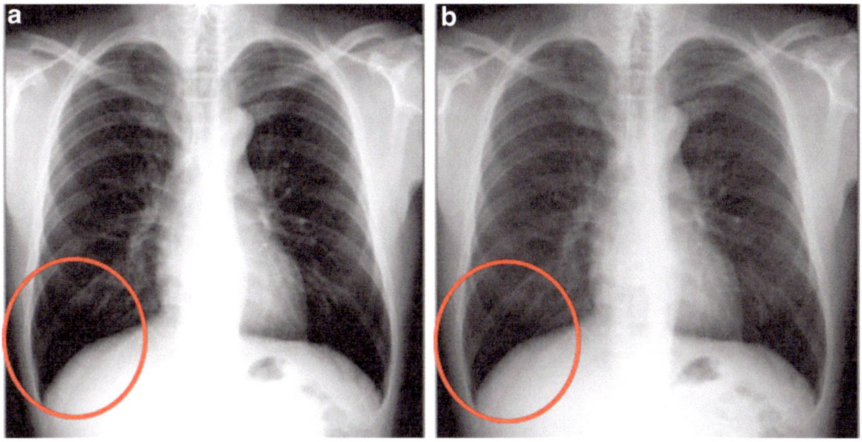

Fig. 4.3 DRC depicts small vessels in the right lower lobe. This technique improves visibility of dense peripheral tissues by applying varying degrees of contrast within an identical image. (**a**) DRC on and (**b**) DRC off. DRC, dynamic range compression

4.1.2 Spatial Frequency Filtering

Frequency filters process an image in the frequency domain based on the Fourier transform. The operator usually takes an image and a filter function in the Fourier domain. This image is then multiplied pixel by pixel with the filter function. Thereafter, the image is retransformed into the spatial domain, where attenuating high frequencies result in a smoother image, whereas attenuating low frequencies enhance the edges. This technique of applying spatial frequency to structures of different sizes within the same image improves visibility. Multifrequency processing, which combines traditional DRC and flat panel (FP), is also available (Fig. 4.4).

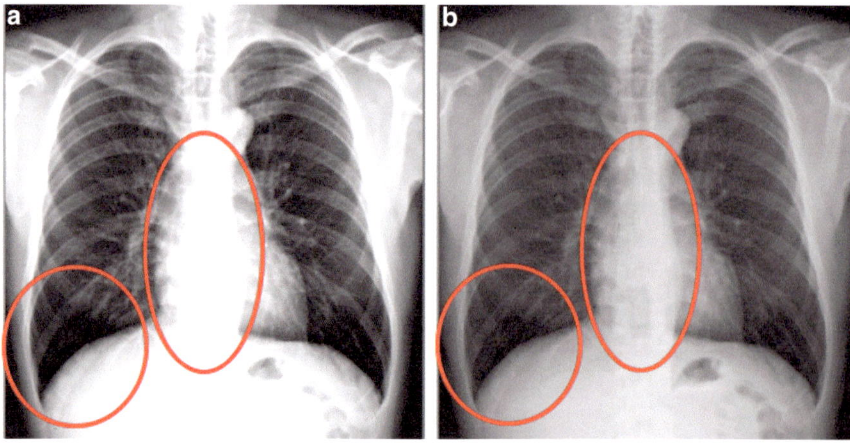

Fig. 4.4 This set of images illustrates the effective use of spatial frequency filter in providing better depiction of the mediastinum while maintaining the contrast of the lungs. (**a**) Without spatial frequency filter and (**b**) with spatial frequency filter

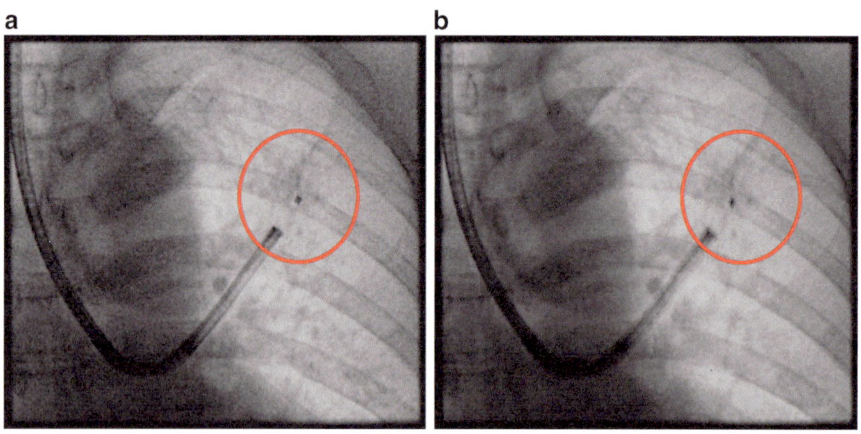

Fig. 4.5 This is an example on how recursive filter works by reducing noise on a clinical chest image. However, the end of the guide sheath is blurred out. (**a**) Without recursive filter and (**b**) with recursive filter

4.1.3 Recursive Filter

This filter calculates output values based on the latest input. Execution of this filter is very easy, but it lacks flexibility and sometimes results in recognizing a subject's motion as persistence of image (Fig. 4.5).

4.2 Tomosynthesis

4.2.1 A New Tomography Method

In conventional x-ray, the regions of interest (ROI) are sometimes difficult to set because of cluttering of signals from above and below. Conventional tomography has been previously used, especially in orthopedics, to produce one image per x-ray projection, which is time-consuming. Furthermore, image flow is sometimes produced and leads to low diagnostic quality.

The new technique of tomosynthesis combines tomography and synthesis to reduce the effects of tissue overlap and to reduce image artifacts by reconstructing optional tomographic planes with only one data acquisition. This technique may also be applied for the thoracic region, not as an equivalent of computed tomography (CT), but to add diagnostic information and value to plain chest radiograph [1–4]. Tomosynthesis may be clinically applied to detect tumors that are near the ribs, those that are obscured by the heart, those in the mediastinum, and those in the subphrenic region (Figs. 4.6 and 4.7).

4.2.2 Theory and Acquisition Technique

Principle: Conventional x-ray radiography is a two-dimensional imaging method; sometimes, ROIs are difficult to visualize because of overlapped tissues above and below. Tomosynthesis is a three-dimensional (3D) imaging technique that may resolve the effects of overlapping tissues [5–7]. With this technique, images are

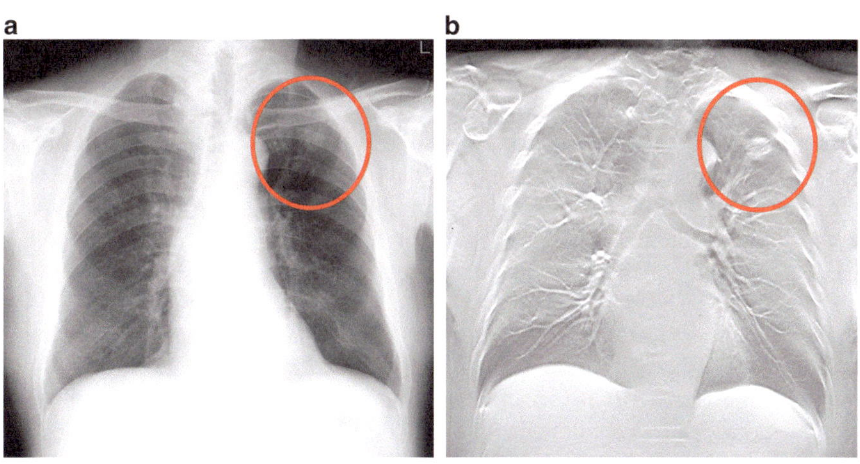

Fig. 4.6 Images of lung diseases. (**a**) Chest x-ray and (**b**) tomosynthesis

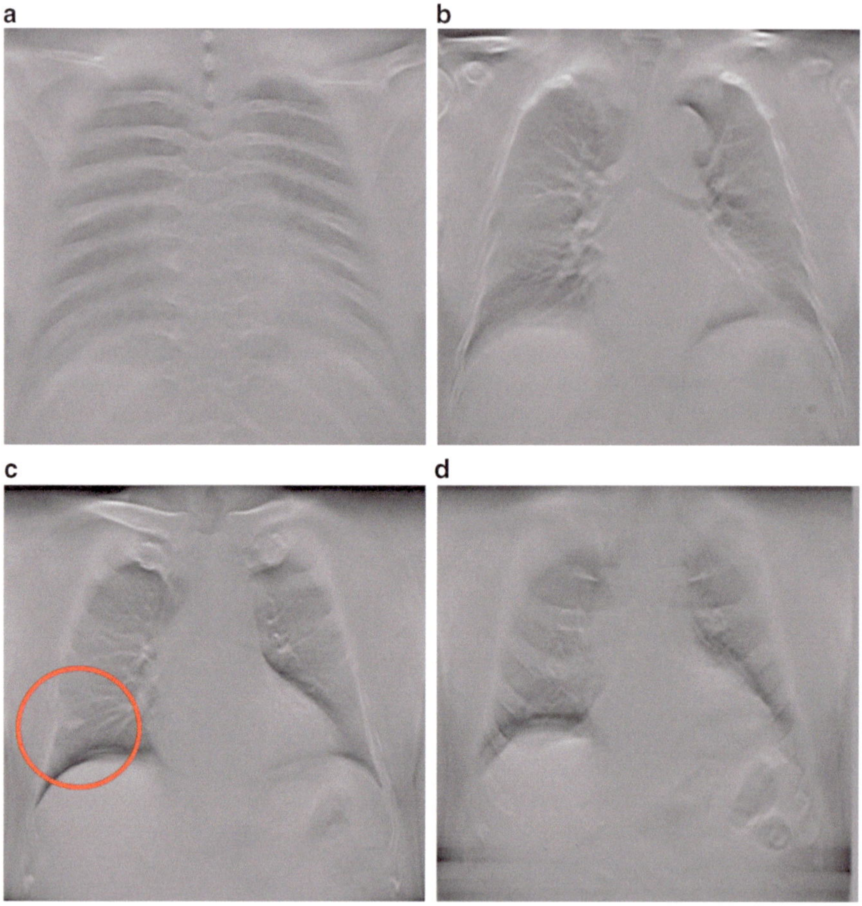

Fig. 4.7 Images of tomosynthesis at different depth. Chest tomosynthesis clearly depicts (**a**) the vertebral body and ribs, (**b**) the bifurcation of trachea, (**c**) a pulmonary lesion, and (**d**) the ribs

acquired at different angles of the x-ray source to delineate structures at different views. The off-axis data acquisition shifts the shadows of the overlapped objects in the images. By shifting and adding the acquired projections, 3D imaging improves the visibility of the target at a particular height by blurring the target of the other heights. No additional data acquisitions are required to improve the visibility of objects at a given height.

Reconstruction methods: Reconstruction algorithms are divided into three categories, namely, back projection algorithms, filtered back projection (FBP), and iterative algorithms (IR) [8]. Back projection algorithms are often referred to as shifted and added (SAA), in which projection images taken at different angles are shifted and added at a certain depth to produce an image. FBP algorithms, which are used for image reconstruction of cone-beam CT, generally provide great precision.

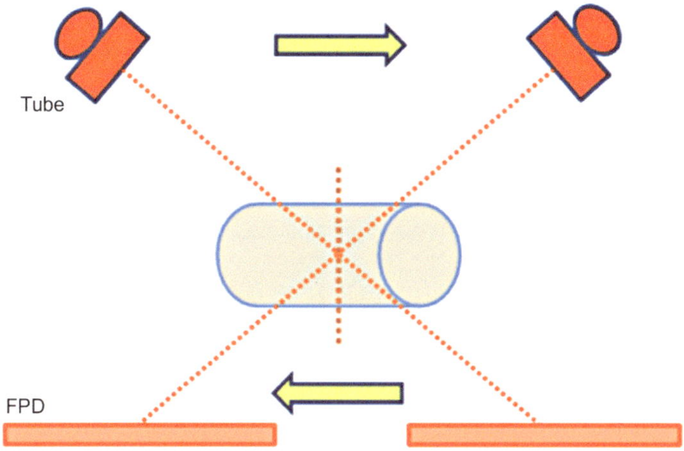

Fig. 4.8 Theory and principle of tomosynthesis

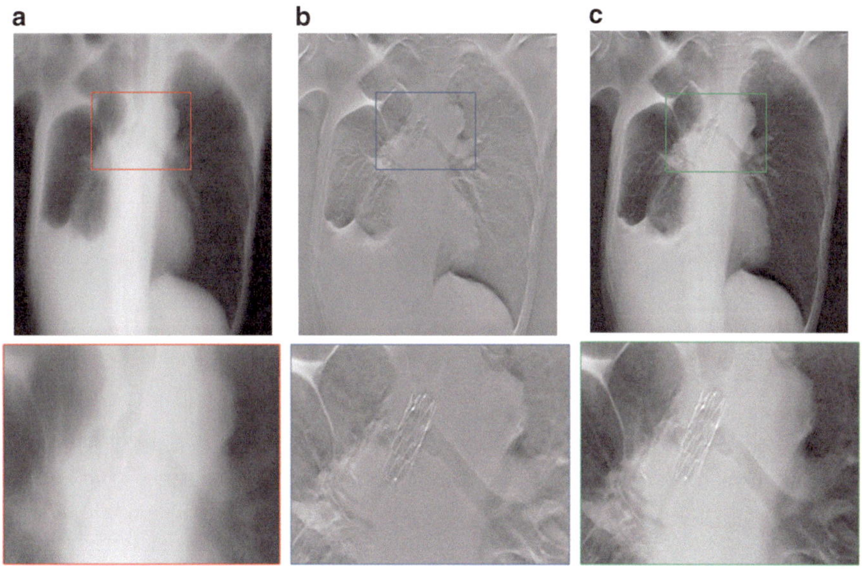

Fig. 4.9 Images of tomosynthesis reconstructed with different function and parameter. (**a**) Shifted and added (SAA), (**b**) FBP (thickness+_), and (**c**) FBP (thickness+_ (DC2))

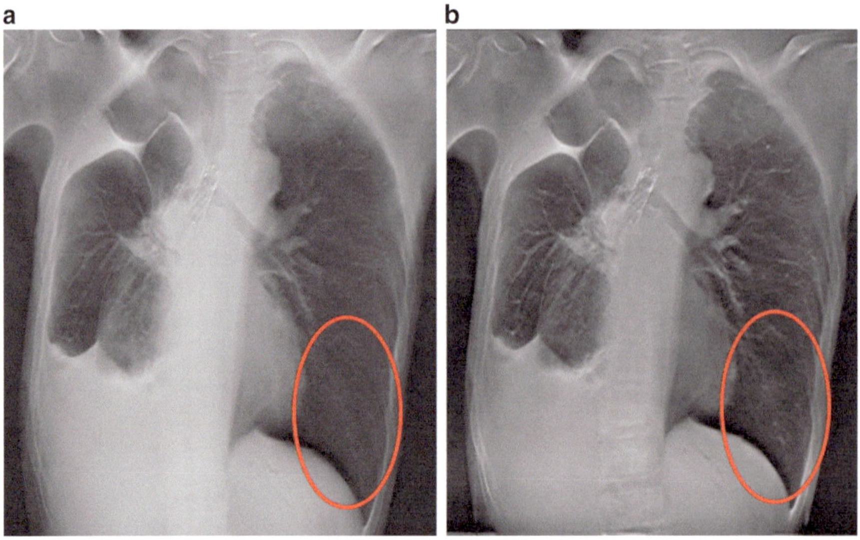

Fig. 4.10 Tomosynthesis imaging (chest) comparison between FBP and IR. (**a**) FBP and (**b**) IR

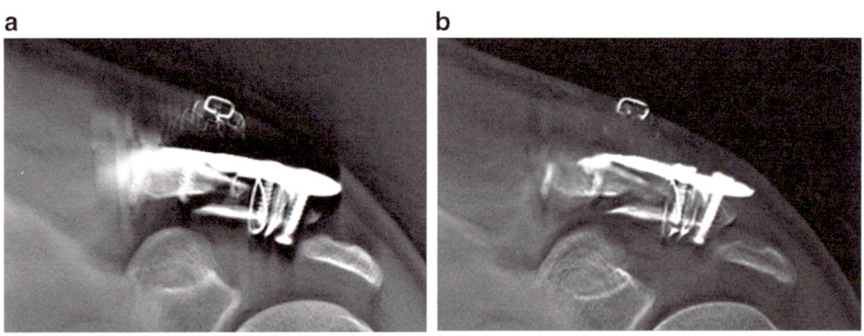

Fig. 4.11 Tomosynthesis imaging (bone) comparison between FBP and IR. (**a**) FBP and (**b**) IR

While x-ray tube rotates from right to left, FBP shifts from left to right (Fig. 4.8). A series of low-dose exposures are done during rotation to create a series of images at a particular height (Fig. 4.9). With IR, the data are processed in a continuous loop where calculations are performed to create different images; projection data are then processed and compared with assumed ideal models to improve the image. When added to dose reduction, IR can reduce streaking and metal artifacts (Figs. 4.10 and 4.11).

References

1. McAdams HP, Samei E, Dobbins 3rd J, Tourassi GD, Ravin CE. Recent advances in chest radiography. Radiology. 2006;241(3):663–83.
2. Dobbins 3rd JT, McAdams HP. Chest tomosynthesis: technical principles and clinical update. Eur J Radiol. 2009;72(2):244–51. doi:10.1016/j.ejrad.2009.05.054. Epub 2009 July.
3. Vikgren J, Zachrisson S, Svalkvist A, Johnsson AA, Boijsen M, Flinck A, Kheddache S, Båth M. Comparison of chest tomosynthesis and chest radiography for detection of pulmonary nodules: human observer study of clinical cases. Radiology. 2008;249(3):1034–41. doi:10.1148/radiol.2492080304. Epub 2008 Oct 10.
4. Johnsson AA, Vikgren J, Svalkvist A, Zachrisson S, Flinck A, Boijsen M, Kheddache S, Månsson LG, Båth M. Overview of two years of clinical experience of chest tomosynthesis at Sahlgrenska University Hospital. Radiat Prot Dosim. 2010;139(1–3):124–9. doi:10.1093/rpd/ncq059. Epub 2010 Feb 24.
5. Dobbins 3rd JT, Godfrey DJ. Digital x-ray tomosynthesis: current state of the art and clinical potential. Phys Med Biol. 2003;48(19):R65–106. Review.
6. Newman L. Developing technologies for early detection of breast cancer: a public workshop summary. Washington, DC: National Academies Press (US); 2000.
7. Bansal GJ, Young P. Digital breast tomosynthesis within a symptomatic "one-stop breast clinic" for characterization of subtle findings. Br J Radiol. 2015;3:20140855.
8. Gomi T, Hirano H. Clinical potential of digital linear tomosynthesis imaging of total joint arthroplasty. J Digit Imaging. 2008;21:312–22, ISSN 0897-1889.

Chapter 5
Quality Control in X-Ray Fluoroscopy and Digital Tomography

Takumi Iwase and Yuzuru Kouno

Abstract Quality control (QC) is a procedure to guarantee safe manipulation of equipment and is usually performed using phantoms designed for daily management. All medical radiological imaging have to be maintained to perform safe examinations, to provide quality radiographs, and to control radiation exposure. Daily equipment management or quality assurance (QA)/QC is promising for this purpose. Collecting and analyzing QC data over a long period should be effective in detecting and responding to early signs of problems.

Keywords Quality control • Quality assurance

5.1 Introduction

All medical radiological imaging have to be maintained sufficiently to perform safe examination, to provide quality radiographs, and to control radiation exposure. Daily equipment management or quality control/quality assurance (QC/QA) is promising for this purpose. Collecting and analyzing QC data over a long period should be effective in detecting and responding to early signs of problems. In this chapter, we would like to introduce a specially designed phantom for the purposes of QA and QC.

T. Iwase • Y. Kouno (✉)
Department of Radiological Technology, National Cancer Center Hospital,
5-1-1, Tsukiji Chou-ku, Tokyo 104-0045, Japan
e-mail: ykouno@ncc.go.jp

T. Izumo et al. (eds.), *Respiratory Endoscopy*,
DOI 10.1007/978-981-287-916-5_5

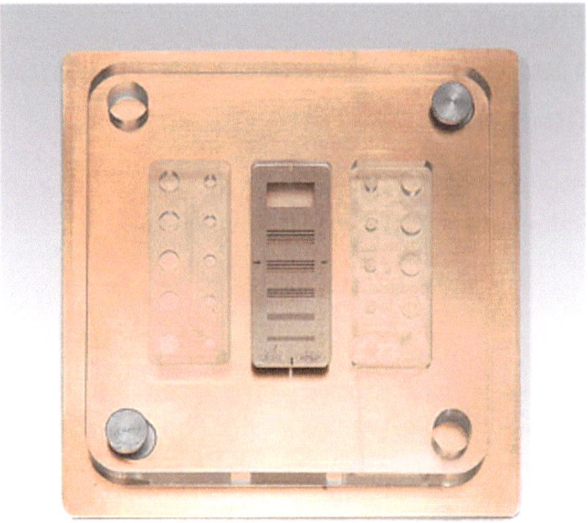

Fig. 5.1 The Japanese Society of Gastrointestinal Imaging phantom is made of acryl, copper, and lead

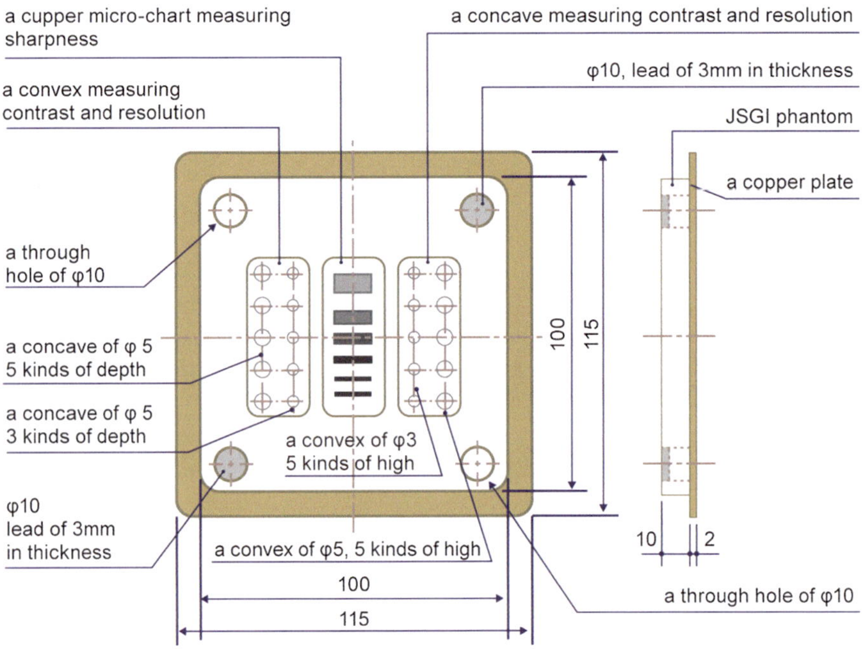

Fig. 5.2 The Japanese Society of Gastrointestinal Imaging phantom measures 11.5 × 11.5 × 1.2 cm

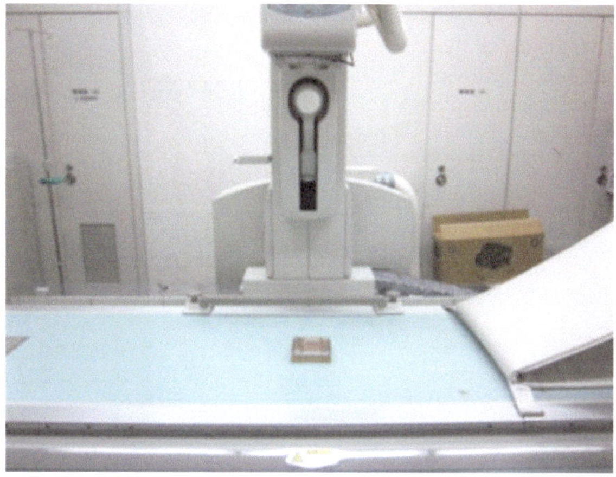

Fig. 5.3 The Japanese Society of Gastrointestinal Imaging phantom and x-ray fluoroscope

5.2 The Japanese Society of Gastrointestinal Imaging (JSGI) Phantom

The JSGI phantom is a quick, easy, and precise measurement tool that may assist in the daily management of x-ray imaging systems. It is characterized by common measurements in computed radiography (CR), digital radiography (DR), and flat panel detector (FPD). The properties and specifications of this phantom are shown in Figs. 5.1 and 5.2. To use this phantom (Fig. 5.3), irradiation fields must be in the range of 110 × 110–115 × 115 mm. For the evaluation of fluorography and radiography, contrast and sharpness are graded according to five ranks. Both fluorography and radiography conditions should be recorded.

Analysis methods: Fig. 5.4 shows a radiography taken by the JSGI phantom. Uneven acryl parts are used to evaluate contrast resolution of an image intensity. Square wave μ chart is used to evaluate sharpness. Using four circles in the corner, the minimum and maximum values of dynamic range can be determined. Dynamic range is the ratio between the largest and smallest values of a changeable quality (Fig. 5.5). Contrast transfer function (CTF) is to be calculated using the μ chart data, which modulate the amplitudes and phases of the electron diffraction pattern (Fig. 5.6). The standard deviation (σ) can be used to quantify noise directly, which is the relationship in quantum-limited imaging, where noise (σ) is proportional to the square root of the dose (Fig. 5.7). The calculated values enable tracking of the age of deterioration of the equipment. However, it is worth mentioning that the radiographies used for the analysis went through a number of image processing methods, and the calculated values should be treated as reference.

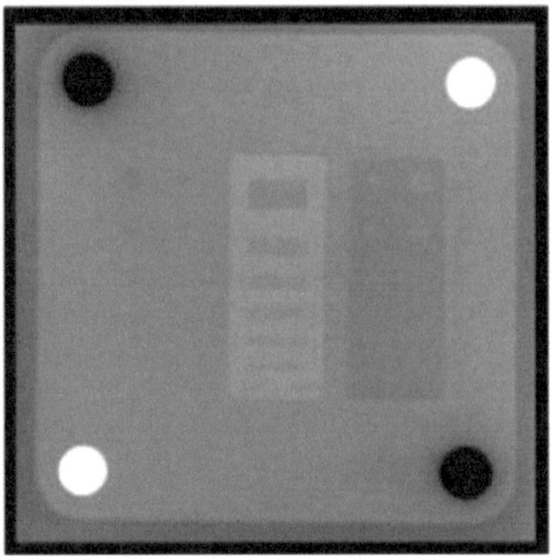

Fig. 5.4 Radiography of with the use of the Japanese Society of Gastrointestinal Imaging phantom

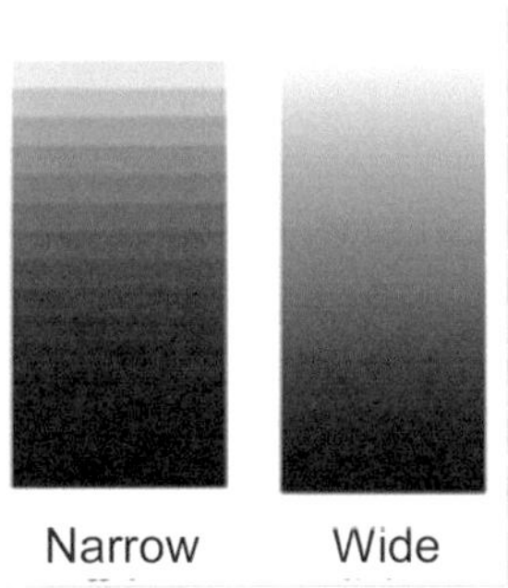

Fig. 5.5 Dynamic range

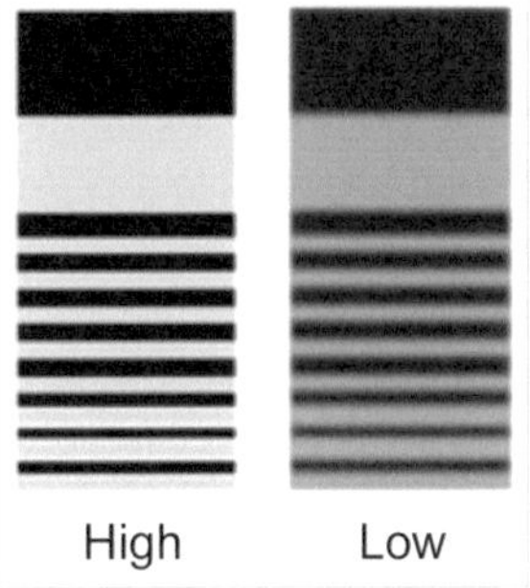

Fig. 5.6 Contrast transfer function (CTF)

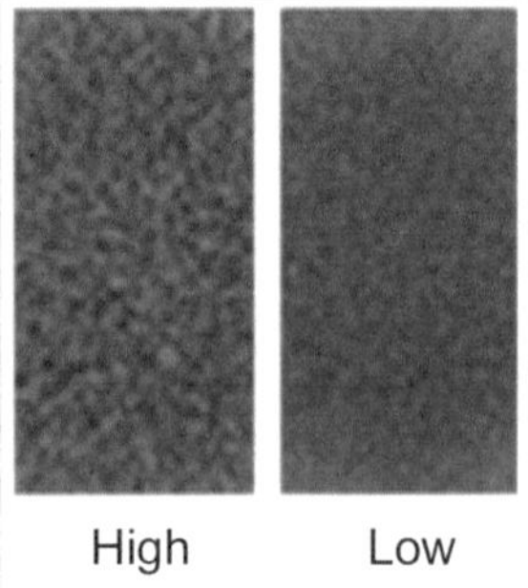

Fig. 5.7 Image noise: standard deviation

Bibliography

1. Nihon Shokakan Gazou Kenkyukai. JSGI Phantom Toriatsukai Setsumeisho Vol.7. 2012

Chapter 6
Computed Tomography Imaging to Bronchoscopic Navigation

Hirobumi Nagasawa and Yuzuru Kouno

Abstract Advancements in multi-detector row computed tomography (MDCT) make volume data available. Furthermore, workstations enable multi-planar reconstruction (MPR), curved planar reconstruction (CPR), and volume rendering (VR) of images. Three-dimensional (3D) computed tomography (CT) imaging should contribute pre-operation planning and reading of physicians.

Keywords Three-dimensional computed tomography • Navigation system • Virtual bronchoscopy

6.1 Introduction

Advancements in multi-detector row computed tomography (MDCT) make volume data available (Fig. 6.1). Furthermore, workstations enable multi-planar reconstruction (MPR) (Fig. 6.2), curved planar reconstruction (CPR), and volume rendering (VR) (Fig. 6.3) of images.

MPR: Volume data are built by adding the axial slices; the workstation will cut slices through the volume in different planes.
CPR: This technique enables flexible multi-planar reformatting along the course of a target artery.
VR: This technique displays samples in a three-dimensional (3D) field without first fitting geometry to the samples (Fig. 6.3).

3D-CT imaging contributes to pre-operation planning and reading of physicians.

H. Nagasawa • Y. Kouno (✉)
Department of Radiological Technology, National Cancer Center Hospital,
5-1-1, Tsukiji Chou-ku, Tokyo 104-0045, Japan
e-mail: ykouno@ncc.go.jp

T. Izumo et al. (eds.), *Respiratory Endoscopy*,
DOI 10.1007/978-981-287-916-5_6

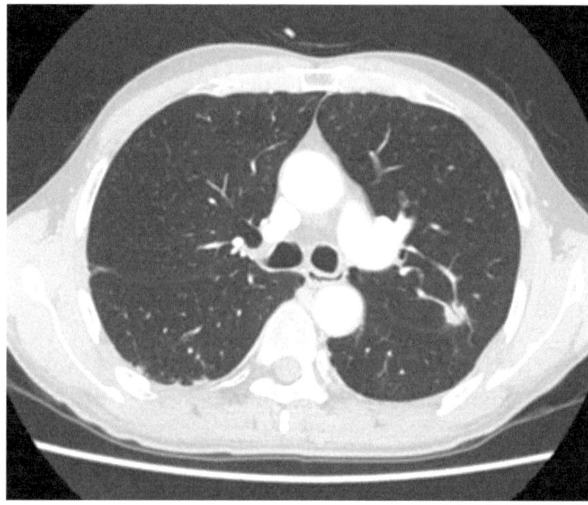

Fig. 6.1 Two-dimensional axial computed tomography image

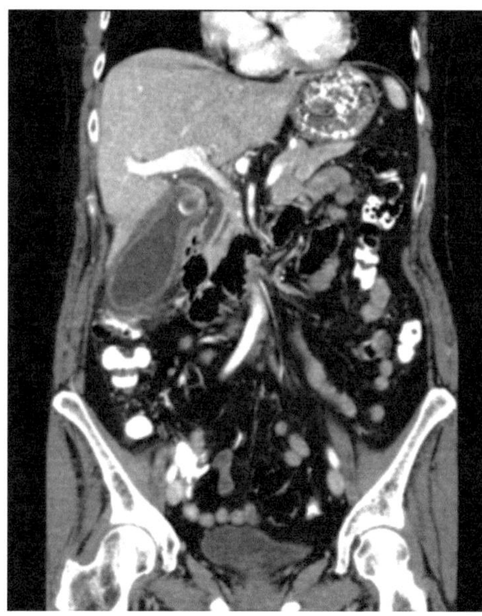

Fig. 6.2 Multi-planar reconstruction (MPR)

6.2 Virtual Bronchoscopy and Its Use

The user can follow the path of the bronchoscope on a navigation map. Zooming in and out on the map can be done with ease. The navigation map may reduce the difference between novices and skilled physicians on their techniques, such as the duration of bronchoscopy, contact with airway wall, etc. In addition, automation in some systems facilitates routine examinations. When a bronchoscope returns to a

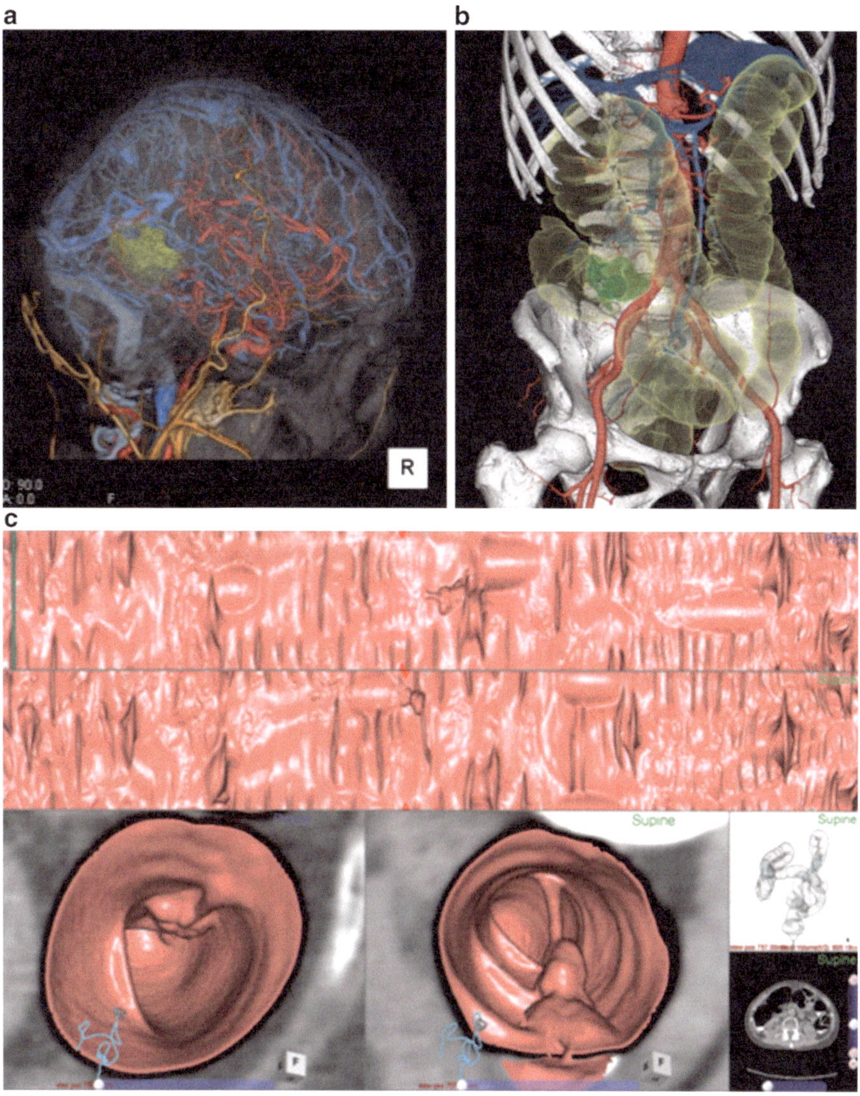

Fig. 6.3 Volume rendering on CT. (**a**) 3D-CT mapping for brain cancer surgery, (**b**) 3D-CT mapping for colon cancer surgery, and (**c**) spreaded images of CT colonography. *CT* computed tomography, *3D* three-dimensional

position that has been used for a given patient, it will automatically display the previous images (Fig. 6.4).

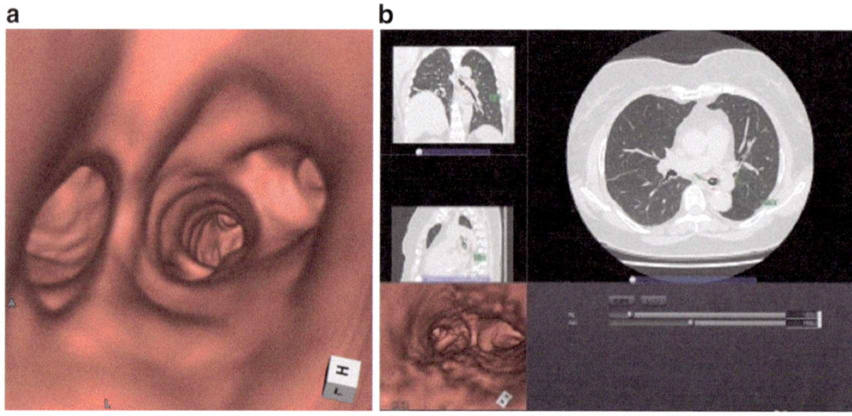

Fig. 6.4 CT bronchoscopy. (**a**) Virtual bronchoscopy. (**b**) Virtual bronchoscopy and simulation

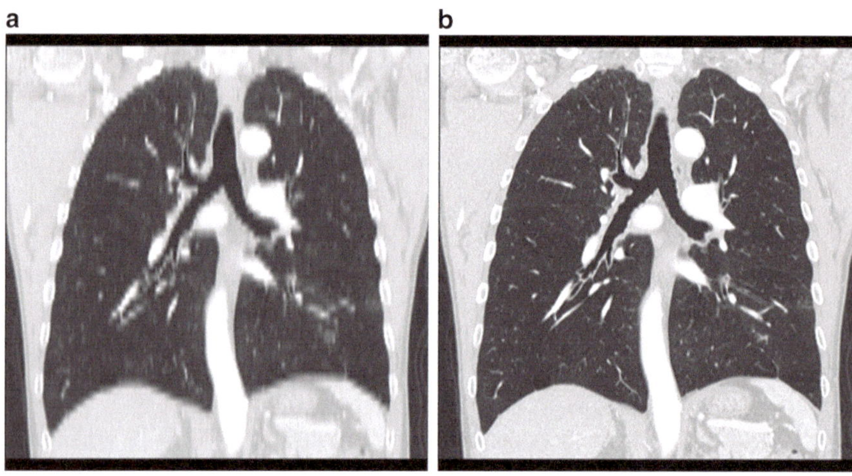

Fig. 6.5 Correlation among MPR image qualities, *slice thickness*, and slice interval. (**a**) Slice thickness of 5 mm and slice interval of 5 mm and (**b**) *slice thickness* of 1 mm and slice interval of 0.5 mm. *MPR* multi-planar reconstruction

6.3 Parameters for 3D-CT Acquisition

Figure 6.5 illustrates how slice thickness and interval cause some effects on MPR imaging.

Small slice thickness (1 mm) and 50 % slice overlap (0.5 mm) reduce stair-step artifacts to a minimum level. Image reconstruction parameters also determine image quality, aside from motion and CT exposure dose on patients during image acquisition. Each institution must optimize these parameters. Figure 6.6 illustrates how the exposure dose affects image quality.

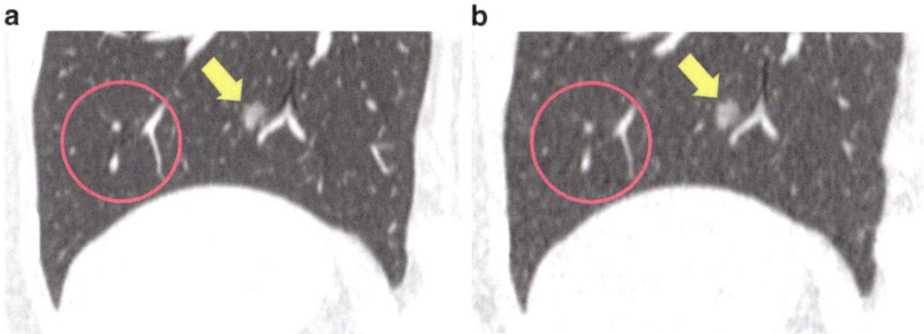

Fig. 6.6 Illustration of how noise from low-dose MPR affects the image quality. MPR imaging using axial CT data at exposure doses of (**a**) 150 mAs and (**b**) 10 mAs. *MPR* multi-planar reconstruction, *CT* computed tomography

Bibliography

1. Koda E, Ito K. 3D volume data – Yasashiku Rinsho ni Chokketsu. Tokyo: Kanehara Shuppan; 2006.
2. Matsumoto Y, Izumo T, Sasada S. Kikanshi-kyo Shindan ni Okeru CT oyobi Workstation no Katsuyo. Rad Fan. 2014;12:69–71.
3. Muramatsu Y, Tsuda Y, Nakamura Y, et al. The development and use of a chest phantom for optimizing scanning techniques on a variety of low-dose helical computed tomography devices. J Comput Assist Tomogr. 2003;27:364–74.
4. Nagasawa H. Kokuritsu Gan Kenkyu Center ni Okeru Zoei CT Kensa no Jissai. Arutei. 2012;60:11–4.
5. Nagasawa H. Aquilion PRIME Symposium 2013; 64 Rei wo Koeru CT no Gijutsu to Rinsho, Kenshin Ryoiki heno Oyo. INNERVISION. 2013. Supplement 7.
6. Sekiguchi R, Nakaya Y, Ishihara T et al. Multi Slice CT niyoru Kansaibo-gan Kensaku; Jido Satsueiho; Real Prep. no Jissenteki Katsuyoho. Eizo-jyouhou (M). 2000;32:916–19
7. Suzuki M, et al. CT Colonography niyoru Daichogan Kenshin Clinical Report. Case 2 Kokuritsu Gan Kenkyu Center Gan Yobo · Kenshin Kenkyu Center 1 Shisetsu Shoukai kara Mae-shochi made. Innervision. 2011;26(1):64–7.
8. Tsujioka K. Multi Slice CT wo Riyo-shita [Saizen no] Sanjigen Gazo Sakuseiho. In: Gazo S, editor. Manual. Tokyo: Sangyo Kaihatsu Kiko; 2006. p. 14–20.
9. Yasuo M. Virtual Kikanshi-kyo navigation. Shinshu Ishi. 2012;60(4):211–3.

Part II
Edition for Doctors

Chapter 7
Fluorographic and Radiographic Conditions in Bronchoscopy Using X-Ray Fluoroscopy

Yuichi Nagai, Takehiro Izumo, and Yuzuru Kouno

Abstract Fluorographic and radiographic conditions have some parameters to optimize, namely, x-ray tube voltage (kV), x-ray tube current (mA), fluoroscopic time (f/s), pulse width (msec), etc. Among them, the latter two are particularly important to compatibly achieve qualified images and appropriate radiation exposure. Fluoroscopic procedures pose a potential risk of radiation-induced cancer. Long-time procedure might cause mild erythema (Shope. Radiographics 16(5):1195–1199, 1996; Valentin. Ann ICRP 30 (2):7–67, 2000; Balter et al. Radiology 254(2):326–341, 2010). Not only system performance but fluorographic and radiographic conditions displayed on the operator console should be monitored throughout the clinical treatment.

Keywords X-ray fluoroscopy • Fluoroscopic time • Pulse width

7.1 Introduction

It is important to compatibly achieve qualified images and appropriate radiation exposure. To achieve this goal, the parameters should be determined according to the need rather than following the manufacture's recommendation. In cases of pediatric patients, for example, priority should be on minimizing the radiographic exposure time and set as such. For qualitative diagnosis, priority should be on the image quality rather than on the moderate radiation exposure.

Y. Nagai
Department of Radiology, National Hospital Organization East Saitama National Hospital, 4147, Kurohama, Hasuda, Saitama 349-0196, Japan

T. Izumo
Department of Respiratory Medicine, Japanese Red Cross Medical Center, 4-1-22 Hiroo, Shibuya-ku, Tokyo 150-8935, Japan

Y. Kouno (✉)
Department of Radiological Technology, National Cancer Center Hospital, 5-1-1, Tsukiji Chou-ku, Tokyo 104-0045, Japan
e-mail: ykouno@ncc.go.jp

T. Izumo et al. (eds.), *Respiratory Endoscopy*,
DOI 10.1007/978-981-287-916-5_7

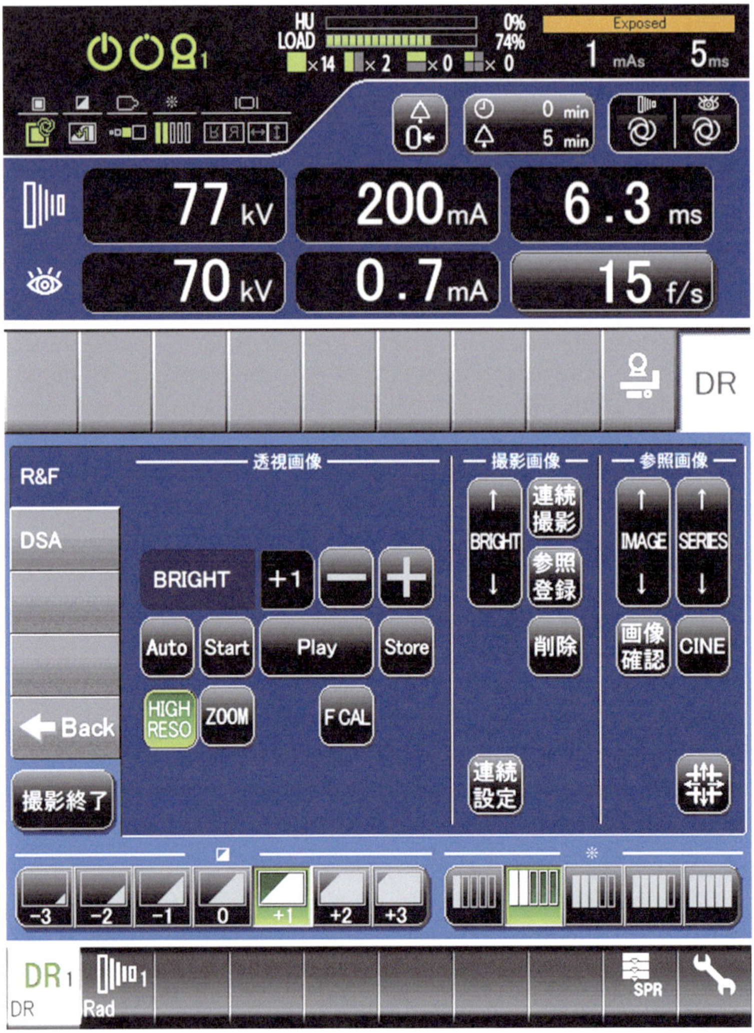

Fig. 7.1 An example display of fluorographic and radiographic conditions

Figure 7.1 indicates an example of fluorographic and radiographic conditions displayed on the operator console.

7.2 X-Ray Fluoroscopic Parameters

X-ray tube voltage or tube voltage in short is applied across anode and cathode making a high electric field. This causes electrons to be emitted and move from cathode to anode.

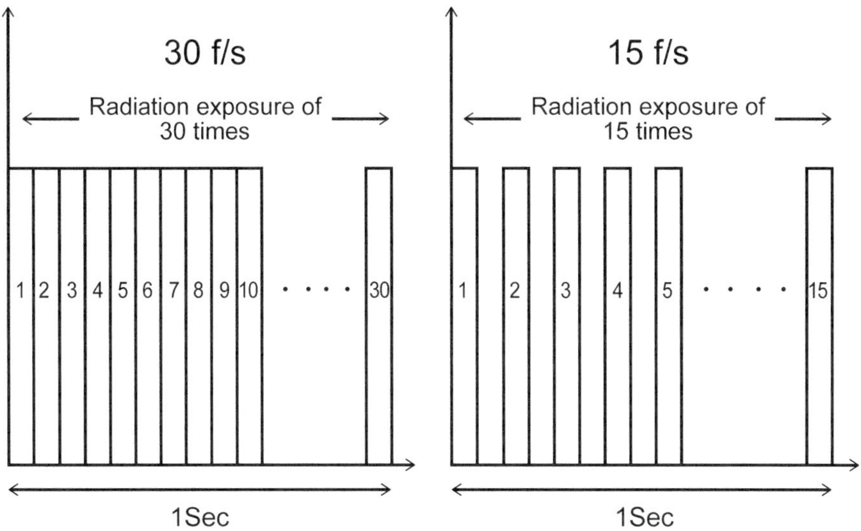

Fig. 7.2 X-ray pulse characteristics (frame/second)

The increase in tube voltage increases the average photon energy and affects the image contrast owing to x-ray blooming and the scatter. Appropriate tube voltage should be chosen according to the patient size.

Tube current, which is the electrical current that flows through the tube, determines radiation dose and image quality. Pulse x-ray is able to reduce the radiation exposure to a great extent producing a sequence of short x-ray pulses instead of continuous x-ray. However, the shorter the pulse, the quality of the image degrades accordingly.

X-ray pulse makes it possible for examination without exposing unnecessary radiation characterized by the term of frame per second (Fig. 7.2) and pulse width (Fig. 7.3). Reducing the number of frames per second above a standard level, the image lag will appear. On the other hand, reducing the pulse width above a level will degrade image granularity.

7.3 Radiographic Parameters

In general, radiographic exposure amounts to ten times as much as that of x-ray fluoroscopy, and the parameters are carefully chosen by the user. In cases under general anesthesia, efforts must be made to minimize radiation exposure time by increasing tube current. This will help to produce unblurred distinct radiography.

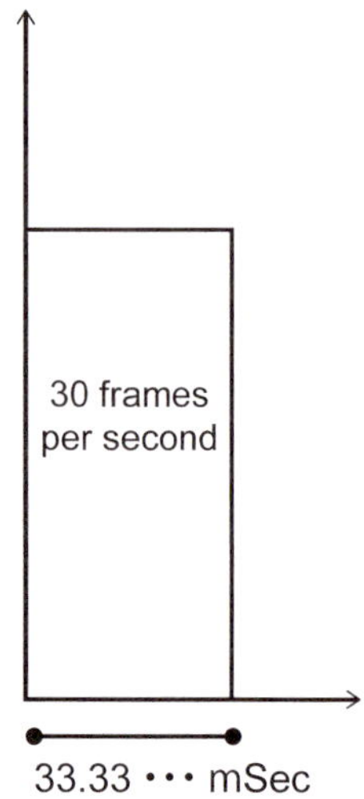

Fig. 7.3 X-ray pulse characteristics (pulse width)

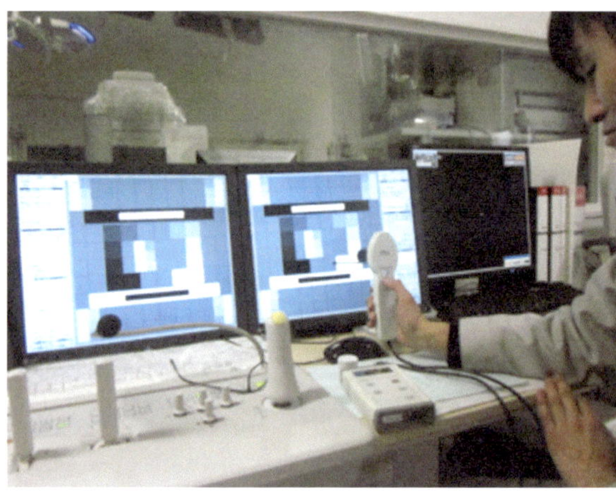

Fig. 7.4 Imaging display brightness check

7.4 Medical Imaging Display System

Quality of each monitor, from checking to calibration, is necessary according to the guideline. Each monitor must be properly calibrated to satisfy the same standard. Figure 7.4 illustrates Society of Motion Picture and Television Engineers (SMPTE) patterns shown on the medical imaging display. Figure 7.5 is a recording and analyzing sheet for this purpose.

PTW CD T54003D

Monitor 1	Illuminance
Measuring point	Brightness
1	320.5
2	220.1
3	147.7
4	94.1
5	62.4
6	40.7
7	24.5
8	15.0
9	9.0
10	5.1
11	1.6

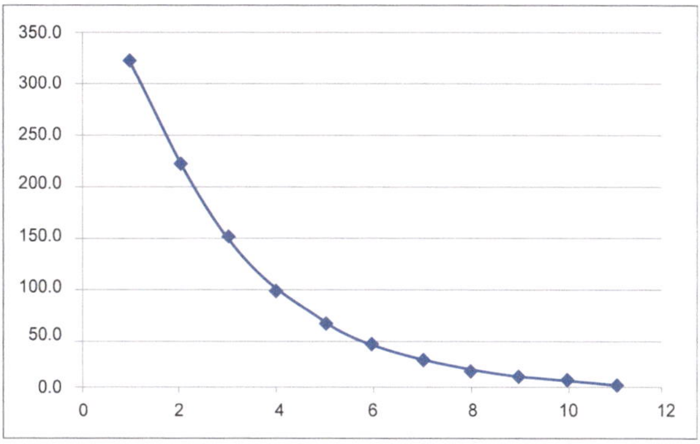

Fig. 7.5 Imaging display recording and analyzing sheet

References

1. Shope TB. Radiation-induced skin injuries from fluoroscopy. Radiographics. 1996;16(5):1195–9.
2. Valentin J. Avoidance of radiation injuries from medical interventional procedures. Ann ICRP. 2000;30(2):7–67.
3. Balter S, Hopewell JW, Miller DL, Wagner LK, Zelefsky MJ. Fluoroscopically guided interventional procedures: a review of radiation effects on patients' skin and hair (pdf). Radiology. 2010;254(2):326–41.

Chapter 8
Identification of the Involved Bronchus to Peripheral Pulmonary Lesions on Computed Tomography

Takaaki Tsuchida

Abstract When performing transbronchial biopsy for solitary peripheral lung nodules, identification of the bronchial branches that led to the involved bronchus of the target lesion is essential. The preferred method is seamless reconstruction of the bronchial route from the target lesion to the lobar bronchus with the use of serial chest computed tomography (CT) images with slice thickness of 2 mm or less. Changing the orientation of the CT images will enable easy reconstruction of the endobronchial branches.

Keywords Bronchial branch • Computed tomography • Peripheral pulmonary lesion • Small airway

8.1 Indications

When performing transbronchial biopsy of focal peripheral lung lesions, it is essential to review the CT images and identify the involved bronchi beforehand. Otherwise, nonspecific searching for the bronchial branch that will lead to the target would prolong procedure time and may cause unwanted bronchial damage.

8.2 Preparation

- CT images with slice thickness of 2 mm or less and reconstructed seamlessly from the target lesion to the lobar bronchus
- Workstation or any image viewer
- Pencil and paper

T. Tsuchida (✉)
Department of Endoscopy, Respiratory Endoscopy Division, National Cancer Center Hospital, 5-1-1, Tsukiji, Chou-ku, Tokyo 104-0045, Japan
e-mail: ttsuchid@ncc.go.jp

T. Izumo et al. (eds.), *Respiratory Endoscopy*,
DOI 10.1007/978-981-287-916-5_8

8.3 Reading the Bronchial Branches

Virtual endoscopic images can be easily reconstructed from serial CT images by changing the direction of the CT slices on the image viewer. Three-dimensional (3D) spatial recognition may vary among individuals; therefore, it is recommended that each person performs bronchial branch reading using CT image orientations that are easy for him/her to understand. In general, the directions that enable easy endobronchial reconstruction from CT images are shown below.

8.3.1 Directions for Changing the Orientation of Axial CT Images Based on the Location of a Lesion

1. For lesions located in the right upper lobe, the CT images may be rotated 90° counterclockwise. In this case, the right lung is depicted on the lower part of the screen.
2. For lesions located in the middle lobe, lingula, right lower lobe, or left lower lobe, the CT images may be horizontally reversed.
3. For lesions located in the left upper lobe, the CT images may be rotated 90° clockwise. In this case, the left lung is depicted on the lower part of the screen.
4. For lesions located in the right or left subsegment S6a, use the original orientation of the CT images.

When performing bronchial branch reading, find the peripheral or segmental/subsegmental bronchus involved in the target lesion first then continue tracing its route toward the center or lobar bronchus. As there are individual differences in spatial awareness, you may also follow the branch from the peripheral side first then read the branching from the center after identifying the branch that leads to the lobar bronchus. As an example, we will perform branch reading of a lesion located in the left lower lobe.

8.3.2 Change the Orientation of the Axial CT Images

1. As mentioned above, change the orientation of the CT image according to the location of the lesion (Fig. 8.1).
2. Focus on the target branch in the adjusted CT image (Fig. 8.2).

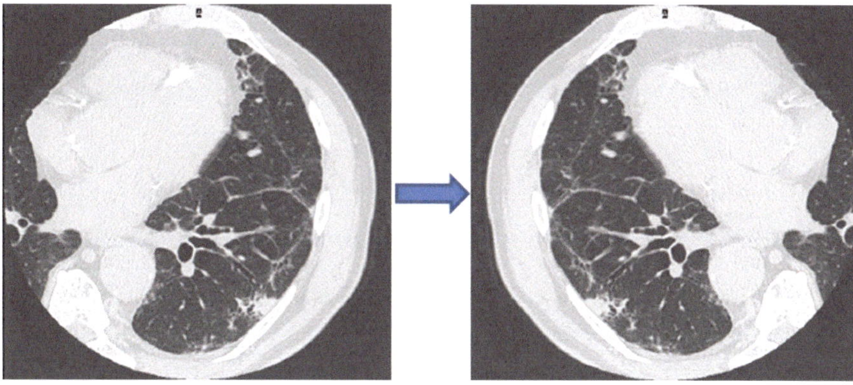

Fig. 8.1 Reverse the image horizontally if a lesion is located in the left lower lobe

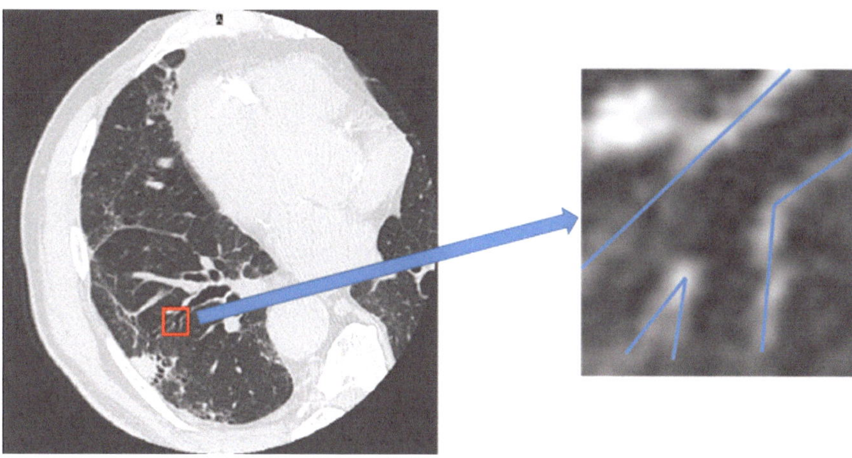

Fig. 8.2 Focus on the target branch, which is the left B9 in this case

8.3.3 Manual Drawing of Virtual Bronchoscopy View

1. Draw the peripheral bronchial branches of the target branch (Fig. 8.3).
2. If the resulting drawing of the bifurcation is not located in the center, rotate the orientation of the virtual bronchoscopy view (Fig. 8.4).

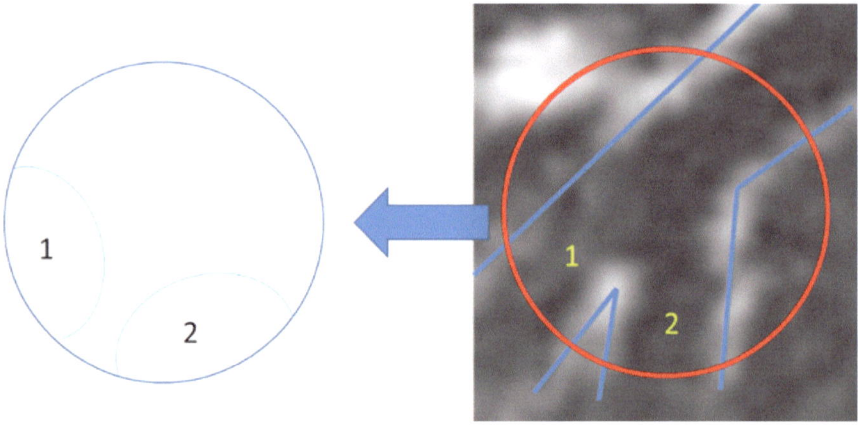

Fig. 8.3 Draw a virtual bronchoscopy view of the bifurcation of the left B9 to left B9a and left B9b

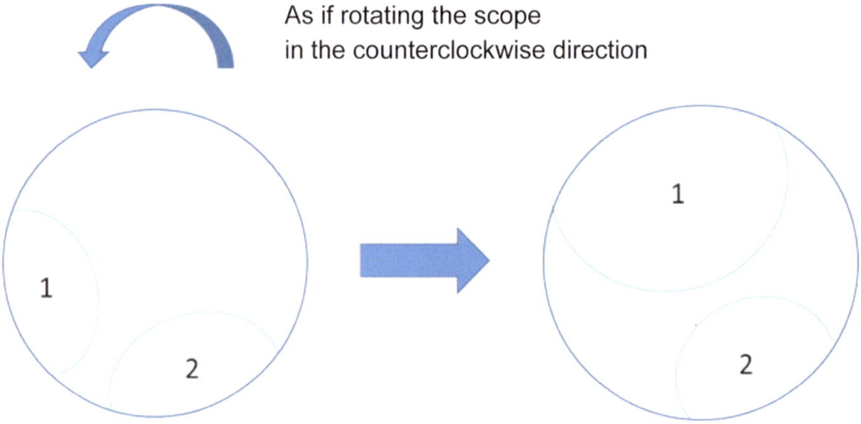

Fig. 8.4 Adjust the orientation of the virtual bronchoscopy view

8.3.4 Trace the Bronchial Route on Serial Axial CT Images While Drawing the Virtual Bronchoscopy Views

1. Identify the involved subsegmental bronchus and make a drawing of the expected bronchoscopic view (Fig. 8.5).
2. Focus on the involved orifice while following its course on serial axial CT images from the periphery to the center until it reaches a bifurcation. At every bifurcation encountered on CT reading, draw the corresponding orifice(s) on another virtual bronchoscopy view. Repeat the steps until a segmental bronchus is reached.
3. Consolidate these virtual bronchoscopy drawings and use them when you perform transbronchial biopsy (Fig. 8.6).

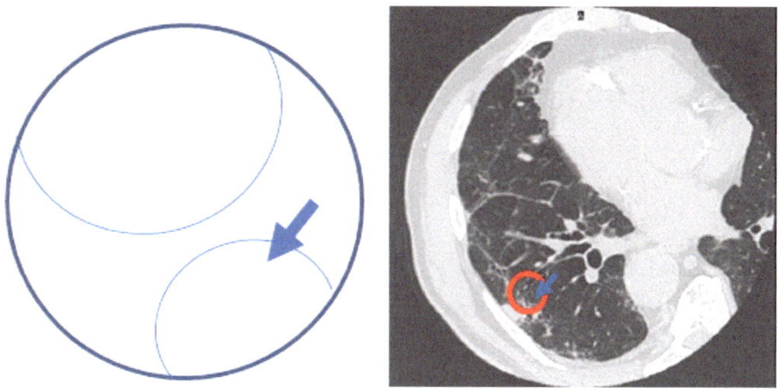

Fig. 8.5 Draw a virtual bronchoscopy view of the peripheral bronchial branch that leads to the lesion (*blue arrow*)

8.4 Some Limitations and Pointers

If you cannot find the involved bronchus, you can start the branch reading from the nearest pulmonary artery to the target lesion. If you find a bronchus running parallel to the artery, change the branch reading from artery to bronchus.

8.5 Efficiency

There is no evidence that the accuracy and time required for transbronchial biopsy are improved by branch reading. Whether by drawing or imagination, every bronchoscopist is required to plan the bronchial route from CT images before starting the procedure. In general, drawing virtual bronchoscopy images may be more reliable than recall of branch reading by imagination.

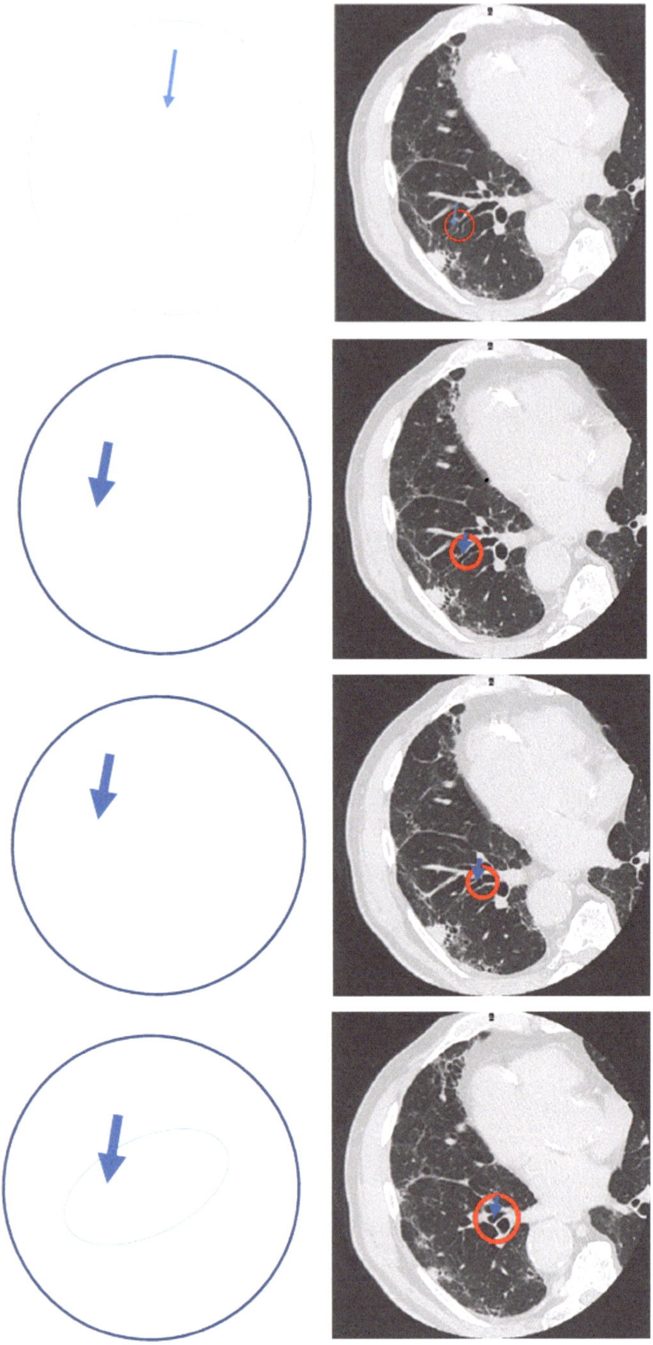

Fig. 8.6 Drawings of virtual bronchoscopy views at every bifurcation from the peripheral to the central, respectively

Chapter 9
Anesthesia for Bronchoscopy

Masahiro Katsurada and Takehiro Izumo

Abstract Adequate pre-procedural laryngopharyngeal anesthesia is important for smooth insertion of the bronchoscope through the pharynx and vocal cords. Moderate to deep intravenous sedation during bronchoscopy is almost always recommended for patient comfort and for the beneficial effects of retrograde amnesia.

Keywords Anesthesia • Bronchoscopy • Lidocaine intoxication • Lidocaine allergy • Sedation

9.1 Indications

Topical laryngopharyngeal anesthesia is an essential procedure for all bronchoscopic examinations in order to decrease the pain associated with bronchoscope insertion through the vocal cords. The method and dose of anesthesia vary among facilities. In this guidebook, we will introduce the anesthesia technique that we use at our facility (Table 9.1). A history of drug allergy should be elicited, and an alternative medication should be considered, as necessary (refer to Sect. 9.4).

9.2 Preparation

1. *Laryngopharyngeal anesthesia using lidocaine spray* (Fig. 9.1):
   (a) 5 mL of 4 % lidocaine
   (b) Jackson nebulizer

M. Katsurada
Department of Respiratory Medicine, Kobe University Graduate School of Medicine, Kobe, Japan

T. Izumo (✉)
Department of Respiratory Medicine, Japanese Red Cross Medical Center, 4-1-22 Hiroo, Shibuya-ku, Tokyo 150-8935, Japan
e-mail: drtake1118@gmail.com

T. Izumo et al. (eds.), *Respiratory Endoscopy*,
DOI 10.1007/978-981-287-916-5_9

Table 9.1 Anesthesia and sedation for bronchoscopy

Preliminary medication	Pethidine hydrochloride (Opystan®) 35 mg/1 mL is injected intravenously at the following doses:
	Weight >50 kg → 0.5 mL
	Weight ≤50 kg → 0.25 mL
	Age >80 years old → 0.25 mL
	Age ≤80 years old → 0.5 mL
Local anesthesia before bronchoscopy	A total of 5 mL of 4 % lidocaine is applied using a Jackson spray to anesthetize the pharyngeal and laryngeal areas
Sedation before bronchoscopy	Midazolam 10 mg/2 mL (Dormicum®) is diluted in 8 mL of saline to make a 10-mL solution; 2–3 mL of this diluted solution is administered intravenously as follows:
	Weight >50 kg → 3 mL
	Weight ≤50 kg → 2 mL
	Age >80 years old → 2 mL
	Age ≤80 years old → 3 mL
Local anesthesia and sedation during bronchoscopy	If severe coughing occurs, 1–2 mL of 2 % lidocaine is injected through the working channel of the bronchoscope. Additional 1–2 mL of diluted midazolam solution may be administered intravenously

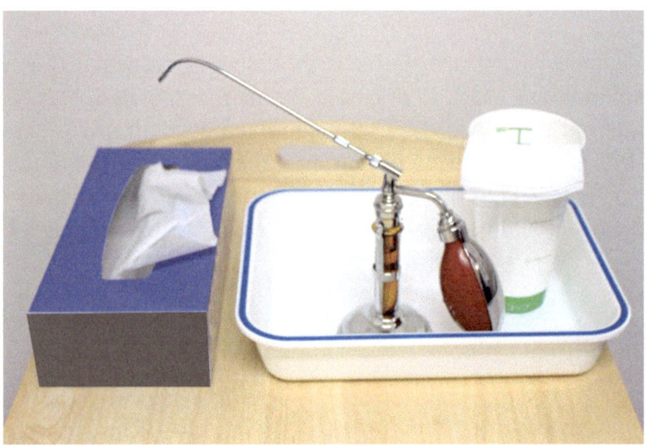

Fig. 9.1 Preparation for laryngopharyngeal anesthesia

(c) Gauze
(d) Kidney basin or cup

2. *Sedatives and analgesics*:

(e) Pethidine hydrochloride, 35 mg/1 mL (Opystan®)
(f) Midazolam, 10 mg/2 mL (Midazolam®)

3. *Anesthesia during bronchoscopy*:

(g) 1-mL aliquots of 2 % lidocaine

9.3 Actual Procedure

Instruct patients not to eat or drink anything 4 h prior to the procedure. Before administration of topical anesthesia, secure and ensure patent venous access. In the endoscopic examination room, ask the patient to be seated, and apply lidocaine spray using Jackson nebulizer for laryngopharyngeal anesthesia (Fig. 9.1). To anesthetize the entire pharynx to the larynx/glottis adequately, ensure clear vision of the pharynx so that the nozzle of the Jackson nebulizer is able to reach the deeper end of the pharynx while taking care to avoid mucosal contact and trauma.

Ask the patient to thrust out his or her chin slightly, and tilt the head upward to secure an open airway. To ensure clear vision of the pharynx, ask the patient to advance his or her tongue. Expectedly, the patient may draw back the tongue on a reflex after stimulation of the pharynx and by the bitter taste of lidocaine; in this case, the operator should stand directly in front of the patient and gently hold the tip of the tongue with gauze. Since there are some patients with strong pharyngeal or cough reflex upon first application, avoid spraying deeply at the start; instead, gently anesthetize the superficial part of the pharynx first then gradually proceed into the deeper parts, such as the inferior part of the pharynx, the larynx, and the area near the vocal cords. Application of lidocaine spray should be done simultaneous with deep and slow inhalation. After two to three sprays, ask the patient to spit out the pooled fluid in the oral cavity into a kidney basin or cup in order to decrease lidocaine absorption into the body, as well as to prevent cough induced by pooling of fluid in the oral cavity (Fig. 9.2).

Adequate laryngopharyngeal anesthesia needs patient cooperation. Therefore, a patient should be made to understand its importance for a smooth bronchoscopy and that this part of the procedure may be the most, but last, painful experience. It would also be necessary to explain to the patient what to expect during application of topical anesthesia, such as an uncomfortable feeling in the throat, hoarseness, or difficulty in swallowing; in the latter case, therefore, assure and advise your patient not to forcibly try to swallow because this can lead to aspiration and cough.

When application of laryngopharyngeal anesthesia is completed, place the patient in a supine position on the examination table and attach the pulse oximeter and automatic blood pressure monitor. After this, the mouth piece may be inserted, and administration of oxygen per nasal cannula may be started at 2–4 L/min to achieve a SpO_2 of at least 90 %. Cover the patient's eyes with gauze to prevent lidocaine or any fluid from getting onto the eyes. Thereafter, administer intravenous pethidine hydrochloride (35 mg/mL) and midazolam (10 mg/2 mL) according to Table 9.1. At our hospital, we mix 10 mg/2 mL of midazolam with 8 mL of normal saline to make a 10-mg/10-mL (1 mg/1 mL) solution (Fig. 9.3).

After induction of sedation, insert the bronchoscope. If laryngopharyngeal anesthesia is effective, insertion would be easy because the vocal cords are open. Once the bronchoscope is inserted into the trachea and as you proceed down the bronchial branches, apply 1-mL aliquots of 2 % lidocaine intermittently through the working channel of the bronchoscope to anesthetize the entire tracheobronchial mucosa. At

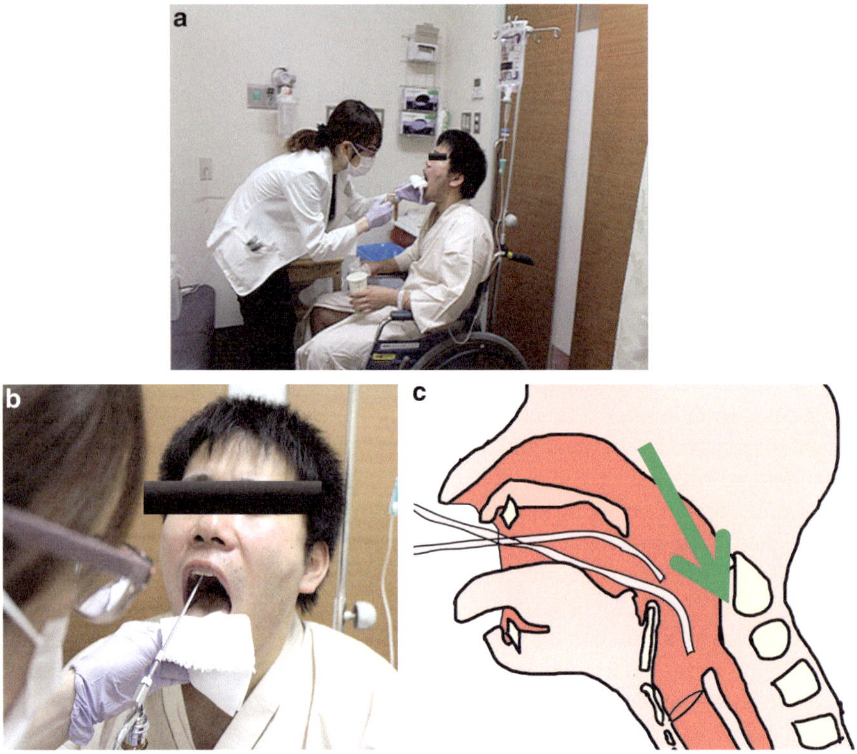

Fig. 9.2 Application of 5 mL of 4% lidocaine for laryngopharyngeal anesthesia. (**a**) The doctor stands in front of a seated patient; (**b**) the doctor should be able to visualize the pharyngeal area during application of anesthesia; (**c**) position and adjust the Jackson nebulizer nozzle tip as illustrated as you proceed with application of lidocaine spray from the superficial to the deeper areas of the laryngopharynx. First, apply minimal lidocaine spray on the pharynx. Then, slant the nozzle gradually in the direction of the arrow to anesthetize the posterior pharynx and the vocal cords

our facility, we use a 10-mL syringe pre-filled with 1 mL of lidocaine plus 9 mL of air to deliver topical anesthesia through the bronchoscope; this way, we are able to push out any remaining lidocaine in the working channel and propel the liquid adequately onto the intended area for anesthesia. Of note, it is important to advise the patient that cough may be expected during the first few applications of lidocaine but will gradually subside as anesthesia starts to take effect. One alternative is the use of catheter spray, which may induce less cough than a syringe spray. Anesthesia is usually administered on the upper lobar bronchi first, so as to allow the lidocaine solution to gravitate to and anesthetize the lower lobar bronchi.

After bronchoscopy, we intravenously administer 2.5 mL of flumazenil 0.5 mg/5 mL to antagonize the effects of midazolam. However, please note that a prolonged sedative effect may still be expected due to residual midazolam in the body.

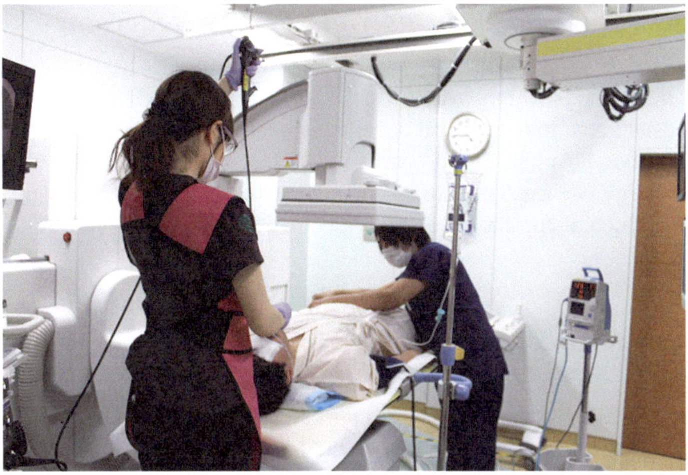

Fig. 9.3 Administration of intravenous sedation. Connect the patient to a pulse oximeter before administration of intravenous sedation prior to bronchoscopy

9.4 Precautions and Countermeasures

9.4.1 Atropine Sulfate

Although atropine sulfate has been considered effective for the suppression of bronchial secretion and for prevention of bronchoconstriction, its added value could not be demonstrated by recent studies. In fact, the British Thoracic Society guidelines and the American College of Chest Physicians (ACCP) consensus statement recommended against the use of atropine due to a potential for tachycardia [1, 2]. In Japan, its utilization has been decreasing, and it is currently not used at our hospital.

9.4.2 Lidocaine Intoxication

Lidocaine intoxication presents with central nervous and cardiovascular symptoms, such as impaired responsiveness, disturbance of consciousness, tremors, hypotension, bradycardia, impaired myocardial contractility, and ventricular arrhythmia. It is caused by administration of lidocaine at doses that exceed 7 mg/kg [2], which is about 17.5 mL of 2 % lidocaine for a 50-kg individual. Therefore, it is always necessary to mind the cumulative dose of lidocaine that you administer during bronchoscopy. Once a patient manifests with symptoms suggestive of lidocaine intoxication, the procedure must be stopped, and countermeasures, such as oxygen administration, maintaining secure venous access, and adequate fluid administration, should be started immediately. Diazepam should be given for remarkable tremors and spasms.

9.4.3 Anesthesia for Patients with Allergy to Lidocaine

In Japan, lidocaine is widely used for laryngopharyngeal anesthesia, but the ACCP consensus statement indicated that cocaine, benzocaine, and tetracaine may also be used [2]. At our hospital, 1 % procaine is used as an alternative for patents with lidocaine allergy; we use 5 mL for laryngopharyngeal anesthesia and 1-mL aliquots for tracheobronchial anesthesia, as described in Sect. 9.3.

9.5 Advantages of Lidocaine

Although studies on lidocaine for local anesthesia during bronchoscopy are few, a randomized controlled trial, which compared lidocaine spray with saline solution spray, demonstrated significantly decreased frequency of coughing and dose of sedatives needed during bronchoscopy in the lidocaine group [3].

References

1. British Thoracic Society Bronchoscopy Guidelines Committee aSoSoCCoBTS. British Thoracic Society guidelines on diagnostic flexible bronchoscopy. Thorax. 2001;56 Suppl 1:i1–21.
2. Wahidi MM, Jain P, Jantz M, Lee P, Mackensen GB, Barbour SY, et al. American College of Chest Physicians consensus statement on the use of topical anesthesia, analgesia, and sedation during flexible bronchoscopy in adult patients. Chest. 2011;140(5):1342–50. doi:10.1378/chest.10-3361.
3. Antoniades N, Worsnop C. Topical lidocaine through the bronchoscope reduces cough rate during bronchoscopy. Respirology. 2009;14(6):873–6. doi:10.1111/j.1440-1843.2009.01587.x.

Chapter 10
Processing Samples

Takaaki Tsuchida and Takehiro Izumo

Abstract Poor handling of specimens may result to a negative study even if enough samples were taken correctly. Avoid smearing dry specimens with two glass slides. Do not grind specimens if these are wet enough. In such cases, draw the specimen with two slide glasses.

Keywords Specimen • Bronchoscopy • Guide sheath flush

10.1 Purpose of Specimen Handling

Biopsy specimens should be handled correctly for proper pathologic evaluation and testing for DNA mutation.

10.2 Preparation of Transbronchial Biopsy/Cytology Specimens (Fig. 10.1)

1. Specimen bottles with formalin
2. Thin tweezers
3. Nitrocellulose papers with square cut sections that are 5-mm wide
4. Glass slides
5. Glass slide bottles with fixing alcohol
6. Plastic tubes with small amount (about 2 ml) of saline
7. Several pieces of gauze

T. Tsuchida (✉)
Department of Endoscopy, Respiratory Endoscopy Division, National Cancer Center Hospital, 5-1-1, Tsukiji, Chou-ku, Tokyo 104-0045, Japan
e-mail: ttsuchid@ncc.go.jp

T. Izumo
Department of Respiratory Medicine, Japanese Red Cross Medical Center, 4-1-22 Hiroo, Shibuya-ku, Tokyo 150-8935, Japan

T. Izumo et al. (eds.), *Respiratory Endoscopy*,
DOI 10.1007/978-981-287-916-5_10

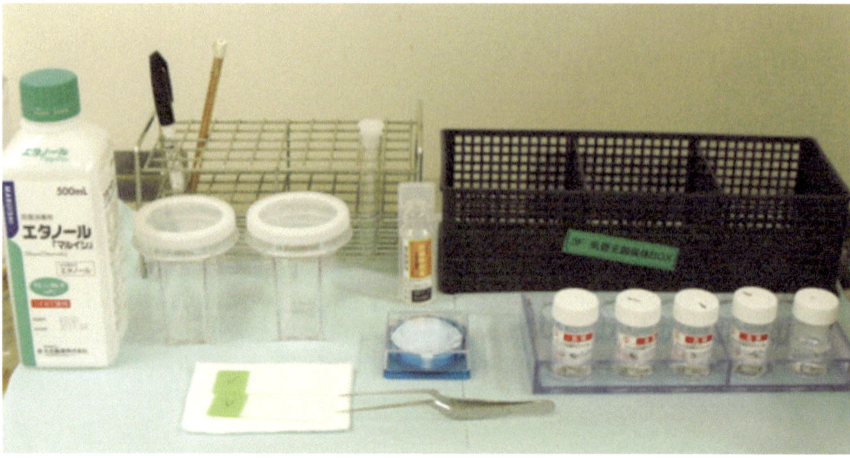

Fig. 10.1 Preparation of transbronchial biopsy/cytology samples

10.3 The Actual Procedure

1. Preparation of transbronchial biopsy specimens
   Using thin tweezers, transfer specimens obtained by forceps on nitrocellulose paper (Fig. 10.2) before placing in a formalin bottle (Fig. 10.3).
2. Handling of the brush samples:
   (a) Smear the tip of the brush on a pair of glass slides (Fig. 10.4).
   (b) Put one glass slide in a bottle containing the fixing alcohol (Fig. 10.5).
   (c) The other glass slide is air-dried for rapid on-site examination (Fig. 10.6). If rapid on-site cytology is not necessary, no additional glass slide is needed.
   (d) Wash the brush tip in a plastic tube with saline as a liquid sample (Fig. 10.7).
3. Handling of transbronchial needle aspiration samples:
   (a) Push out the needle aspiration specimen on a glass slide (Fig. 10.8).
   (b) If there are core tissue specimens available, pick these up with thin tweezers and transfer on nitrocellulose paper before placing in a formalin bottle.
   (c) After removing the core tissues from the glass slides, make slide preparations with the use of squash preparation or wedge method (Fig. 10.9).
   (d) During the smear preparation, any liquid component protruding from the edge of the bonding glass slides should be removed with gauze.
   (e) If the liquid component of the specimen is not enough, make slide preparations using squash method.

Fig. 10.2

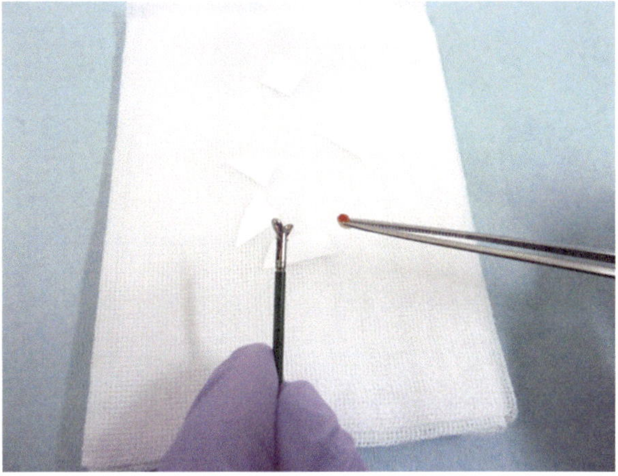

Fig. 10.3

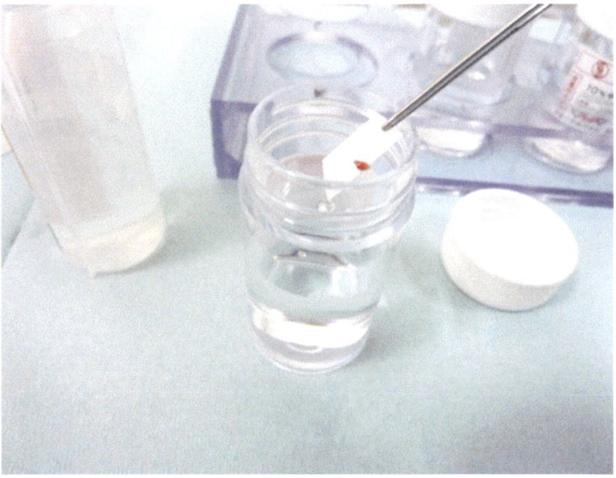

Fig. 10.4

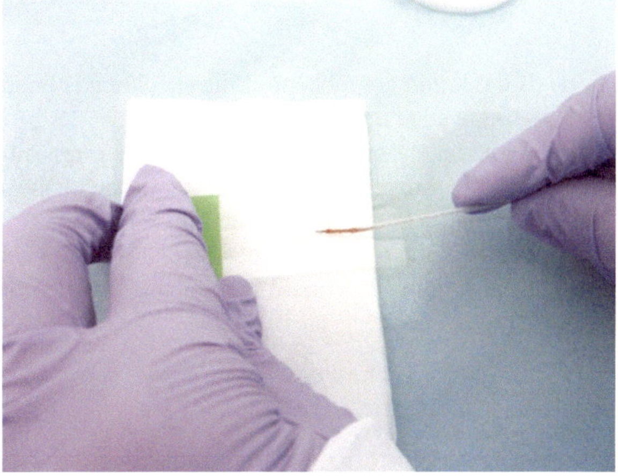

Fig. 10.5

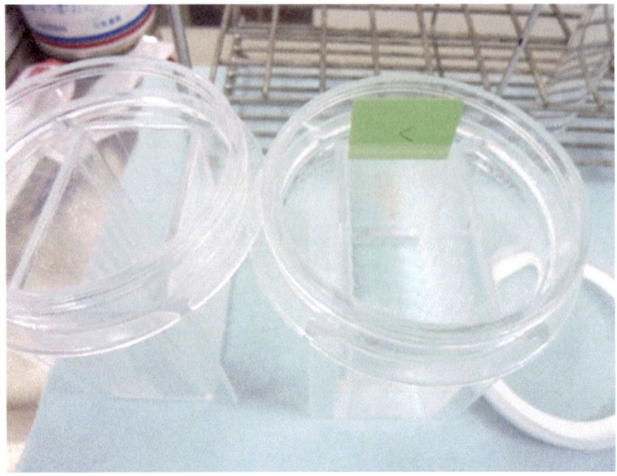

Fig. 10.6

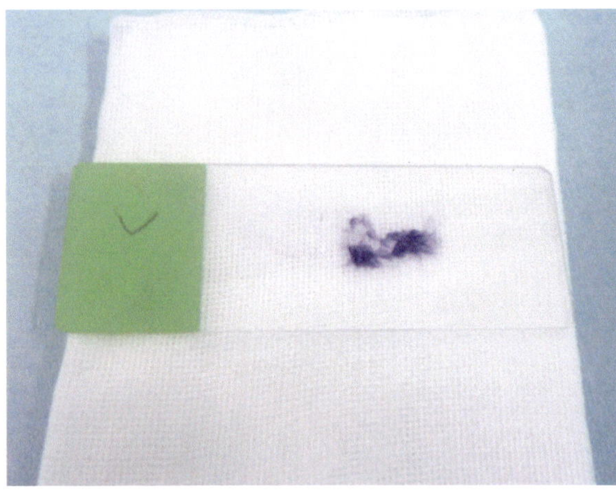

(f) If the liquid component of the specimen is enough, make slide preparations using wedge method.
(g) Immediately put the slide preparations into a bottle with fixing alcohol. If rapid on-site cytology is necessary, one of the slide preparations should be air-dried without fixing (Fig. 10.10).
(h) Push out the remaining specimens inside the needle with 2 ml of saline into a plastic tube as a liquid specimen (Figs. 10.11 and 10.12).

Fig. 10.7

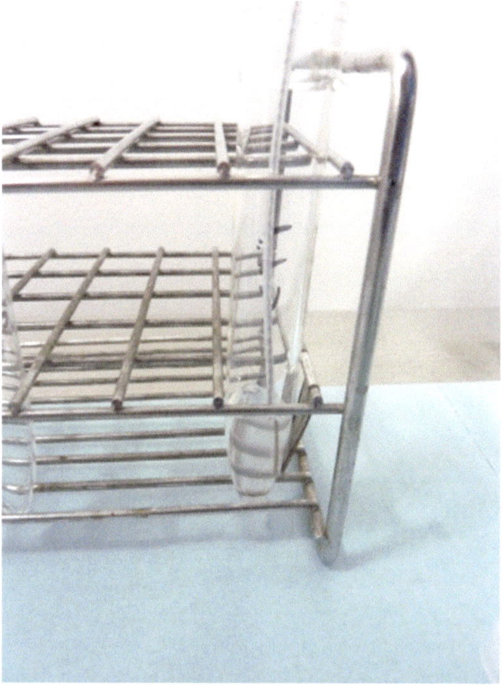

Fig. 10.8

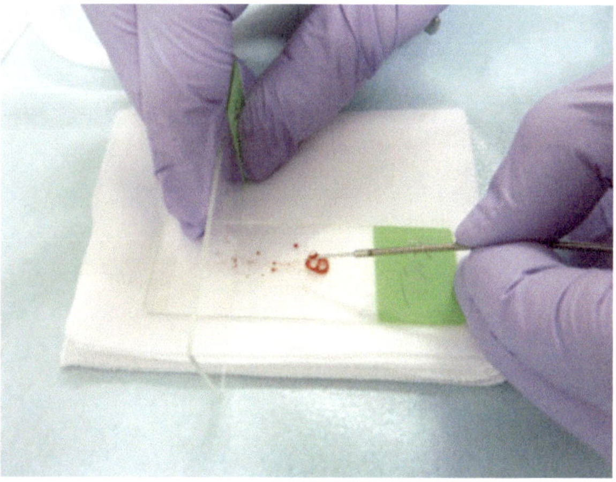

Fig. 10.9

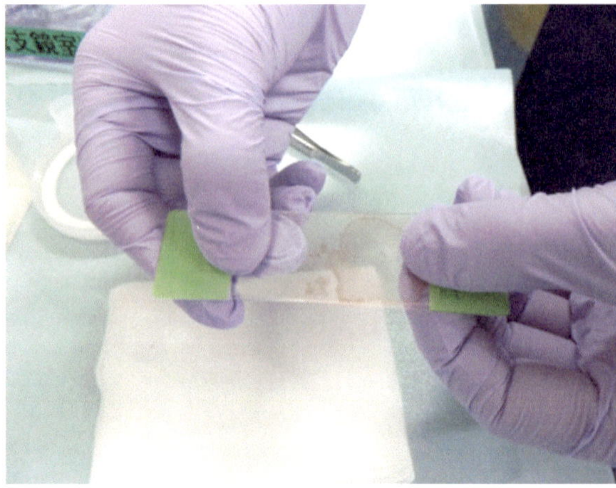

Fig. 10.10

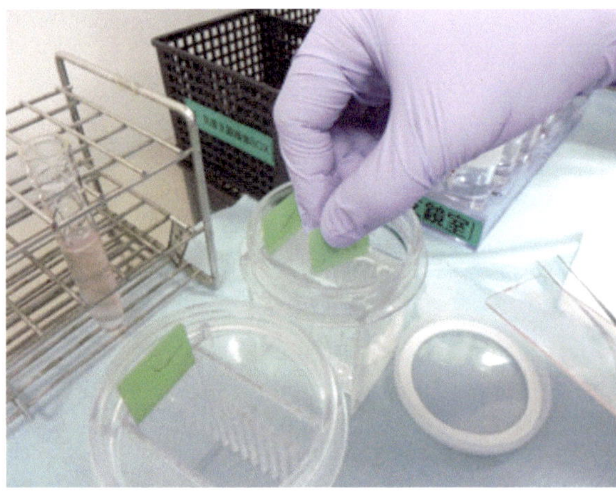

Fig. 10.11

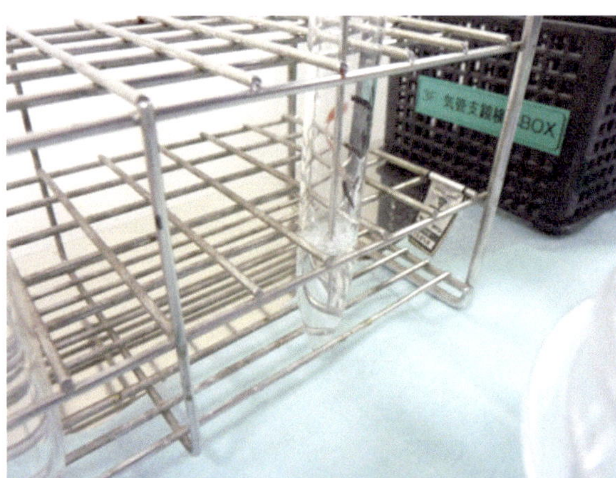

Fig. 10.12

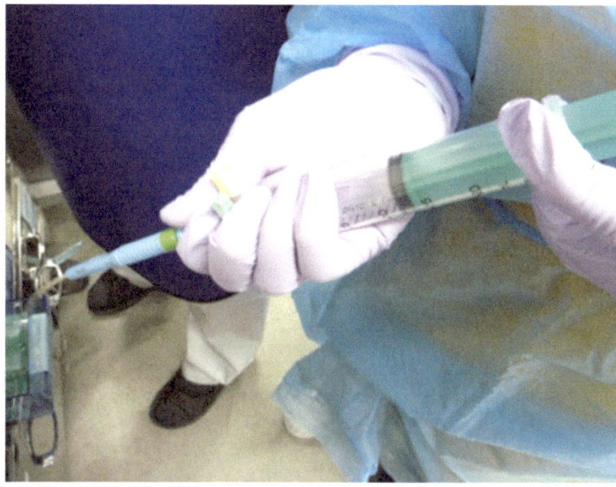

Fig. 10.13

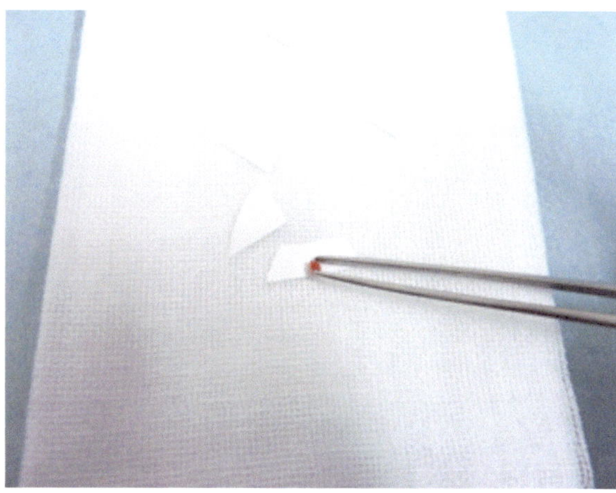

10.4 Limits and Measures

Depending on the way of sample preparation, proper pathologic diagnosis may become difficult even if the sample was obtained correctly:

1. A small transbronchial biopsy specimen that contains the diagnostic cells may get dislodged and stick to the back of the lid of the specimen bottle (Fig. 10.13). This may be prevented by placing the specimen on nitrocellulose paper.
2. Glass slide preparations dry quickly; this makes microscopic evaluation on Papanicolaou staining difficult. When preparing glass slide samples for cytology, do the smears quickly and immediately put the slide into the bottle with fixing alcohol.

10.4.1 Advantages and Disadvantages of Smear Sample and Liquid Sample

1. Smear sample is quick to dry and makes diagnosis by Papanicolaou staining difficult.
2. During slide preparation, crushing the cells by performing the smear strongly will make diagnosis difficult.
3. Liquid cytology samples may be difficult to evaluate microscopically when there is cell swelling.

Bibliography

1. Izumo T, Sasada S, Matsumoto Y, et al. Radial endobronchial ultrasound and guide sheath for peripheral pulmonary lesions. J Jpn Soc Respir Endosc. 2014;36:392–7.

Chapter 11
Rapid On-Site Cytology Evaluation

Takaaki Tsuchida and Takehiro Izumo

Abstract It is important for bronchoscopists and cytologists to keep in mind that rapid on-site cytology evaluation is intended not only to distinguish between benign and malignant diagnoses but also to select a sampling device.

Keywords ROSE • Transbronchial biopsy • Transbronchial needle aspiration • Lymph node • Peripheral pulmonary lesions

11.1 Purpose of Rapid On-Site Cytology Evaluation (ROSE)

To determine whether the collected specimens are sufficient for routine cytology examination

To determine whether the collected specimens are taken from the target lesion

Serves as a guide for selecting sampling devices

11.2 Preparation for ROSE

1. Diff-Quik® stain:

   - Diff-Quik® staining kit (Sysmex, Kobe, Japan) (Fig. 11.1)
   - A bottle of tap water
   - Bottles with fixing alcohol and staining solutions
   - Dryer
   - Microscope

T. Tsuchida (✉)
Department of Endoscopy, Respiratory Endoscopy Division, National Cancer Center Hospital, 5-1-1, Tsukiji, Chou-ku, Tokyo 104-0045, Japan
e-mail: ttsuchid@ncc.go.jp

T. Izumo
Department of Respiratory Medicine, Japanese Red Cross Medical Center, 4-1-22 Hiroo, Shibuya-ku, Tokyo 150-8935, Japan

T. Izumo et al. (eds.), *Respiratory Endoscopy*,
DOI 10.1007/978-981-287-916-5_11

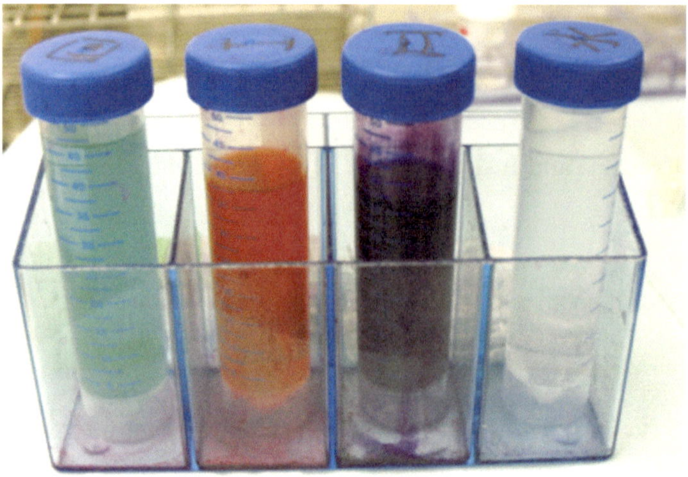

Fig. 11.1 Diff-Quik® staining kit

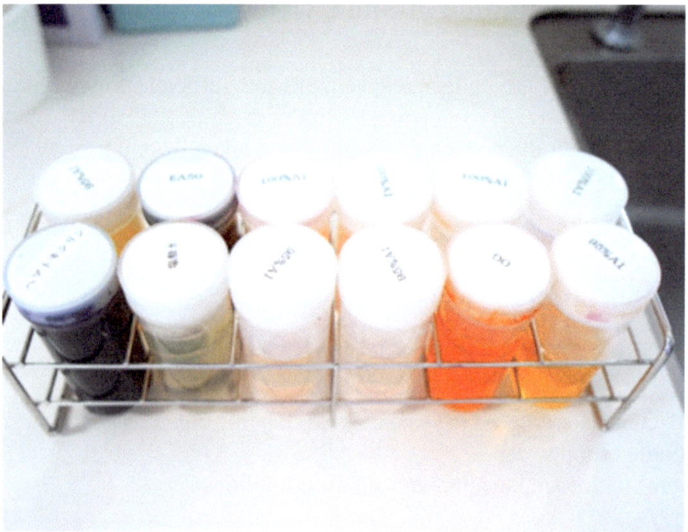

Fig. 11.2 A portion of the rapid Papanicolaou staining set

2. Rapid Papanicolaou stain (Fig. 11.2):

- Ninety-five percent ethanol
- One-hundred percent ethanol
- Hydrochloric acid
- Gill's hematoxylin
- OG-6

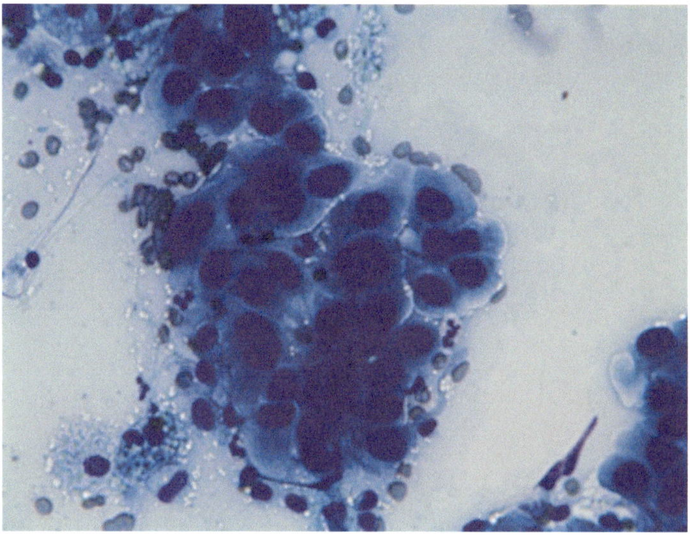

Fig. 11.3 Slide preparation stained by Diff-Quik®

- EA50
- Xylene
- Mounting medium
- Cover glasses
- Microscope

11.3 Procedure for ROSE

1. Diff-Quik® stain (Fig. 11.3):
    (a) Use cold air to dry the glass slides that contain the brush smears or imprints of specimens.
    (b) Dip the sample on the glass slide in the fixing alcohol of the staining kit for 10 s.
    (c) Stain for 20 s in solution I of the staining kit.
    (d) Stain for 20 s in solution II of the staining kit.
    (e) Rinse the stained slide preparation with water, and apply hot air to dry.
    (f) Observe by microscopy.
2. Rapid Papanicolaou stain (Fig. 11.4):
    (a) Fix the slide preparation in 95 % ethanol for 1 min or more.
    (b) Rinse with running water for a few seconds.
    (c) Stain for 90 s in Gill's hematoxylin.
    (d) Rinse with running water.

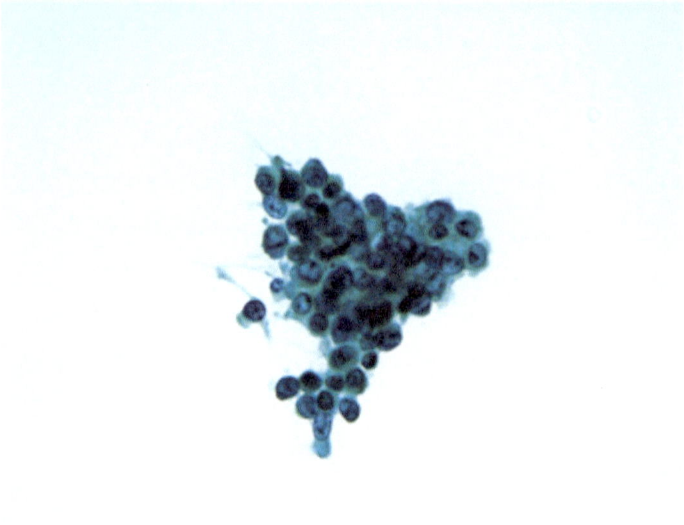

Fig. 11.4 Slide preparation stained by rapid Papanicolaou

(e) Put the slide preparation in and out of hydrochloric acid for ten times.
(f) Rinse with running water.
(g) Dip in 95 % ethanol for a few seconds.
(h) Stain for 60 s in OG-6.
(i) Dip in 95 % ethanol for two times to wash out unnecessary OG-6.
(j) Stain for 90–120 s in EA50.
(k) Dip in 100 % ethanol for three times to wash out unnecessary EA50 and to dehydrate sufficiently.
(l) Permeate the slide preparation with xylene for three times.
(m) Seal with a cover glass.
(n) Observe on microscopy.

11.4 Case Presentation

1. We performed transbronchial biopsy of a tumor located in the right S^2a to S^6a of the lung (Fig. 11.5a).
2. The finding on radial endobronchial ultrasound (R-EBUS) was "within" (Fig. 11.5b).
3. We tried brushing cytology at first, but Diff-Quik® stain showed abundance of ciliated columnar cells (Fig. 11.6).
4. Correlating the R-EBUS and ROSE findings, we estimated that the tumor was located outside the bronchial subsegment in which the guide sheath has been inserted. Therefore, we chose an aspiration needle to further obtain samples.

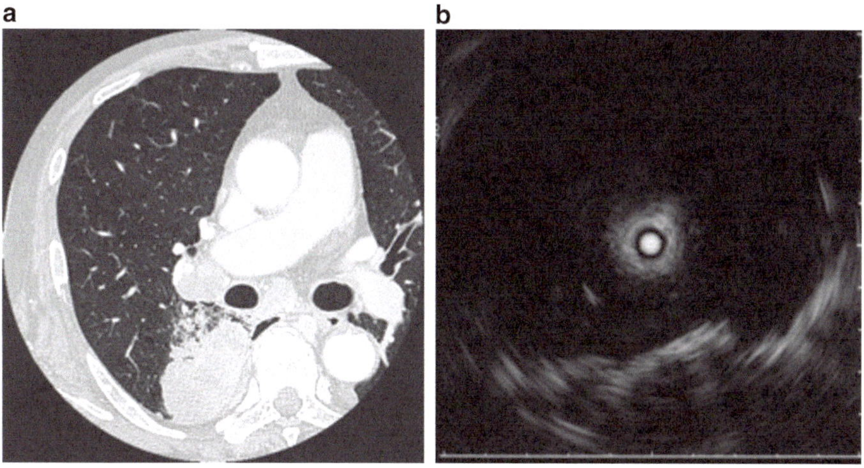

Fig. 11.5 Representative case. (**a**) Computed tomography shows tumor at right S^6. (**b**) Radial EBUS findings show “within”

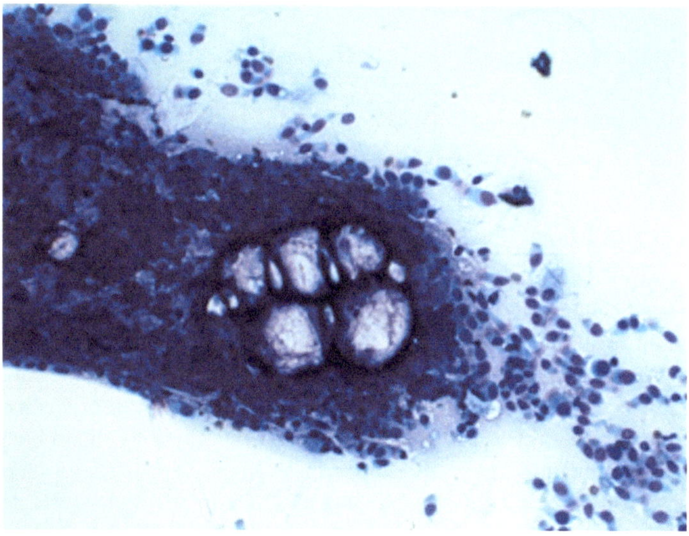

Fig. 11.6 Slide preparation of brushing cytology stained by Diff-Quik®

5. The ROSE of the transbronchial needle aspiration (TBNA) sample was suspicious for small-cell cancer (Fig. 11.7).
6. In this case, results from the biopsy specimens by forceps and brushing cytology were negative. Only the result of TBNA showed small-cell carcinoma. As in this case, R-EBUS showed “within” even if the lesion was located outside the bronchial wall; sometimes, in such situations, sufficient material cannot be obtained from the lesion with the use of forceps or brush. When ROSE shows inconclusive

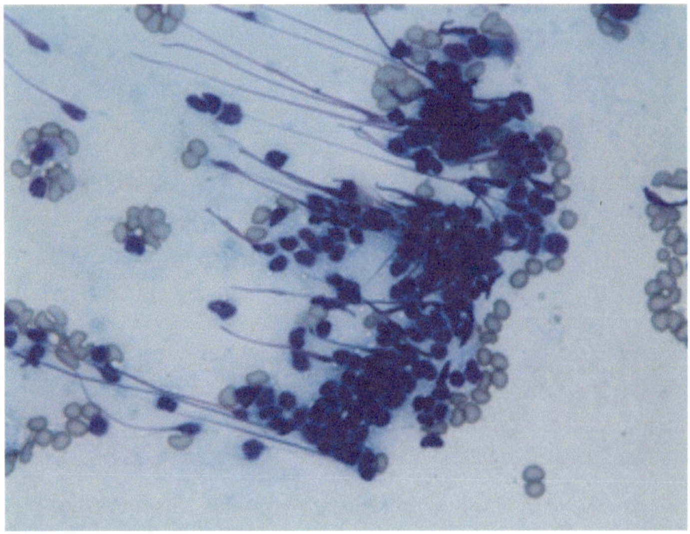

Fig. 11.7 Slide preparation of transbronchial needle aspiration sample stained by Diff-Quik®

findings in a case that is clinically highly suspicious for malignancy, we choose to add TBNA or to use a thicker guide sheath and thicker forceps even if R-EBUS suggests that the sampling devices are "within" the lesion.

11.5 Limits and Measures

There are advantages and disadvantages for the Diff-Quik® stain and rapid Papanicolaou stain. Diff-Quik® stain is a simple procedure, and handling of the chemicals is easier. On the other hand, it is limited by the difficulty in examining the cytoplasm, especially in the presence of abundant mucus and blood cells. If Diff-Quik® stain is chosen for ROSE, one should make it a point to obtain better specimens and to pay attention to sample processing. Rapid Papanicolaou stain enables easier evaluation of the cytoplasm and nucleus and is relatively less affected by the presence of mucus and blood cells. On the other hand, the procedure is complicated, and handling of the chemicals must be strict. Moreover, since highly volatile solvents are used, it is necessary to pay attention to ventilation.

ROSE plays important roles in determining whether a lesion was sufficiently sampled and in guiding bronchoscopists in selecting appropriate and additional devices for biopsy. When cytopathologist or pathologists conduct ROSE, it may be usual to simply read the slides as only "negative." However, we underscore the importance of checking whether the ROSE findings include peripheral lung or bronchial epithelium. When puncturing lymph nodes during EBUS-TBNA, correct determination of adequacy of material, based on the number of lymphocytes and macrophages, also needs to be requested. If sarcoidosis or sarcoid reaction is suspected, it is important to convey this fact to person in charge of the ROSE.

11.6 Performance

According to a prospective study by Uchida et al. [1] on 657 cases, ROSE improved the diagnostic rate of transbronchial biopsy by 16 % (from 74.4 to 90.3 %).

Reference

1. Uchida S, Imamura F, Takenaka A, et al. Improved diagnostic efficacy by rapid cytology test in fluoroscopy-guided bronchoscopy. J Thorac Oncol. 2006;1:314–8.

Chapter 12
Type and Selection of Flexible Bronchoscope

Shinji Sasada

Abstract Diagnostic bronchoscopy for peripheral pulmonary lesions is not yet established. At present, the method varies according to the preferences of the physicians. A new middle-range diameter bronchoscope with a large working channel (prototype thin 1T scope) combines the function of a large scope and a thin or ultrathin scope to enable farther reach to the periphery while maintaining the ability to collect adequate specimen.

Keywords Bronchoscopy • Peripheral pulmonary lesions • Tissue sampling • New middle-range diameter bronchoscope with a large working channel (prototype thin 1T scope)

12.1 The Development of the Bronchoscope

The very first prototype of the bronchoscope was the one used by Gustav Killian (Germany) in 1897 to remove bronchial foreign body using a rigid laryngoscope [1]. Thereafter, in 1907, Chevalier Jackson (USA) improved the form of the current rigid bronchoscope for use in endobronchial foreign body extraction and tracheobronchial stent placement [2]. In 1966, Shigeto Ikeda (National Cancer Center, Japan) developed the first prototype of the flexible fiberoptic bronchoscope, which is currently being used commonly worldwide. Since then, the function of the flexible bronchoscope has evolved to enable bending the tip up and down and to include a working channel for insertion of instruments, such as biopsy forceps or brush, along with the observation window. With the strong flexibility of the fiberoptic bronchoscope, it has become possible to approach difficult to reach bronchial branches, such as the right B1 and B2, the left B1+2, and the bilateral B6.

S. Sasada (✉)
Department of Respiratory Medicine, Tokyo Saiseikai Central Hospital,
1-4-17, Mita, Minato-ku, Tokyo 108-0073, Japan
e-mail: sasastaf@hotmail.co.jp

T. Izumo et al. (eds.), *Respiratory Endoscopy*,
DOI 10.1007/978-981-287-916-5_12

Table 12.1 Various types of flexible bronchoscopes

	Outer diameter of the distal tip (mm)	Outer diameter of the shaft (mm)	Inner diameter of working channel (mm)	Details
Olympus video bronchoscope 260 series				
BF-260	4.9	4.9	2.0	Standard
BF-1T260	5.9	6.0	2.8	Large channel
BF-6C260	5.9	5.7	2.0	High vision
BF-P260F	4.0	4.4	2.0	Thin
BF-XP260F	2.8	2.8	1.2	Ultrathin
BF-F260	5.5	5.4	2.0	Autofluorescence
BF-UC260FW	6.9	6.3	2.2	Convex-type EBUS
Olympus video bronchoscope 290 series				
BF-Q290	4.8	4.9	2.0	Standard
BF-1TQ290	5.9	6.0	3.0	Large channel
BF-H290	6.0	5.7	2.0	High vision
BF-P290	4.2	4.1	2.0	Thin
BF-XP290	3.1	2.8	1.2	Ultrathin
Pentax video bronchoscope				
EB-1572K	5.5	5.1	2.0	Standard
EB-1972K	6.3	6.2	2.8	Large channel
EB-1170K	3.8	3.7	1.2	Thin
Fuji video bronchoscope				
EB-530H	5.4	4.9	2.0	Standard
EB-530T	5.8	5.9	2.8	Large channel
EB-530P	3.8	3.8	1.2	Thin
EB-530US	6.7	6.3	2.0	Convex-type EBUS
Prototype (Olympus)	5.1	5.1	2.6	Middle-range diameter with a large channel

12.2 Types of Flexible Bronchoscopes

Various types of the flexible fiberoptic bronchoscope are available. The large-diameter bronchoscope with high resolution, such as the high-definition scope, is used for visible, endobronchial lesions; the small-diameter bronchoscope has been developed to biopsy peripheral pulmonary lesions, and the convex scanning ultrasound bronchoscope has been developed for the purpose of hilar and mediastinal lymph node biopsy (Table 12.1).

12.3 The Current State of Peripheral Pulmonary Lesion Diagnosis

Recently, a meta-analysis on the diagnostic yield of bronchoscopy for peripheral pulmonary lesions has been reported [3]. Particularly, the use of endobronchial ultrasound (EBUS) and/or virtual bronchial navigation (VBN) has resulted in improved diagnostic rates, with a pooled sensitivity as high as 70% [4, 5].

12.4 Choice of Bronchoscope for Peripheral Pulmonary Lesions

In general, there are currently two available sizes of the bronchoscope. First is the thick or large-diameter bronchoscope that has an outer diameter of 6 mm and an inner diameter of 2.8–3.0 mm (BF-1T260/BF-1TQ290; Olympus, Tokyo, Japan). The second is the thin or small-diameter bronchoscope that has an outer diameter of 4.0 mm and an inner diameter 2.0 mm (BF-P260F/BF-P290; Olympus, Tokyo, Japan). Bronchoscopes used for peripheral pulmonary lesions are selected depending on the size and site of the lesion. The thick bronchoscope can use larger devices, which is advantageous in providing larger biopsy specimens, but insertion to more peripheral subsegmental bronchi is limited. On the other hand, the thin bronchoscope has excellent operability for the peripheral subsegmental bronchi but is limited by the use of small biopsy devices.

With these facts in mind, what bronchoscope is the best for the diagnosis of peripheral pulmonary lesions? Surely, everyone has this question in everyday clinical practice. It would seem like a conquest to be able to reach as far peripheral as possible, but this practice would immediately stagnate if the procedure is not diagnostic.

12.5 New Middle-Range Diameter Bronchoscope with a Large Working Channel: Prototype Thin 1T Scope

We have been studying how to solve the problem mentioned in Sect. 12.4. For that challenge, we deduced that the answer was to develop a scope with "thin outer diameter and thick inner diameter" in order for us to reach a lesion as close as possible and to obtain tissue at the same time. Therefore, in collaboration with Olympus Corporation, we developed a "prototype thin 1T scope," which is a middle-range diameter bronchoscope with a large working channel (Fig. 12.1), specifically, an

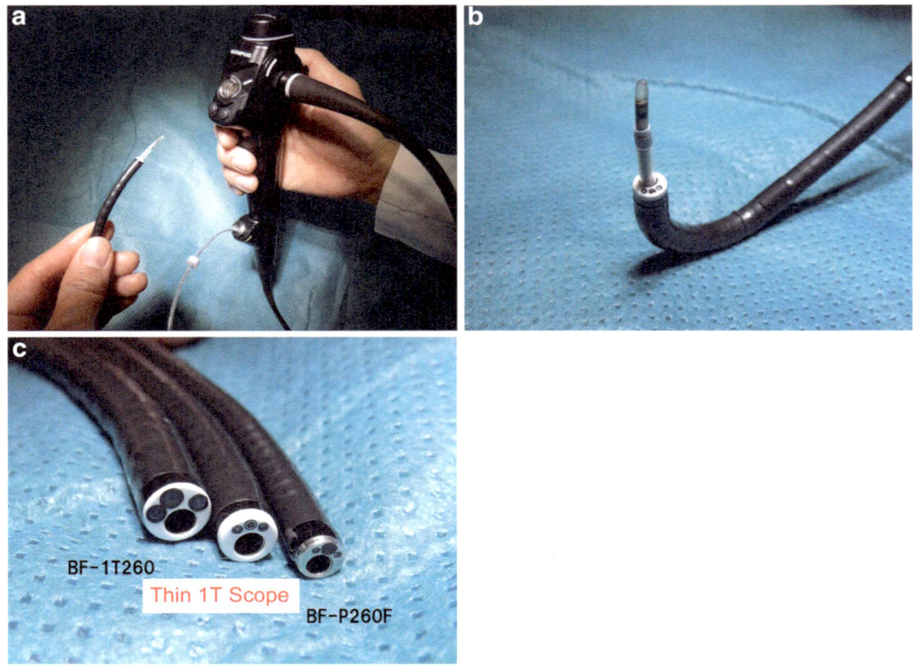

Fig. 12.1 (**a**) The middle-range diameter bronchoscope with large channel (prototype thin 1T scope, Olympus). (**b**) A large guide sheath (K-203, Olympus) with radial EBUS probe can be inserted through the working channel of the prototype thin 1T scope. (**c**) Comparison of the bronchoscope tips: BF-1T260 (*left*, 5.9 mm OD and 2.8 mm WC), thin prototype of the conventional scope (*center*, 5.1 OD and 2.6 mm WC), and BF-P260F (*right*, 4.0 OD and 2.0 mm WC). The tip of the prototype thin 1T scope is tapered. *EBUS* endobronchial ultrasound, *OD* outer diameter, and *WC* working channel

Classifications	①Peripheral-small lesions	② Central-small lesions	③ Large lesions
	If the lesion was ≦30 mm and adjacent to the visceral pleura, or if the nodule was very small (solid ≦10mm or pure GGO ≦ 15mm) and located in the outer half of the hemi-thorax	If the lesion was ≦30 mm and not adjacent to the visceral pleura	If the lesion was > 30 mm
	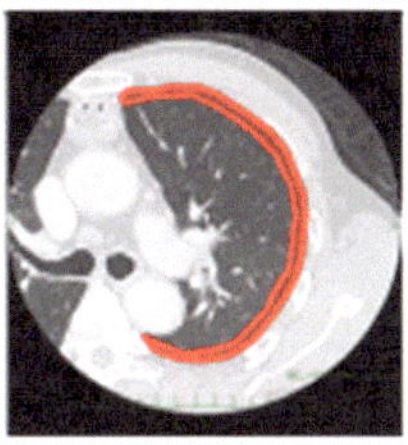	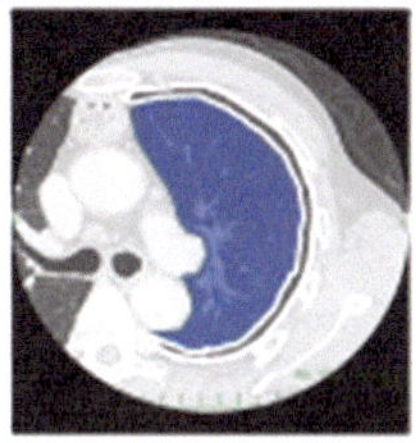	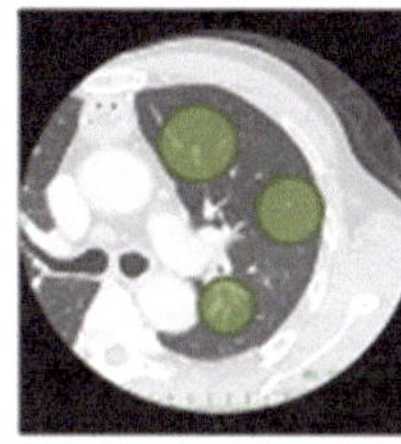
Accuracy with prototype thin IT scope	72.0%	96.3%	94.4%
Recommendations	BF-P260F or BF-P290 Small GS (K201)	Prototype thin IT scope or Large scope Large GS (K203) GS-TBNA	Prototype thin IT scope or Large scope Large GS (K203) GS-TBNA

Fig. 12.2 Classification and selection criteria of bronchoscope for peripheral pulmonary lesions

outer diameter of 5.1 mm and an inner diameter of 2.6 mm [6]. The optical system of this new bronchoscope adopted the hybrid system; the bending angle of the tip is up to 180° flexion and 130° extension. With these features, it is possible to use a large-diameter guide sheath (GS) kit (K-203, Olympus, Tokyo, Japan).

12.6 Experience on the Use of the Prototype Thin 1T Scope

Seventy patients with peripheral pulmonary lesions who underwent diagnostic bronchoscopy with EBUS-GS using the prototype scope from September 2013 to November 2013 at the National Cancer Center, Japan, were analyzed [6]. Diagnostic performance of the procedure was analyzed and compared among three groups of peripheral pulmonary lesions: "peripheral-small" lesions (less than 30 mm and adjacent to the visceral pleura), "central-small" lesions (less than 30 mm and not adjacent to the visceral pleura), and "large" lesions (more than 30 mm). Sixty patients (85.7 %) had malignant disease. Diagnosis was established in 61 of 70 patients (87.1 %); the respective yields for "central-small" and "large" lesions were significantly higher than that for "peripheral-small" lesions (96.3 %, 94.4 %, 72 %;

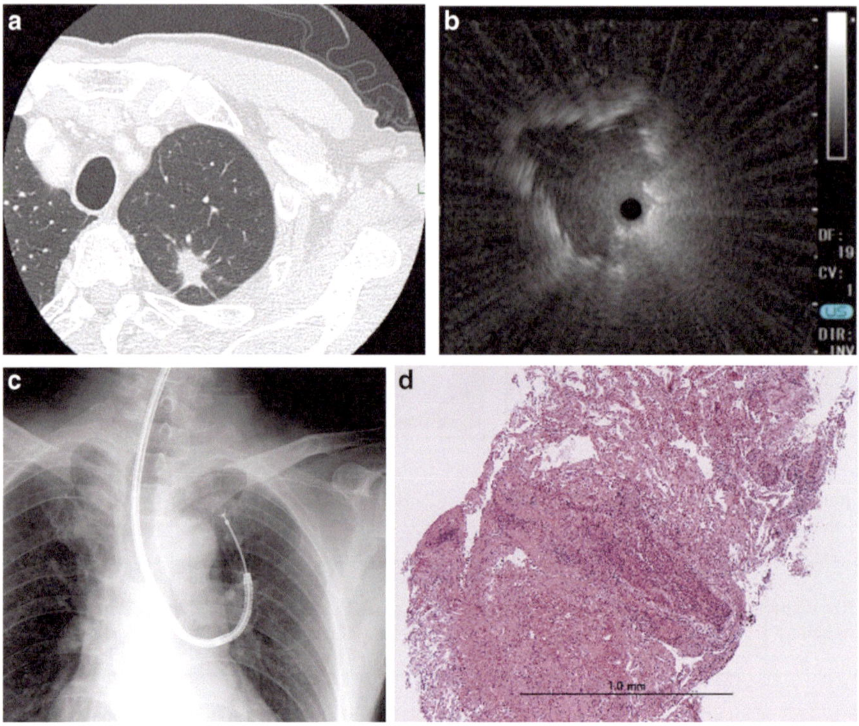

Fig. 12.3 A case of a 72-year-old man who was admitted because of abnormal shadow on chest radiograph. (**a**) Computed tomography scan shows a solid tumor, measuring 18 mm in the largest diameter, in the left S1+2; this was classified as "central small." (**b**) The radial EBUS probe was advanced into the left B1+2a bronchus, following virtual bronchoscopic navigation, and demonstrated low-echoic signals located adjacent to the probe. (**c**) Fluoroscopy imaging during endobronchial ultrasound with a guide sheath procedure. (**d**) Histopathologic evaluation of the transbronchial biopsy specimen shows squamous cell carcinoma (hematoxylin–eosin stain, ×40)

$P=0.0026$) (Fig. 12.2). These diagnostic accuracies were achieved regardless of other clinical and procedural factors, such as lesion size, feature (ground glass opacity or solid), EBUS-probe location (within or outside), or operator skill (Figs. 12.3, 12.4, and 12.5). There were no major post-procedural complications.

The new scope was much better compared to the large-diameter bronchoscope, because the tip of the new scope has a tapered structure, which enables the scope to be wedged deeper into the bronchus. Based on our data, bronchoscopy had a high diagnostic yield, similar to that of percutaneous needle biopsy and surgical lung biopsy, for lesions not adjacent to the pleura. The prototype thin 1T scope combined the functions of the large scope and thin or ultrathin scope in terms of reachability and specimen collection ability (Fig. 12.6).

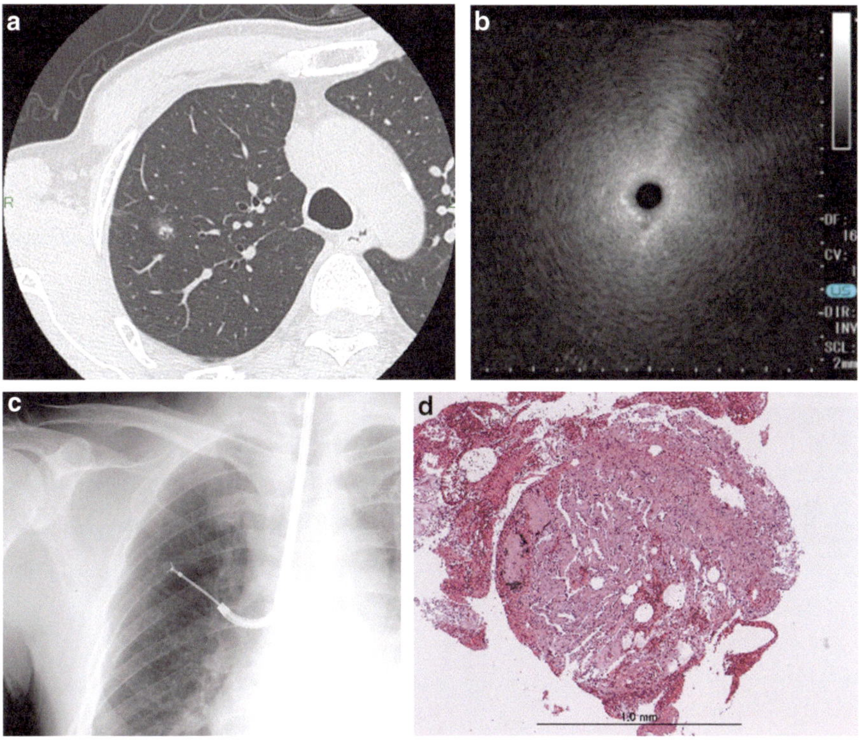

Fig. 12.4 A case of a 66-year-old man with abnormal shadow in the right upper lobe on chest radiograph. (**a**) Computed tomography scan shows a 12-mm, part-solid ground glass opacity nodule that is located away from the visceral pleura; this was classified as "central small." (**b**) The EBUS image through the right B2b reveals *Blizzard sign*, which shows coarse hyperechoic signals. (**c**) Fluoroscopy imaging during endobronchial ultrasound with a guide sheath procedure. (**d**) Histopathologic evaluation of the transbronchial biopsy specimen shows adenocarcinoma with lepidic growth pattern (hematoxylin–eosin stain, ×40)

12.7 Clinical Significance of Choosing an Optimal Bronchoscope

In recent years, with the increase in lung oncogenic driver mutations, such as mutant EGFR gene, ALK fusion type of cancer gene, etc., cases that require adequate tissue samples for both pathologic diagnosis and genotyping have been rapidly increasing [7]. Furthermore, there have been new EGFR mutation-positive resistant strains (e.g., T790M, c-MET amplification, HGF activation), for which third-generation EGFR tyrosine kinase inhibitors (TKI) and MET inhibitors can be used; particularly, osimertinib (AZD9291) is highly active for lung cancer patients with EGFR T790M mutation and who develop disease progression despite therapy with EGFR

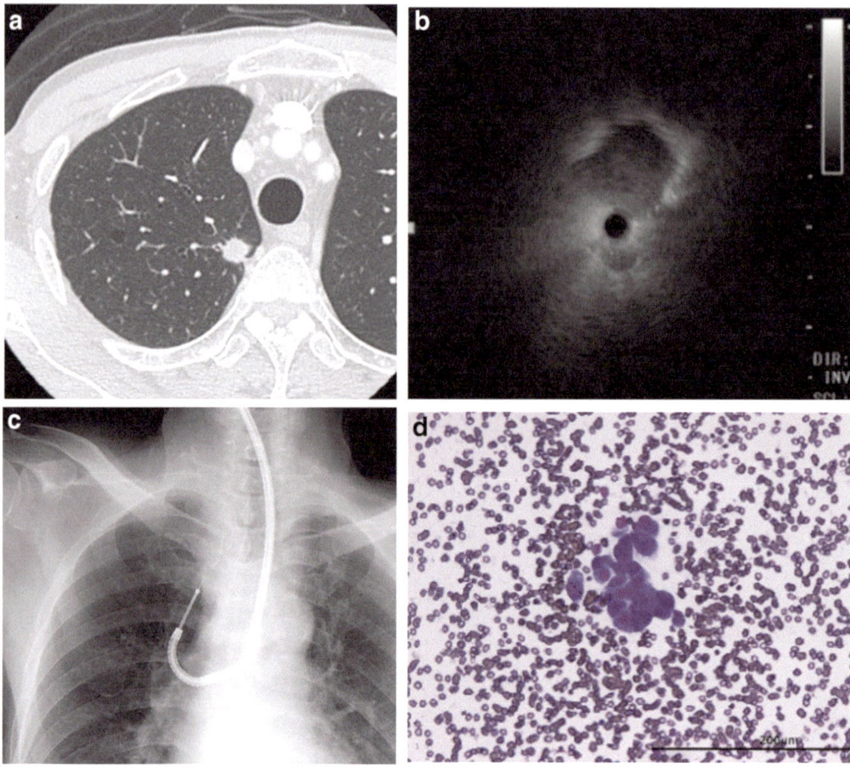

Fig. 12.5 A case of 75-year-old man with chest abnormal shadow in right upper lobe. (**a**) Computed tomography scan shows a 9-mm solid tumor that is located adjacent to the visceral pleura; this was classified as "peripheral-small." (**b**) The EBUS image through the right B1a reveals low-echoic lesion located adjacent to the probe. (**c**) Fluoroscopy imaging during GS-TBNA procedure. (**d**) Cytologic specimen from GS-TBNA shows adenocarcinoma (Papanicolaou stain, ×100). GS-TBNA, transbronchial needle aspiration through a guide sheath

TKI [8]. According to a phase I trial with expansion cohorts, nivolumab, a fully human immunoglobulin G4 programmed death 1 immune checkpoint inhibitor antibody, may be given and is generally well tolerated in patients with advanced solid tumors. In fact, nivolumab monotherapy produced durable responses and encouraging survival rates in patients with heavily pretreated NSCLC [9]. With all these promising lung cancer treatments available, the necessity of obtaining enough tumor samples after recurrence (re-biopsy) is underscored, and bronchoscopy is one of the valuable tools for this purpose. Therefore, the choice of an optimal scope is important. The prototype thin 1T scope is preferable for re-biopsy.

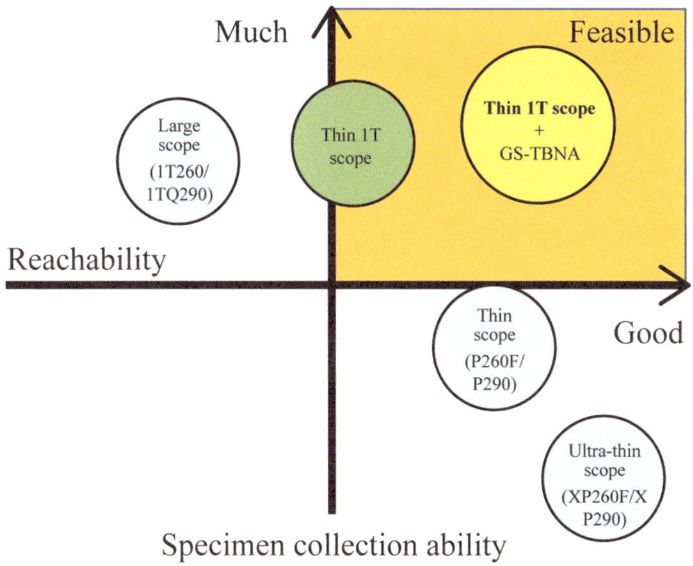

Fig. 12.6 Positioning of the various bronchoscopes used in peripheral pulmonary lesion diagnosis. The prototype thin 1T scope has an intermediate function between the large scope and the thin or ultrathin scope, in terms of having both of reachability and specimen collection ability. It does not deviate significantly from the essential purpose of doing diagnostic bronchoscopy

References

1. Killian G. Meeting of the Society of Physicians of Freiburg Dec. 17, 1897. Munchen Med Mschr. 1898;45:378.
2. Jackson C. Foreign bodies in the trachea, bronchi and esophagus. Laryngoscope. 1907;15:527.
3. Wang Memoli JS, Nietert PJ, Silvestri GA. Meta-analysis of guided bronchoscopy for the evaluation of the pulmonary nodule. Chest. 2012;142:385–93.
4. Kurimoto N, Miyazawa T, Okimasa S, et al. Endobronchial ultrasonography using a guide sheath increases the ability to diagnose peripheral pulmonary lesions endoscopically. Chest. 2004;126:959–65.
5. Ishida T, Asano F, Yamazaki K, et al. Virtual bronchoscopic navigation combined with endobronchial ultrasound to diagnose small peripheral pulmonary lesions: a randomised trial. Thorax. 2007;131:549–53.
6. Sasada S, Izumo T, Chavez C, et al. A new middle-range diameter bronchoscope with large channel for transbronchial sampling of peripheral pulmonary lesions. Jpn J Clin Oncol. 2014;44:826–34.
7. Lindeman NI, Cagle PT, Beasley MB, et al. Molecular testing guideline for selection of lung cancer patients for EGFR and ALK tyrosine kinase inhibitors: guideline from the College of American Pathologists, International Association for the Study of Lung Cancer, and Association for Molecular Pathology. J Thorac Oncol. 2013;8:823–59.
8. Jänne PA, Yang JCH, Kim DW, et al. AZD9291 in EGFR inhibitor–resistant non–small-cell lung cancer. NEJM. 2015;372:1689–99.
9. Gettinger SN, Horn L, Gandhi L, et al. Overall survival and long-term safety of Nivolumab (anti–programmed death 1 antibody, BMS-936558, ONO-4538) in patients with previously treated advanced non–small-cell lung cancer. J Clin Oncol. 2015;33:2004–12.

Chapter 13
Latest in Bronchoscopy (High-Vision Scope with Rotation Function)

Takehiro Izumo

Abstract Rotation function of a bronchoscope enables easier selection of bronchi and use of Endobronchial Watanabe Spigot (EWS®). High-vision scope facilitates a clearer assessment of endobronchial mucosa by narrow band imaging, compared with and in addition to conventional white light bronchoscopy.

Keywords High-vision scope • Rotation function • Narrow band imaging • Autofluorescence imaging

13.1 Introduction

Conventionally, manipulation of a bronchoscope entailed up-and-down movement of the lever at the handle, as well as other motions, such as flexion/extension of the wrist or shifting the examiner's position. However, accurate diagnosis of a peripheral lung lesion by bronchoscopy requires precise selection of the bronchial route. In the past, approaching difficult-to-reach bronchial segments, such as the left B^6, right B^6, left B^{1+2}, left $B^{10}a$, and left $B^{10}c$, necessitated extensive wrist motion or unnatural posture of the bronchoscopist, which limited smooth insertion of devices, including radial endobronchial ultrasound probe, guide sheath, and biopsy forceps. The new bronchovideoscope BF-290 series (Olympus Ltd,; Fig. 13.1a, b) is equipped with a rotation function at the working channel insertion port; in addition, the high-vision scope, which was commonly used as a gastrointestinal videoscope, is now equipped for respiratory endoscopy as BF-H290 (Olympus Ltd).

T. Izumo (✉)
Department of Respiratory Medicine, Japanese Red Cross Medical Center,
4-1-22 Hiroo, Shibuya-ku, Tokyo 150-8935, Japan
e-mail: drtake1118@gmail.com

T. Izumo et al. (eds.), *Respiratory Endoscopy*,
DOI 10.1007/978-981-287-916-5_13

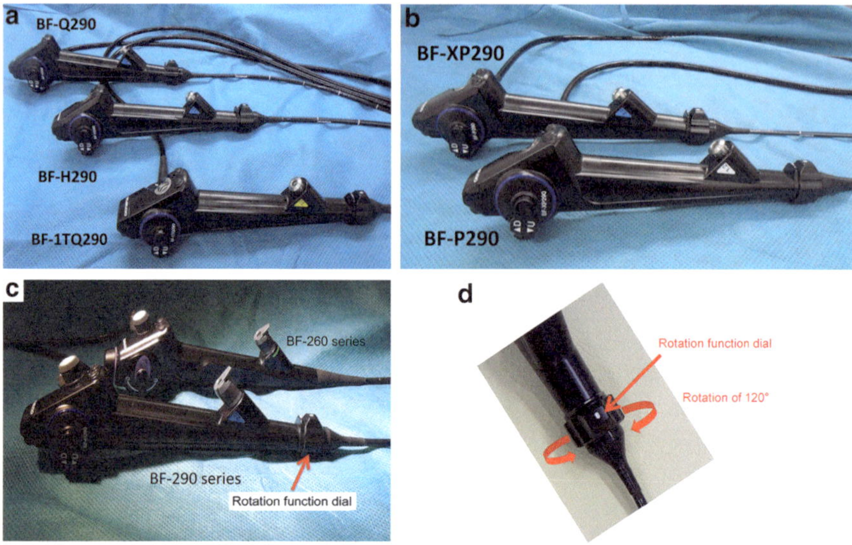

Fig. 13.1 BF-290 series (Olympus, Ltd). (**a**) BF-Q290, BF-H290, BF-1TQ290. (**b**) BF-XP290, BF-P290. (**c**) Comparison of the BF-260 series and the BF-290 series. The BF-290 scopes are newly equipped with a rotation dial at the working channel insertion port (*red arrow*). (**d**) The dial at the working channel insertion port may be rotated up to 120° clockwise and counterclockwise

13.2 Bronchoscope with Rotation Function at the Working Channel Insertion Port

This is a new function of the BF-290 bronchoscope series (Fig. 13.1c). A dial at the working channel insertion port allows clockwise or counterclockwise rotation of 120° (Fig. 13.1d). The rotation mechanism is also useful for fine control of the direction of the scope during selection of the involved bronchi. Most of the scopes in this series (e.g., BF-H290, BF-Q290, BF-P290, and BF-XP290) may be flexed up to 210° to enable easier operability compared with conventional scopes; an exception is BF-1TQ290, which may be flexed only up to 180°. Another advantage of this rotation function is for bronchial occlusion by EWS; this procedure entails alignment of the longitudinal axes of the target bronchus and the EWS, which may be difficult at times. In such cases, the rotation function of this new scope may address this limitation.

13.3 Improvement of Image Quality

Among the BF-290 series, BF-H290 is the first model equipped with a high-definition screen. The quality of white light and narrow band imaging has been improved (Fig. 13.2). Compared with the traditional video endoscopy system (EVIS

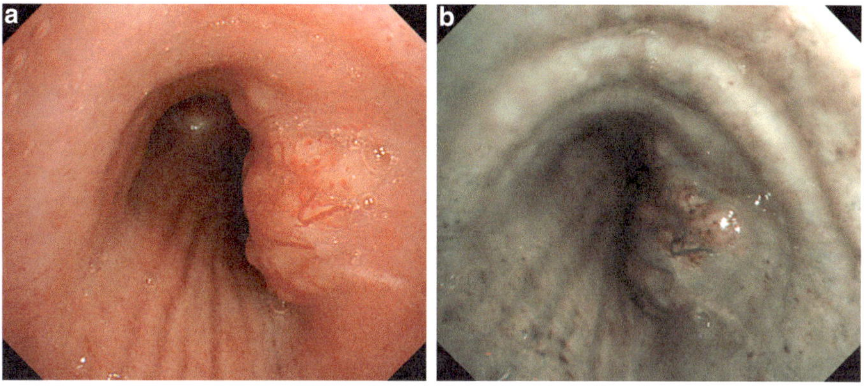

Fig. 13.2 Bronchoscopy using high-resolution scope* on a case of tracheal MALT lymphoma. (**a**) High-resolution image on *white* light bronchoscopy enables a detailed and clearer observation of the lesion. (**b**) NBI clearly shows the direction of blood vessels on the mucosal surface. *MALT* mucosa-associated lymphoid tissue, *NBI* narrow band imaging. * BF-H290; Olympus, Tokyo, Japan

LUCERA SPECTRUM; Olympus Ltd), the new video system (EVIS LUCERA ELITE; Olympus Ltd) of the BF-290 series has improved sensor for noise suppression and rendering high-resolution images; in addition, the amount of light during autofluorescence imaging using BF-260F was also improved. These developments are expected to facilitate better and easier confirmation of the progression of abnormalities in the bronchial mucosa (Fig. 13.3). In particular, the quality and size of the endoscopic images of BF-P290 and BF-XP290 have improved. The conventional thin scopes of the hybrid type used to be inferior in terms of display quality and size, but these have been remarkably improved after introduction of the videoscope (Fig. 13.4). Overall, these advancements on the bronchoscope enable easier operability, especially in the peripheral lung areas.

13.4 Precautions for the Rotation Function

Since the rotation function does not automatically return to the neutral position after use, please be reminded of the changes in the orientation of the scope as you maneuver the rotating dial; after the procedure, you should return it to the neutral position.

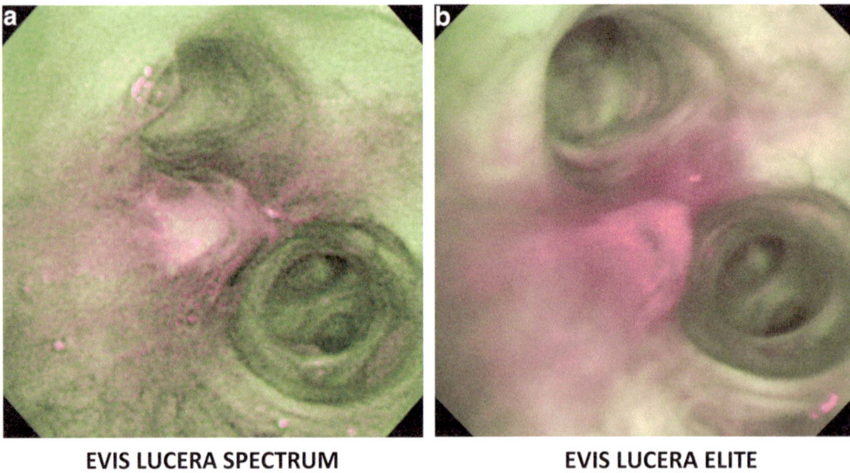

Fig. 13.3 Differences in autofluorescence imaging between the new and old video endoscopy systems in a case of squamous cell cancer on the left upper lobe bronchus. Compared with the (**a**) conventional system*, the (**b**) new system** enables noise suppression to render high-resolution images for easier confirmation of the progression of abnormalities in the bronchial mucosa. * EVIS LUCERA SPECTRUM; Olympus Ltd. ** EVIS LUCERA ELITE; Olympus Ltd

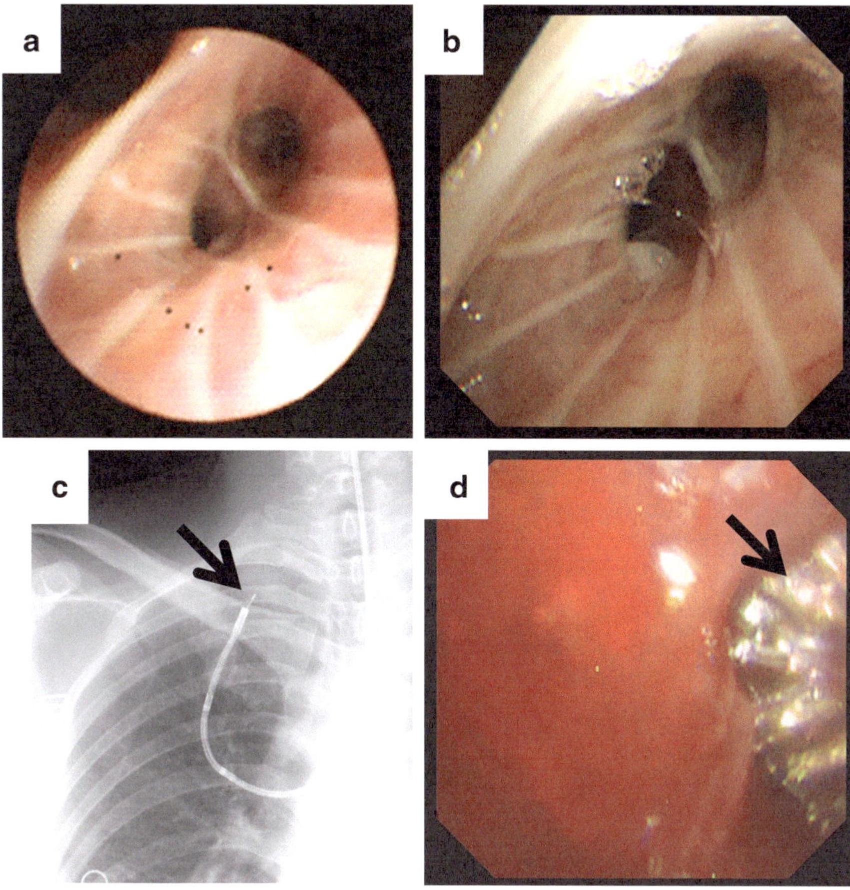

Fig. 13.4 Transbronchial biopsy of a peripheral pulmonary lesion in the right upper lobe. Compared with the (**a**) endoscopic image using BF-XP260F*, the (**b**) endoscopic image using BF-XP290* is remarkably improved in terms of display quality and size. (**c**) Fluoroscopy guidance of transbronchial brushing cytology (*black arrow*) even at the peripheral bronchial subsegments. (**d**) The improved display quality and size of the endoscopic image using BF-XP290* enables visualization of the cytology brush (*black arrow*) at the time of specimen collection. * Olympus Ltd, Tokyo, Japan

Chapter 14
Basic Flexible Bronchoscopy

Shinji Sasada

Abstract Do not forget that every new technology has been born out of a basic procedure that has long been introduced. A fast way to proficiency is to master bronchoscope handling.

Keywords Basic bronchoscopy • Transbronchial biopsy • Transbronchial lung biopsy • Bronchoalveolar lavage

14.1 Introduction

Recently, new technologies, such as endobronchial ultrasound (EBUS) and virtual bronchial navigation (VBN), have been developed to approach peripheral pulmonary lesions. These make it possible to determine the route and biopsy site of a lesion. However, in order to make a diagnosis, it is necessary to obtain a sufficient and appropriate amount of specimen. In fact, determining the bronchial route and biopsy site is not equivalent to making a diagnosis. Therefore, it is essential to master the basic diagnostic procedures before making use of technology. After all, these new technologies are extensions of the basic bronchoscope technology that has long been introduced and used.

14.2 Basic Techniques of Bronchoscopy

Since bronchoscopy is accompanied by patient pain and risk, it is necessary to maintain safety and reliability of the examination. To reduce pain, consider aggressive but adequate pharyngeal anesthesia with sedation. The basic technique begins by directing the tip of the scope toward the target lesion by enough wrist rotation

S. Sasada (✉)
Department of Respiratory Medicine, Tokyo Saiseikai Central Hospital,
1-4-17, Mita, Minato-ku, Tokyo 108-0073, Japan
e-mail: sasastaf@hotmail.co.jp

T. Izumo et al. (eds.), *Respiratory Endoscopy*,
DOI 10.1007/978-981-287-916-5_14

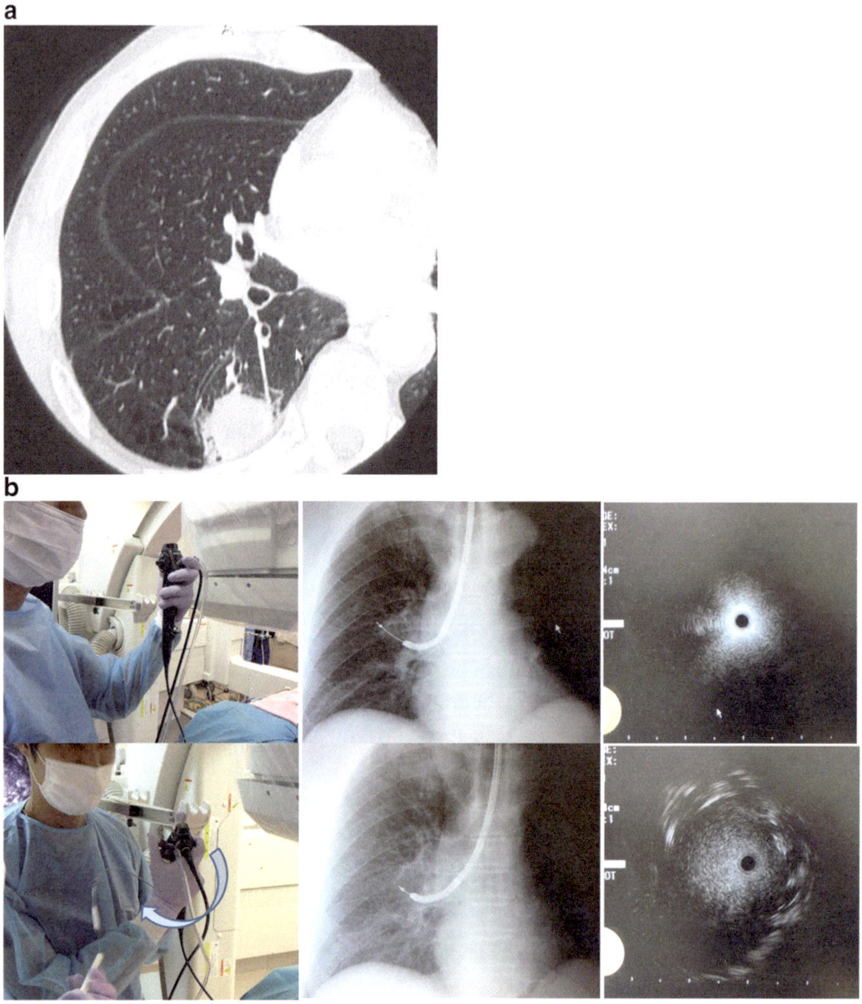

Fig. 14.1 A representative case to show the importance of scope rotation. (**a**) A patient with a lung mass on the right S6 on chest CT. (**b**) During bronchoscopy, initial X-ray fluoroscopy shows that the radial EBUS probe seems to have reached the lesion; however, there was no EBUS signal detected. Aggressive scope rotation to 180° while changing the operating hand from left to right succeeded in detecting a tumor signal on EBUS and subsequent diagnosis

and manipulation of the up-down (flexion-extension) angle; in particular, proper handling of the bronchoscope consists of 70 % rotation and 30 % up-down manipulation (Fig. 14.1). Generally, approaching more angled bronchial bifurcations (e.g., right B1, left B1+2, bilateral B6, etc.) is difficult; this may be overcome by wedging the bronchoscope, fine adjustments of the handle, and changing the operating hand. When performing bronchoscopy for peripheral pulmonary lesions, the approach

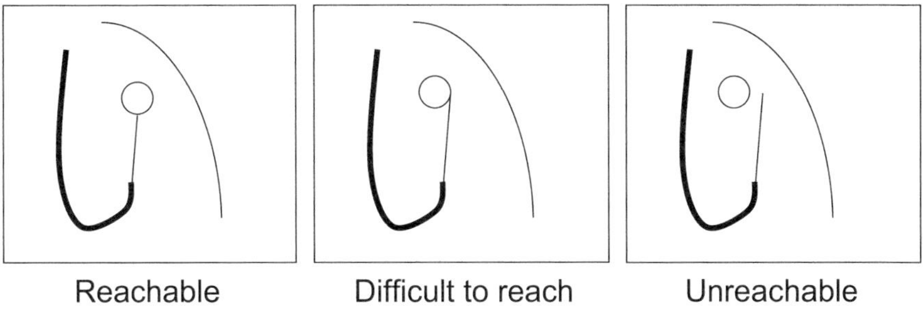

Fig. 14.2 Assessment of the probability to reach a peripheral pulmonary lesion under X-ray fluoroscopy

should mainly be done, while the tip is flexed (up-angle). After arriving at the target lesion, you can adjust the devices by extension (down-angle) manipulation.

14.3 Role of the Assistant

Fluoroscopy-guided biopsy requires an assistant who will use the devices; proper coordination with the operator becomes a key to success. With improper operation of the assistant, diagnostic accuracy may be affected, and unexpected complications may occur.

14.4 Transbronchial Biopsy (TBB)

Prior assessment of the probability to reach a peripheral pulmonary lesion by fluoroscopic biopsy is important. Biopsy devices, such as brush, forceps, etc., are observed as two-dimensional on X-ray fluoroscopy; the choice of biopsy technique should be based on the probability to reach a peripheral pulmonary lesion, such as "reachable," "difficult to reach," and "unreachable" (Fig. 14.2). As described above, the tip of the flexible bronchoscope should be rotated toward the area of the target lesion; otherwise, potentially "reachable" lesions would be determined as "unreachable" (Fig. 14.3). In general, each pulmonary segment may be reached by the same manner of bronchoscope manipulation. According to the chest computed tomography (CT) scan, the direction and degree of the bronchoscope rotation may be simulated (Fig. 14.4).

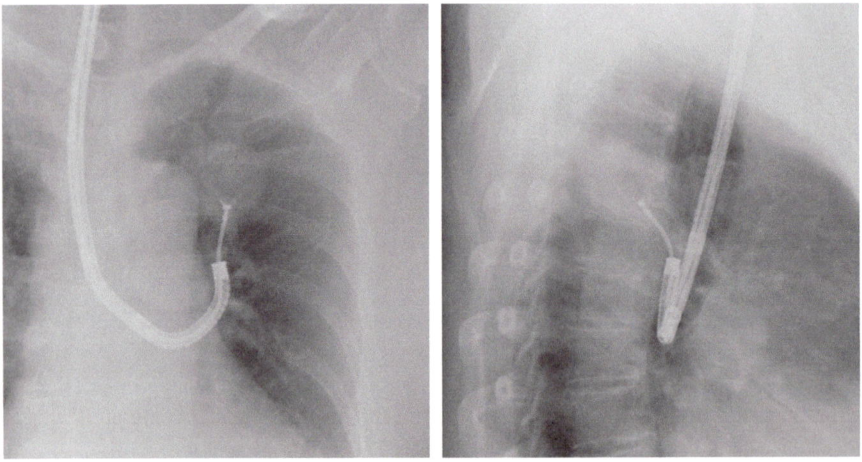

Fig. 14.3 Inappropriate scope operation. Since bronchoscope rotation is not enough, lateral view shows that the tip of the scope is not directed toward the lesion

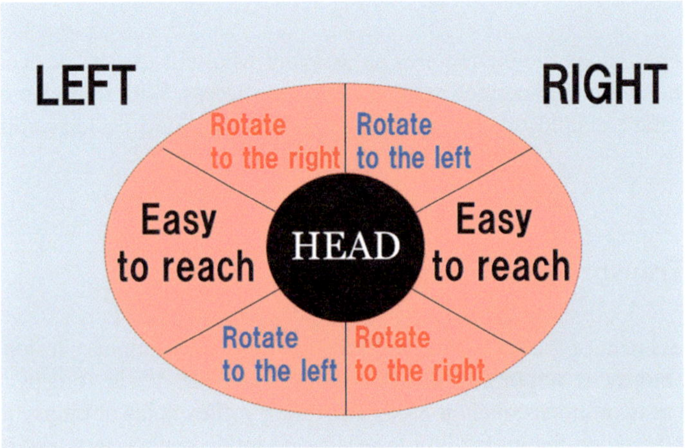

Fig. 14.4 Simulation before examination. Simulate the direction and degree of bronchoscope rotation according to the chest CT scan. For example, for a lesion in the right S3b, rotate the scope to the left

14.4.1 Reachable Lesions

These lesions may be easily reached under fluoroscopy guidance; in addition, check for movement of the X-ray shadow of the tumor while performing biopsy. For tumors in apical segments or those with surrounding inflammation and fibrosis, biopsy may sometimes be difficult. In such cases, it would be better to add trans-bronchial needle aspiration (TBNA) (Fig. 14.5).

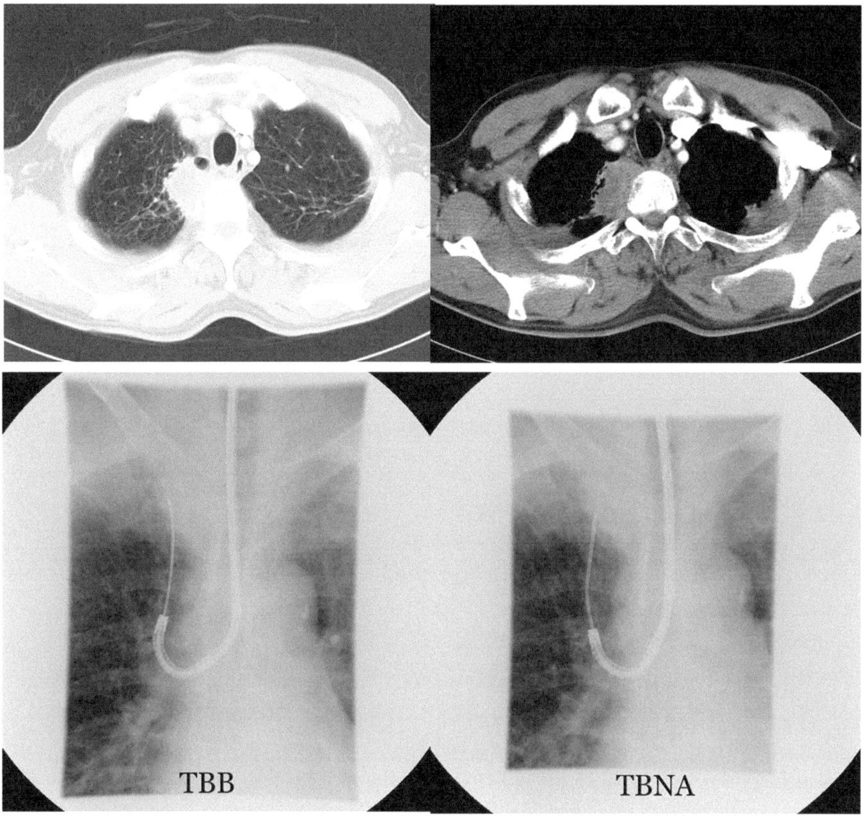

Fig. 14.5 TBNA for an apical tumor with fibrosis. The forceps biopsy (TBB) specimen reveals inflammatory changes with fibrosis only. Additional TBNA specimen shows adenocarcinoma. *TBB* transbronchial biopsy *TBNA* transbronchial needle aspiration

14.4.2 Difficult to Reach Lesions

For these lesions, the affected bronchus may be accessed using the curette, which is used to scrape gently the side of the target lesion under X-ray fluoroscopy. The Sasada transbronchial angled forceps (STAF®, Machida, Tokyo, Japan) is also useful (Fig. 14.6) [1]. As with the other methods, it is better to carry out TBNA in order to make a route for sampling from the bronchi to the lesion.

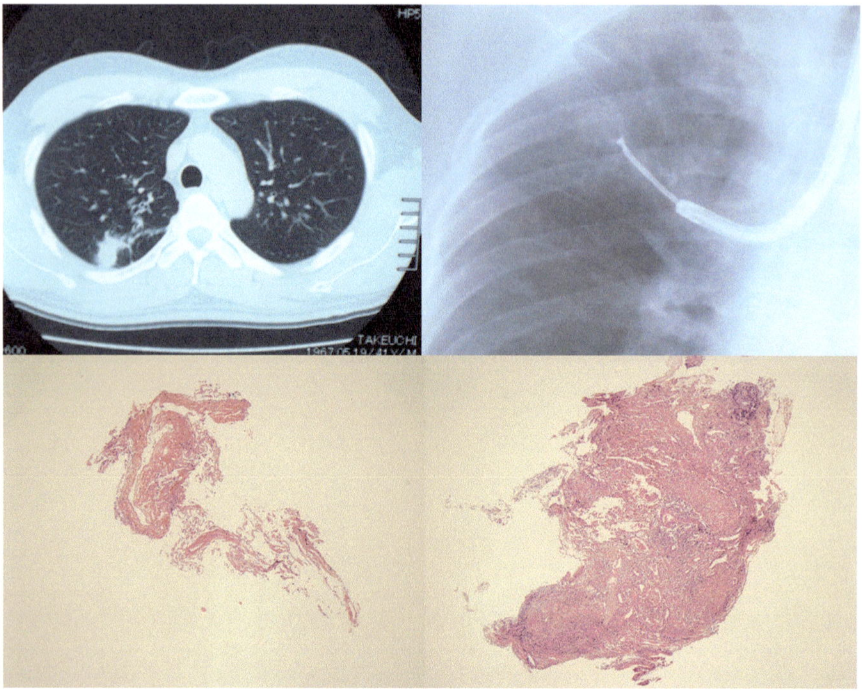

Fig. 14.6 Transbronchial biopsy using the STAF® for tuberculoma. First TBB specimen reveals normal bronchial mucosa, but the fourth specimen reveals epithelioid granuloma with Langerhans giant cells. *TBB* transbronchial biopsy,*STAF* Sasada transbronchial angled forceps

14.4.3 Unreachable Lesions

Try considering the curette and TBNA, as described above. However, if adequate samples or an accurate diagnosis is not obtained, try guided bronchoscopy (e.g., VBN, EBUS, etc.) or consider other approaches, such as transthoracic or surgical.

14.4.4 For Reliable Tissue Collection

1. Simulate the direction and degree of bronchoscope rotation according to the chest CT scan.
2. While rotating the bronchoscope and doing up-down movements of the tip, check for tumor movement under X-ray fluoroscopy while palpating the tumor with the use of biopsy devices (closed biopsy forceps or brush) to determine the biopsy site.

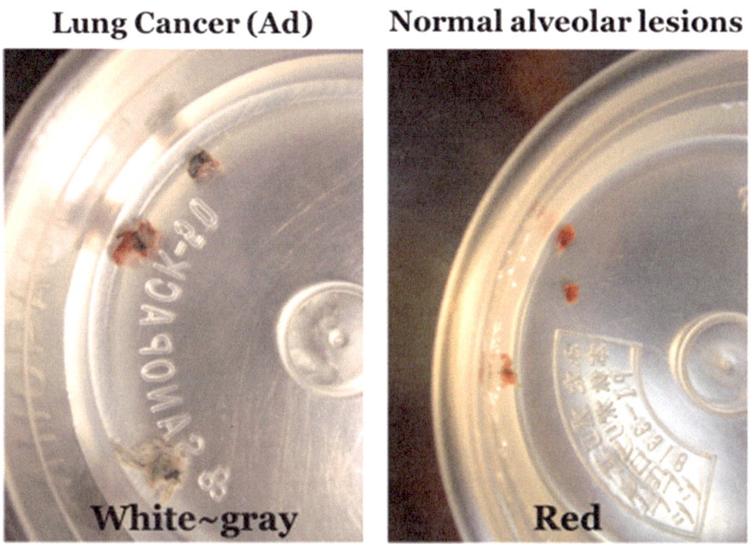

Fig. 14.7 Comparison of gross findings of collected specimens

3. Open and jab the forceps against the biopsy site, and then close it slowly while feeling the resistance of the lesion.
4. After 2–3 s, slowly pull the closed forceps out of the bronchoscope working channel.
5. Check the specimens (size, color, etc.) (Fig. 14.7).

14.5 Transbronchial Lung Biopsy (TBLB)

TBLB is a procedure for collecting bronchoalveolar tissues that are close to the pleura. TBLB is used in the diagnosis of diffuse lung diseases, such as interstitial pneumonia, pulmonary fibrosis, granulomatous disease, various types of infectious pneumonia, and malignant disease.

The actual procedure:

1. Under X-ray fluoroscopy, insert the forceps to a point that is just below the pleura.
2. Pull back the forceps for about 1–2 cm and open the cups during inhalation.
3. During exhalation, press gently while opening the forceps.
4. Close the forceps cups while checking for pleuritic pain.
5. Pull the closed forceps out of the bronchoscope working channel.
6. Check for bronchial hemorrhage or pneumothorax.

As much as possible, choose a bronchus that is perpendicular to the pleura under X-ray fluoroscopy. The preferred biopsy site is about 1 cm from the pleura. When performing biopsy from the lower lobe, it is better for the patient to be breathing lightly during bronchoscopy because large respiratory excursions may be associated with higher risks of complications. The appropriate biopsy number for the upper or lower lobe is around three pieces. Also, we should select fenestrated forceps to prevent crushing of the collected specimens. The collected tissues are expanded with the use of negative pressure from a syringe with saline before fixing it in formalin solution. Re-expansion of the biopsy sample is done because alveolar tissues tend to collapse during biopsy.

14.6 Bronchial Alveolar Lavage (BAL)

14.6.1 Indications

Particularly, BAL is useful for diseases, such as eosinophilic pneumonia, pulmonary alveolar proteinosis, pneumocystis pneumonia, alveolar hemorrhage, cancer lymphangitis, and the like (Figs. 14.8, 14.9, 14.10, 14.11, 14.12, 14.13, 14.14, and 14.15). Specifically, characteristic colors of BAL fluid are seen in pulmonary alveolar proteinosis (white) and alveolar hemorrhage (red). Diseases that show lymphocytosis in the BAL fluid are sarcoidosis, hypersensitivity pneumonitis, idiopathic organizing pneumonia, lymphocytic interstitial pneumonia, and malignant lymphoma. Eosinophilic pneumonia and Churg-Strauss syndrome show significant eosinophilia in the BAL fluid. Bronchial asthma, allergic bronchopulmonary aspergillosis, and drug-induced pneumonia show nonspecific findings. Neutrophilia can be seen especially in acute respiratory distress syndrome. In patients with history of asbestos inhalation, asbestos bodies can be detected (Fig. 14.16).

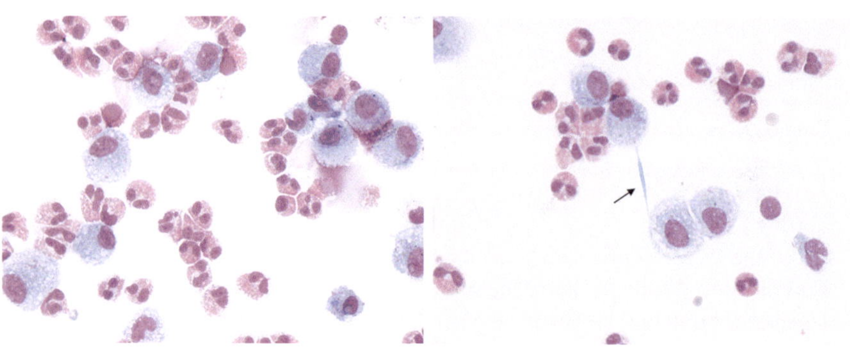

Fig. 14.8 BAL fluid analysis in eosinophilic pneumonia shows Charcot-Leyden crystal (*arrow*), elevated eosinophil fraction of 78.7 %, and CD4/CD8 ratio of 1.69

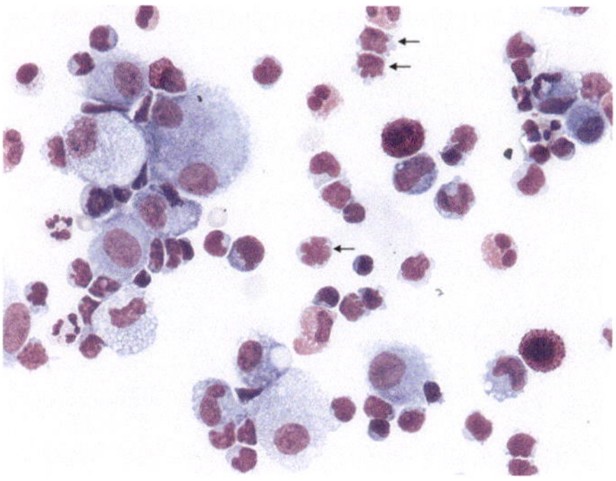

Fig. 14.9 BAL fluid analysis in hypersensitivity pneumonitis shows activated lymphocytes (*arrow*), elevated lymphocyte fraction of 67.7 %, and CD4/CD8 ratio of 0.29

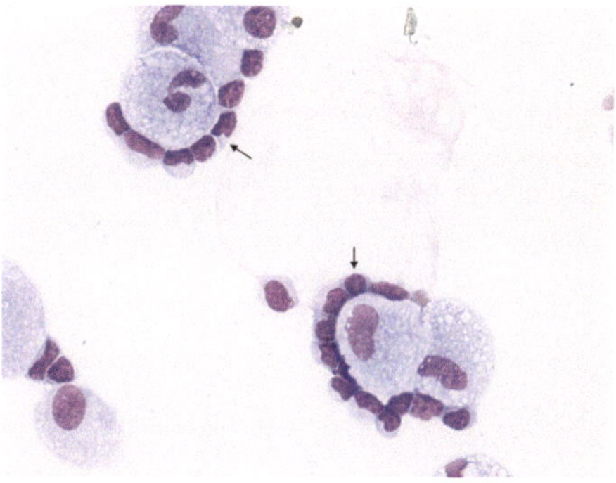

Fig. 14.10 BAL fluid analysis in sarcoidosis shows rosette-like lymphocyte (*arrow*), elevated lymphocyte fraction of 45.5 %, and CD4/CD8 ratio of 6.93

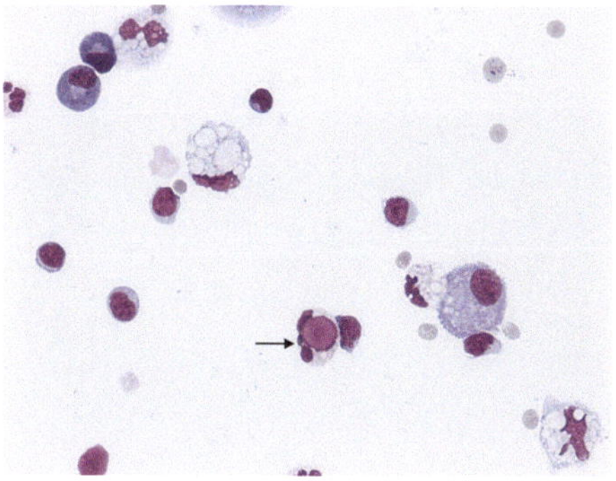

Fig. 14.11 BAL fluid analysis in systemic lupus erythematosus shows LE cell (*arrow*), elevated lymphocyte fraction of 33.5 %, and CD4/CD8 ratio of 0.95

14.6.2 Procedure

Control of the cough is important to obtain better samples during BAL. Although BAL can be performed with the use of the ordinary bronchoscope, patients who have very sensitive cough reflex may be given sedatives, such as midazolam. In addition, it is preferable to provide oxygen inhalation during the procedure. When the bronchoscope is inserted, take care to avoid contamination of the BAL fluid with normal flora and secretions in the oral cavity. Intermittent application of lidocaine

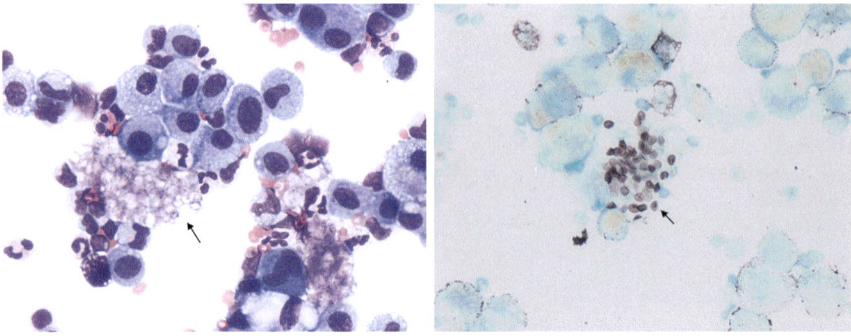

Fig. 14.12 BAL fluid analysis in pneumocystis pneumonia shows bacterial cells (*arrows*); the image on the right shows Grocott staining

Fig. 14.13 BAL fluid analysis in mycosis shows Candida cells (*arrow*)

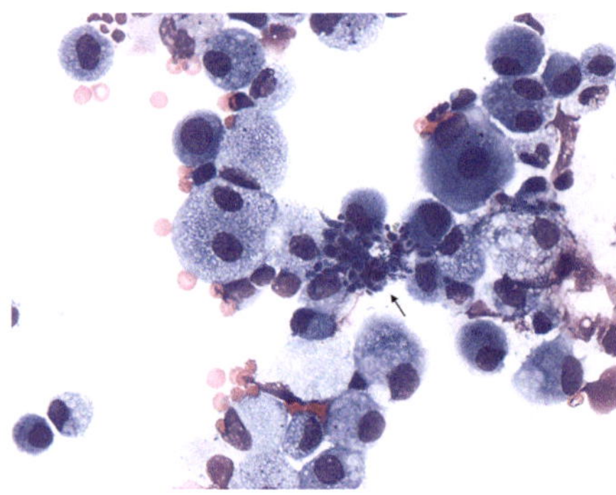

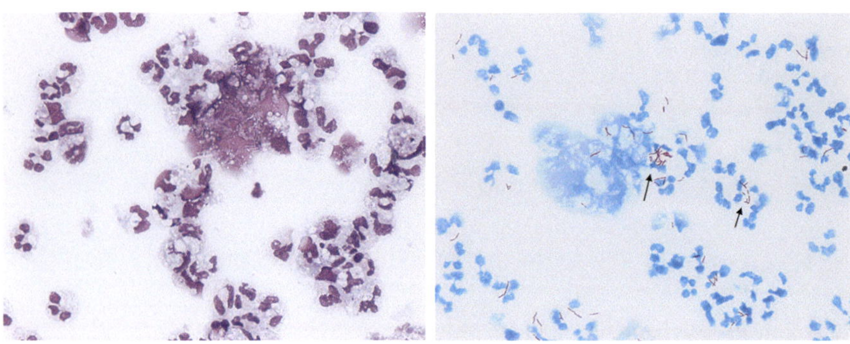

Fig. 14.14 BAL fluid analysis in pulmonary tuberculosis shows bacterial cells (*arrows*); the image on the right shows Ziehl-Neelsen staining. Neutrophil fraction is elevated at 98.3 %

on the bronchial mucosa is needed, but the extra lidocaine should be aspirated before BAL.

A bronchoscope with a diameter of 5–6 mm is preferred. For diffuse lung disease, the middle lobe or lingular segments (through B4 or B5) can be considered to

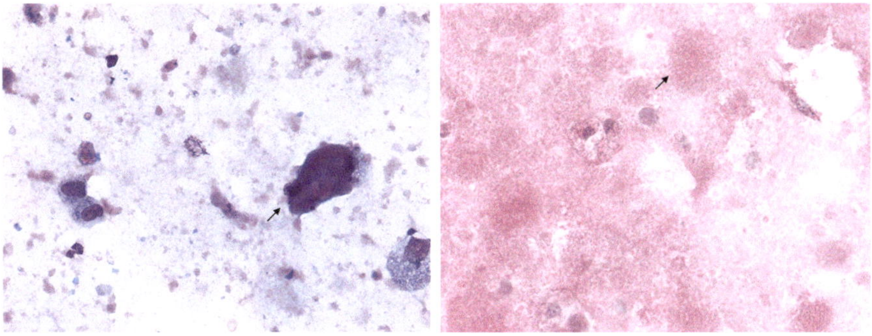

Fig. 14.15 BAL fluid analysis in pulmonary alveolar proteinosis shows foamy macrophages (*arrows*); the image on the right shows PAS staining

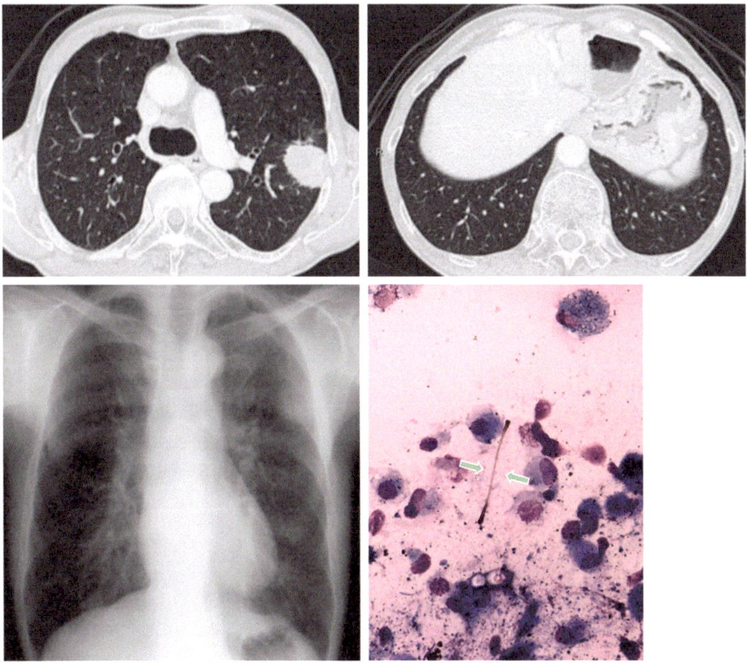

Fig. 14.16 A 58-year-old man, who works in a factory that manufactures iron walls and who has lung adenocarcinoma. Although obvious findings of asbestosis was not seen on chest CT, BAL fluid shows 8.4 asbestos bodies/ml

represent the entire lung; in addition, a bronchoscope can be easily wedged in these bronchi, so fluid recovery is good. In fact, the percentage of BAL fluid recovered is reduced by about 20 % in the lower lobe, compared with that in the middle/lingular segments. In Japan, the standard BAL procedure consists of sequential instillation of three 50-ml aliquots of warm saline through the intended lung segment.

A recommended technique is to slowly instill and withdraw fluid from the working channel of the bronchoscope while keeping the scope in the middle of the lumen. The ideal average recovery rate is about 50–70 % of the total instilled volume. If the BAL fluid recovered is 25 % or less, evaluation and analysis of results would be difficult and may not be accurate.

14.6.3 Complications

In idiopathic pulmonary fibrosis, one of the factors for poor prognosis is acute exacerbation, during which diffuse alveolar damage sets in. Although acute exacerbation after BAL is well known in IPF, the actual frequency is not clear. Another possible complication during BAL is hypoxemia; therefore, prophylactic oxygenation should be on standby. Fever several hours after BAL is considered as chemical pneumonia, but prophylactic antibacterial agents are not always valid. Other possible complications are bleeding, bronchospasm, angina, arrhythmia, pneumothorax, hypotension, and hypercapnia. Most of these are minor, with a frequency of around 5 %.

14.6.4 Contraindications

1. Exacerbation of infectious disease is likely after BAL
2. Within 6 weeks after myocardial infarction
3. Serious arrhythmia
4. Bleeding tendencies
5. Extremely poor general condition

Carefully consider if exacerbation is expected in patients with severe respiratory failure. Administer enough oxygen to keep the SaO_2 90 % or more. For patients in hypercapnic respiratory failure, watch out for further CO_2 accumulation due to administration of high oxygen concentrations. Intubated patients may still undergo BAL, provided that adequate oxygenation is ensured during the procedure. In patients with bronchial asthma, premedication with inhaled short-acting bronchodilator is recommended [2].

References

1. Sasada S, Ogata Y, Kobayashi M, et al. Angled forceps used for transbronchial biopsy in which standard forceps are difficult to manipulate: a comparative study. Chest. 2006;129:725–33.
2. British Thoracic Society Bronchoscopy Guidelines Committee. British Thoracic Society guidelines on diagnostic flexible bronchoscopy. Thorax. 2001;56 Suppl 1:i1–21.

Chapter 15
Tomography-Guided Transbronchial Biopsy for Peripheral Pulmonary Lesions

Takehiro Izumo

Abstract Tomosynthesis is a kind of digital imaging modality that is capable of reconstructing a coronal plane of arbitrary height from a single tomographic scan. Recent research has shown that these tomographic images were superior at detecting nodules compared with chest radiography. Regardless of the procedure (endoscopy, angiography, gastrointestinal fluoroscopy, or surgery), real-time image capture by tomosynthesis is important in making the procedure easier and to improve precision. Normal fluoroscopy is quite capable of confirming positions in a transverse direction but has trouble confirming positions in the anteroposterior direction. Techniques that have real-time imaging capabilities need further development. In addition, making the capture of tomosynthesis images possible by gantry movement in both transverse and lateral directions will certainly increase the amount of freedom allowed to the operator during procedures. Further development and applications of procedures using tomosynthesis are expected.

Keywords Bronchoscopy • EBUS • Tomosynthesis • Transbronchial biopsy

15.1 Introduction

In the field of respiratory medicine, chest radiography and computed tomography (CT) have been the main modalities used for imaging in routine medical care. The word tomosynthesis (SONIALVISION safire series, Shimadzu Ltd., Japan) is coined from "tomography" and "synthesis"; it is a kind of digital imaging modality that is capable of reconstructing a coronal plane of arbitrary height from a single tomographic scan [1]. Recent research has shown that these tomographic images were superior at detecting nodules compared with chest radiography [2]. The exposure dose of a single tomosynthesis is equivalent to several chest radiography scans

T. Izumo (✉)
Department of Respiratory Medicine, Japanese Red Cross Medical Center,
4-1-22 Hiroo, Shibuya-ku, Tokyo 150-8935, Japan
e-mail: drtake1118@gmail.com

T. Izumo et al. (eds.), *Respiratory Endoscopy*,
DOI 10.1007/978-981-287-916-5_15

Table 15.1 Characteristics of each modality

	Chest radiography	Chest tomosynthesis (SONIALVISION safire series)	Chest CT
Examination time	Several seconds	Several tens of seconds	Several minutes
Performance when detecting lesions that are difficult to visualize	Limited capability of showing ground-glass opacity lesions and nodules that overlap with the mediastinum or diaphragm	Capable of showing nodules and ground-glass opacities (inferior to CT) (at the edge of its field of view range)	Capable of showing nodules and ground-glass opacities
System cost	Low	Medium	High
Space requirements for system installation	Small	Medium	Large
Image reconstruction and display	Only displayed in the direction of radiography	Capable of reconstructing any coronal plane section	Capable of reconstruction along any plane
Dedicated system for image reconstruction (workstation)	None	Dedicated workstation	Dedicated (multifunctional) workstation
Exposure dose	Low	Low to medium	Medium to high (low-dose CT = medium)
Imaging range	Medium	Medium (somewhat narrow)	Wide
Metal artifacts	None	Few	Many
Use with bronchoscopy procedures	Only for display of mapping images	Capable of X-ray fluoroscopy (supports procedures in real time)	CT-guided bronchoscopy

or around one-tenth the exposure dose of a chest CT scan, but the system installation space is smaller than that of a chest CT scan. In light of this, tomosynthesis may be positioned between chest radiography and chest CT in the field of respiratory medicine [3, 4]. Table 15.1 shows the respective characteristics of chest radiography, chest tomosynthesis, and chest CT.

15.2 Real-Time Tomosynthesis-Guided Bronchoscopy

Regardless of the procedure (endoscopy, angiography, gastrointestinal fluoroscopy, or surgery), real-time image capture by tomosynthesis is important in making the procedure easier and to improve precision. We have investigated real-time

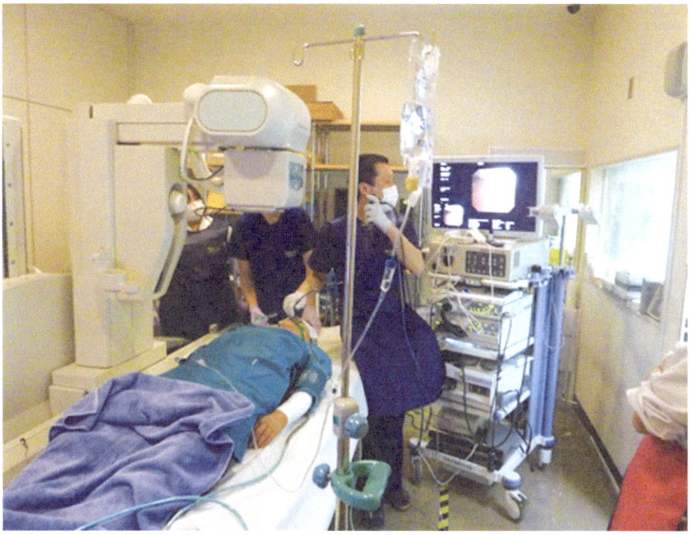

Fig. 15.1 Performing real-time tomosynthesis-guided bronchoscopy

tomosynthesis-guided bronchoscopy, a new technique that enables confirmation of the position of biopsy instruments, such as forceps or needle, inside a lesion, along transverse and anteroposterior directions. Normal fluoroscopy is quite capable of confirming positions in a transverse direction but has trouble confirming positions in the anteroposterior plane. To date, confirming the position of biopsy instruments in the anteroposterior direction has required the use of a C-arm or manual shifting of a patient in the lateral recumbent position during examination. Confirming the position of a lesion is not always easy due to the presence of mediastinal structures. The use of tomosynthesis to capture images will make it very easy to ascertain and correct the positional relationship between a peripheral pulmonary lesion and the biopsy instruments. An illustration of an actual examination setup is shown in Fig. 15.1. The biopsy instrument inside the lesion can be confirmed on the tomosynthesis screen by reconstructing contiguous cross sections in the anteroposterior direction from the back through the anterior chest (Figs. 15.2 and 15.3). However, movement of the gantry in a longitudinal direction along the body for tomosynthesis prevents the operator from standing at the head of the patient during bronchoscopy; instead, the operator needs to be positioned on the side of the patient (Fig. 15.1), making control of the bronchoscope somewhat difficult. Techniques that have real-time imaging capabilities need further development. In addition, making the capture of tomosynthesis images possible by gantry movement in both transverse and lateral directions will certainly increase the amount of freedom allowed to the operator during procedures.

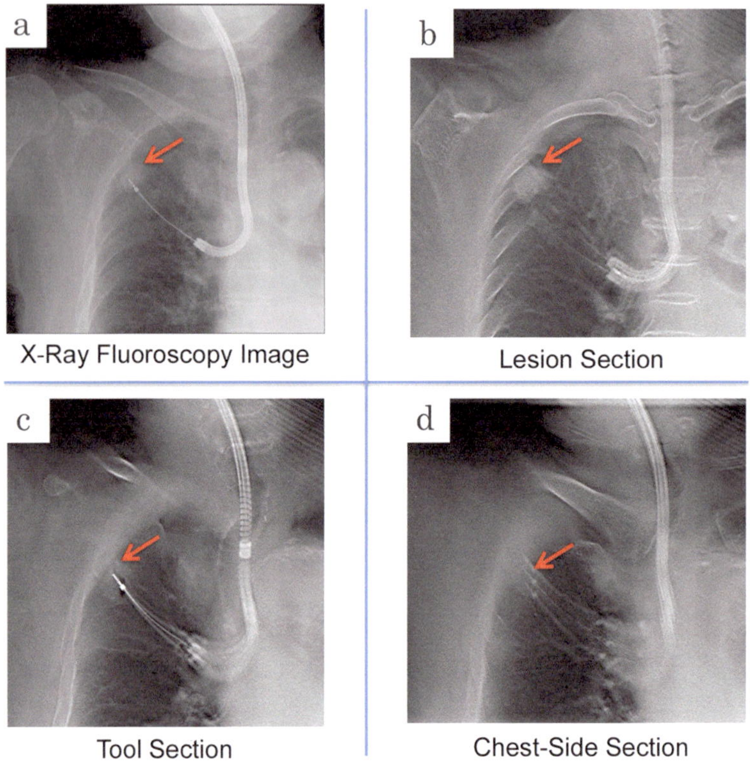

Fig. 15.2 An example of real-time tomosynthesis-guided bronchoscopy procedure shows that the biopsy instrument is not in the target lesion. (**a**) The biopsy instrument appears to be positioned entirely within the lesion on an X-ray fluoroscopy image. (**b**) Tomosynthesis section clearly shows that the biopsy instrument is not inside the lesion. (**c**) Less clear visualization of a lesion when the position of the biopsy instrument is tangential to the anterior portion of the lesion. (**d**) The biopsy instrument is observed in a section that does not show the lesion, which easily confirms that the biopsy instrument is present on the chest side (anterior to the lesion)

15.3 Conclusions

Further improvements on the real-time capabilities of tomosynthesis, a system that integrates digital tomography with fluoroscopy, are required for its applicability in the field of respiratory medicine. Further developments and performance of procedures using tomosynthesis are expected.

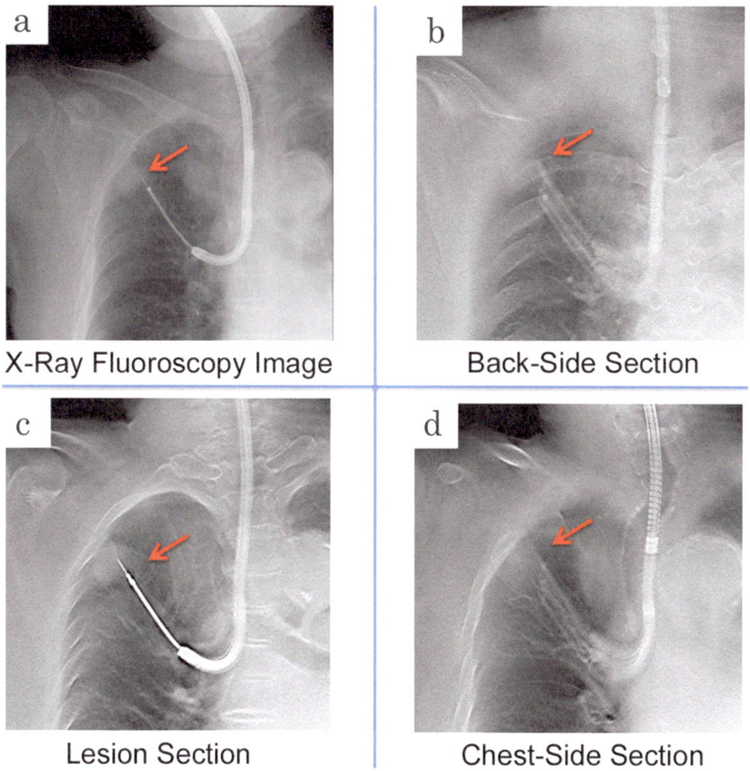

Fig. 15.3 An example of real-time tomosynthesis-guided bronchoscopy procedure shows that the biopsy instrument is in the target lesion. (**a**) The biopsy instrument appears to be positioned entirely within the lesion on an X-ray fluoroscopy image. (**b**) A posterior section on tomosynthesis shows both the lesion and the biopsy instrument similarly. (**c**) Tomosynthesis section (anteroposterior direction) that most clearly shows the lesion and the biopsy instrument inside it. (**d**) An anterior section on tomosynthesis depicts the lesion and biopsy instrument inside it and confirms the same position that was seen on the posterior section

References

1. Yamada Y, Jinzaki M, Hasegawa I, Shiomi E, Sugiura H, Abe T, et al. Fast scanning tomosynthesis for the detection of pulmonary nodules: diagnostic performance compared with chest radiography, using multidetector-row computed tomography as the reference. Invest Radiol. 2011;46(8):471–7. doi:10.1097/RLI.0b013e318217b838.
2. Terzi A, Bertolaccini L, Viti A, Comello L, Ghirardo D, Priotto R, et al. Lung cancer detection with digital chest tomosynthesis: baseline results from the observational study SOS. J Thorac Oncol. 2013;8(6):685–92. doi:10.1097/JTO.0b013e318292bdef.

3. Izumo T, Sasada S, Chavez C, Nagai Y, Kitagawa M, Torii J, et al. The value of chest tomosynthesis in locating a ground glass nodule (GGN) during endobronchial ultrasonography with a guide sheath: a case report. J Thorac Dis. 2013;5(3):E75–7. doi:10.3978/j.issn.2072-1439.2013.04.10.
4. Izumo T, Sasada S, Chavez C, Tsuchida T. The diagnostic utility of endobronchial ultrasonography with a guide sheath and tomosynthesis images for ground glass opacity pulmonary lesions. J Thorac Dis. 2013;5(6):745–50. doi:10.3978/j.issn.2072-1439.2013.11.30.

Chapter 16
Radial Endobronchial Ultrasound Findings

Takehiro Izumo

Abstract It is important to know the typical R-EBUS findings in order to decide the biopsy site; conversely, contrast, gain, and scanning direction need to be set properly before using R-EBUS for image interpretation. For ground glass opacity (GGO) lesions, R-EBUS signals need to be compared with and delineated from the signals of a normal lung.

Keywords Radial endobronchial ultrasound • R-EBUS pattern • Bronchoscopy • Peripheral pulmonary lesion

16.1 Basic Settings of an Ultrasound Device

First of all, when conducting radial endobronchial ultrasound (R-EBUS), the ultrasound device should be set as shown in Table 16.1 and Fig. 16.1 in order to distinguish the R-EBUS signals of a lesion from that of its background. Setting the device is particularly important for ground glass opacity (GGO), which generates ultrasound signals that are very similar with those of the normal lung. The scanning direction is set as NORMAL by default, but the orientation of the R-EBUS image generated would be the same as that of an axial slice computed tomography (CT) image (i.e., as if facing a recumbent patient from the foot). When performing bronchoscopy with R-EBUS guidance, the scanning direction should be set to inverse (INV) in order to match the R-EBUS image with the direction of the lesion [1, 2].

T. Izumo (✉)
Department of Respiratory Medicine, Japanese Red Cross Medical Center,
4-1-22 Hiroo, Shibuya-ku, Tokyo 150-8935, Japan
e-mail: drtake1118@gmail.com

T. Izumo et al. (eds.), *Respiratory Endoscopy*,
DOI 10.1007/978-981-287-916-5_16

Table 16.1 Setting of ultrasound device (EU-ME1®, Olympus)

Gain value (G)	9/19
Contrast value (C)	4/8
Image quality (I)	Image-1
Scanning direction (DIR)	Inverse (INV)

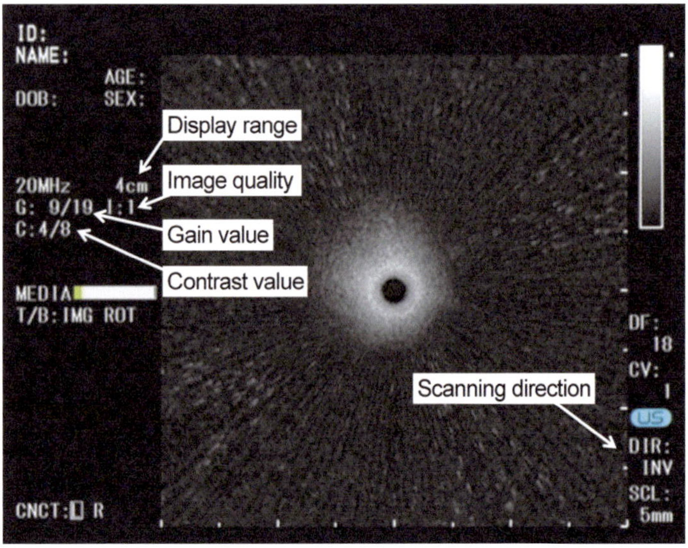

Fig. 16.1 Setting of the ultrasound device

16.2 Typical R-EBUS Findings [3–8]

R-EBUS is a device to confirm the location of a lesion, but this would be difficult if the typical findings are not known. Basically, a solid lesion is visualized as a heterogeneous gray signal, but some air-filled lesions show high-intensity echoes scattered on the inside. GGO presents with blizzard sign, which is an enhancement of high-intensity signals, or mixed blizzard sign, which shows high-intensity signals scattered inside a heterogeneous signal. It is sometimes difficult to distinguish between a blood vessel and a pulmonary parenchymal lesion because the device is not equipped with a Doppler mode. Nevertheless, blood vessels are usually visualized as hypoechoic signals, not heterogeneous. The followings are the most commonly encountered R-EBUS findings:

1. R-EBUS scanning of a peripheral pulmonary lesion using an ultrasound probe that is functioning properly (Fig. 16.2).
2. R-EBUS scanning of a peripheral pulmonary lesion when an ultrasound probe is filled with air bubbles (Fig. 16.3). The absence of signals may give the impression

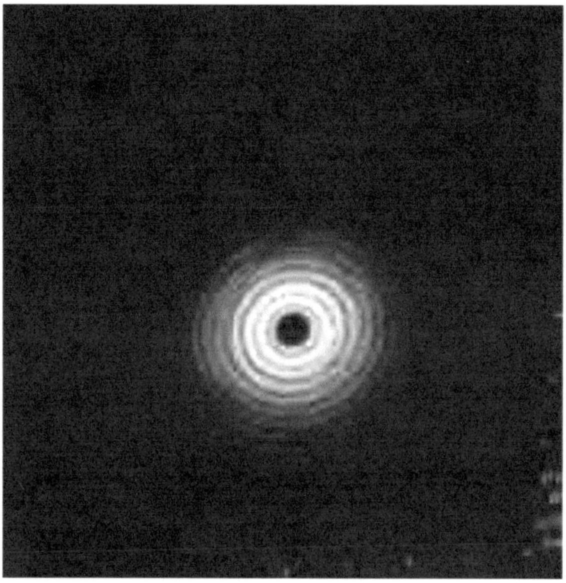

Fig. 16.2 Typical R-EBUS scanning of a peripheral pulmonary lesion shows a heterogeneous circumferential signal around the probe

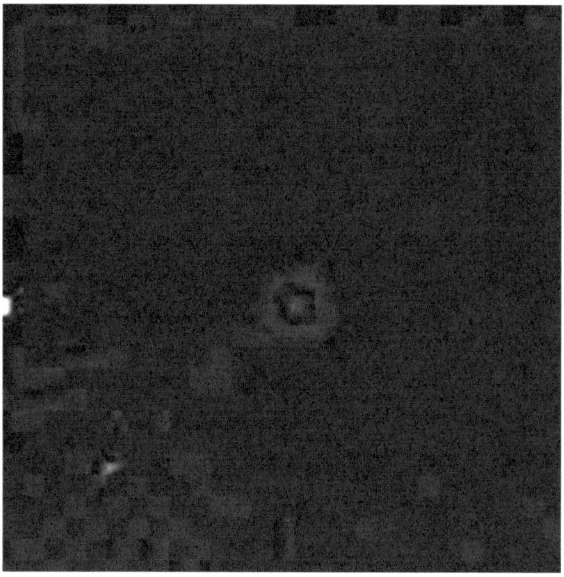

Fig. 16.3 R-EBUS scanning of a peripheral pulmonary lesion shows no signal around the probe. In this case, the probe is filled with bubbles

that the ultrasound probe is damaged. In such case, let the air bubbles come out by holding the probe at 5 cm from its tip and shaking it gently while facing downward.

3. Blood vessels have hypoechoic signals on R-EBUS (Fig. 16.4). Confirm by moving the ultrasound probe back and forth.
4. R-EBUS findings of a solid lesion -1 (Fig. 16.5).

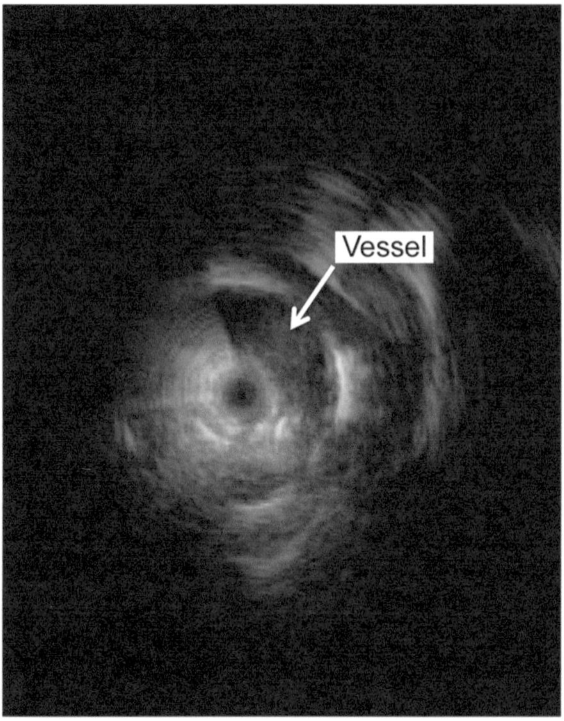

Fig. 16.4 R-EBUS findings of a blood vessel show hypoechoic signals

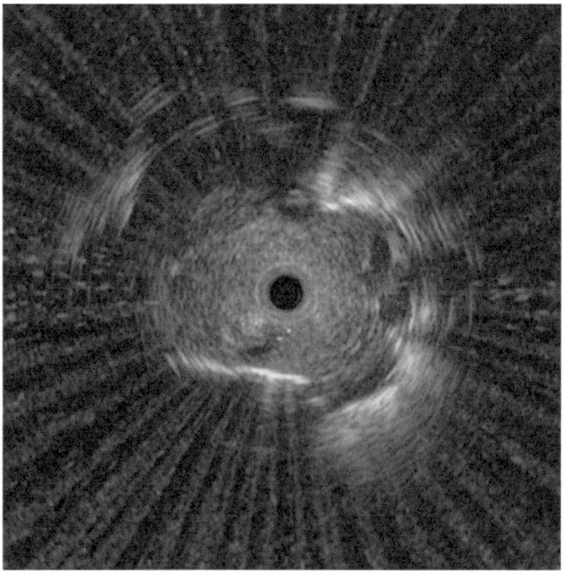

Fig. 16.5 R-EBUS findings of a solid lesion

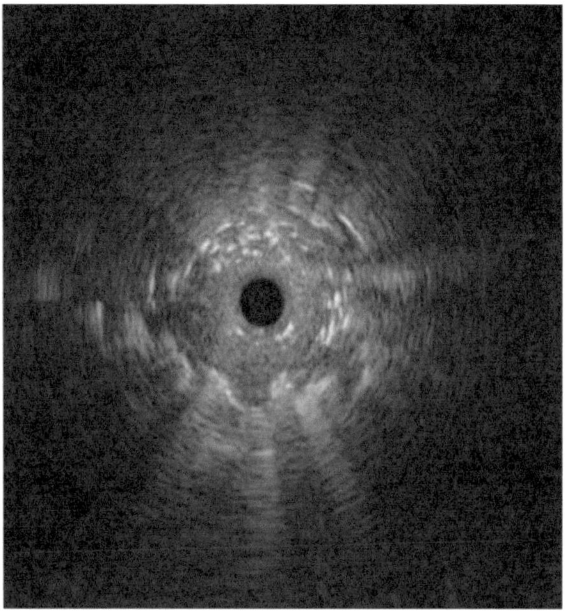

Fig. 16.6 R-EBUS findings of a solid lesion

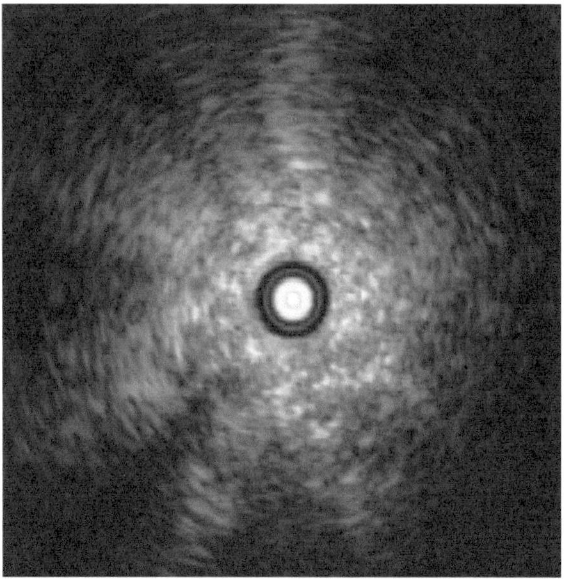

Fig. 16.7 R-EBUS findings of a part-solid ground glass opacity lesion show mixed blizzard sign

5. R-EBUS findings of a solid lesion -2 (Fig. 16.6).
6. R-EBUS findings of a part-solid GGO lesion (mixed blizzard sign, Fig. 16.7).
7. R-EBUS findings of a pure GGO lesion (Fig. 16.8). When the ultrasound probe is inserted into a GGO lesion, the snowstorm appearance that is usually seen in a

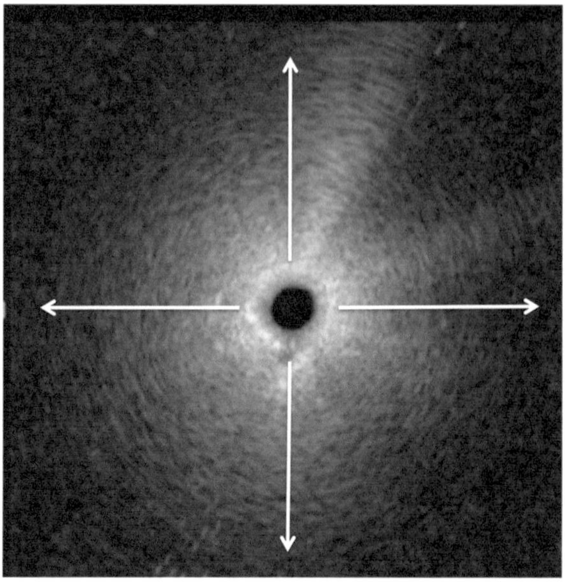

Fig. 16.8 R-EBUS findings of a pure ground glass opacity lesion show blizzard sign or enhancement of the snowstorm appearance (*white arrows*)

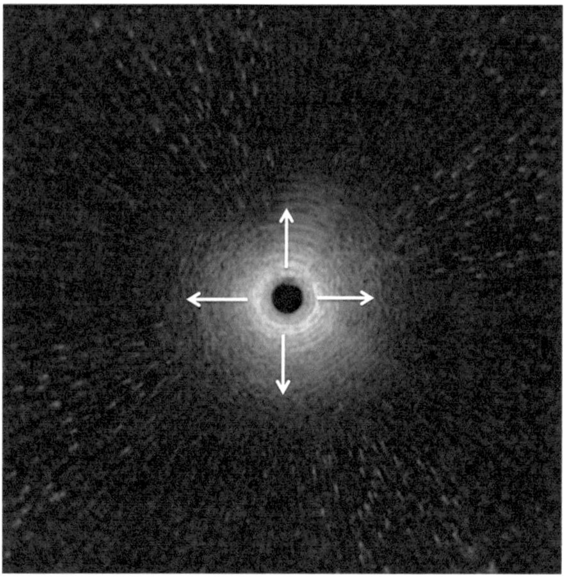

Fig. 16.9 R-EBUS findings of a normal lung show the snowstorm appearance

normal lung will be enhanced (blizzard sign). It is important to detect these subtle differences between pure GGO and normal lung signals.

8. R-EBUS findings of a normal lung (Fig. 16.9).

16.3 Conclusion

It is important to know the typical R-EBUS findings in order to detect the location of a lesion. In the future, the value of locating a small lesion precisely would be underscored, particularly when developing bronchoscopic treatment for peripheral lung lesions. Further discussion on the R-EBUS findings of GGO is necessary [9].

References

1. Kurimoto N, Izumo T. Handbook for radial EBUS/guide sheath bronchoscopy for peripheral pulmonary lesions handbook. Olympus medical systems; 2014.
2. Izumo T, Sasada S, Matusmoto Y, et al. Radial endobronchial ultrasound and guide sheath for peripheral pulmonary lesions. J Jpn Soc Respir Endosc. 2014;36:392–7.
3. Izumo T, Sasada S, Chavez C, et al. The diagnostic utility of endobronchial ultrasonography with a guide sheath and tomosynthesis images for ground glass opacity pulmonary lesions. J Thorac Dis. 2013;5:745–50.
4. Ikezawa Y, Sukoh N, Shinagawa N, et al. Endobronchial ultrasonography with a guide sheath for pure or mixed ground-glass opacity lesions. Respiration. 2014;88:137–43.
5. Kurimoto N, Murayama M, Yoshioka S, et al. Analysis of the internal structure of peripheral pulmonary lesions using endobronchial ultrasonography. Chest. 2002;122:1887–94.
6. Sasada S, Izumo T, Chavez C, et al. Blizzard sign as a specific endobronchial ultrasound image for ground glass opacity: a case report. Respir Med Case Rep. 2014;12:19–21.
7. Chavez C, Sasada S, Izumo T, et al. Image-guided bronchoscopy for histopathologic diagnosis of pure ground glass opacity: a case report. J Thorac Dis. 2014;6:E81–4.
8. Sasada S, Izumo T, Chavez C, et al. A new middle-range diameter bronchoscope with large channel for transbronchial sampling of peripheral pulmonary lesions. Jpn J Clin Oncol. 2014;44:826–34.
9. Izumo T, Sasada S, Chavez C, et al. Radial endobronchial ultrasound images for ground glass opacity pulmonary lesions. Eur Resp J. 2015;45:1661–8.

Chapter 17
Radial EBUS Findings for Ground Glass Opacity: Comparison of Radiologic and Pathologic Findings

Takehiro Izumo

Abstract Radial endobronchial ultrasound (EBUS) findings of ground-glass opacity (GGO) peripheral pulmonary lesions are mainly classified into those with blizzard sign and those with mixed-blizzard sign. It is important to understand that the obtained images may vary depending on which part of the GGO the radial EBUS probe reaches. As the proportion of the solid component of a GGO increases, radial EBUS signals are more likely to present a mixed-blizzard sign. It is important to precisely identify the location of a GGO for development of bronchoscopic treatment modalities in the future.

Keywords Ground-glass opacity • Blizzard sign • Mixed blizzard sign • High-resolution computed tomography • Surgical findings

17.1 Introduction

Until recently, bronchoscopic diagnosis of ground-glass opacity (GGO) lesions has been considered almost impossible. One of the several reasons for this belief may be the difficult visualization of a GGO on X-ray fluoroscopy; for radial endobronchial ultrasound (R-EBUS)-guided biopsies, the characteristic findings of GGO lesions are not well known [1, 2]. Therefore, the diagnostic yield of bronchoscopy for GGO lesions, even with the use of endobronchial ultrasound with a guide sheath (EBUS-GS), has been low at 60–65 %, compared with that for solid lesions [1, 2]. Among the GGO lesions, the diagnostic yield of bronchoscopy for pure GGO lesions (no solid component) was lower compared with that for part-solid GGO lesions. We have previously identified and reported the "blizzard sign" for GGO, a specific R-EBUS finding that was clearly different from that of a normal lung, albeit subtly [3, 4]. Subsequently, we verified our observations by conducting a study on

T. Izumo (✉)
Department of Respiratory Medicine, Japanese Red Cross Medical Center, 4-1-22 Hiroo, Shibuya-ku, Tokyo 150-8935, Japan
e-mail: drtake1118@gmail.com

T. Izumo et al. (eds.), *Respiratory Endoscopy*,
DOI 10.1007/978-981-287-916-5_17

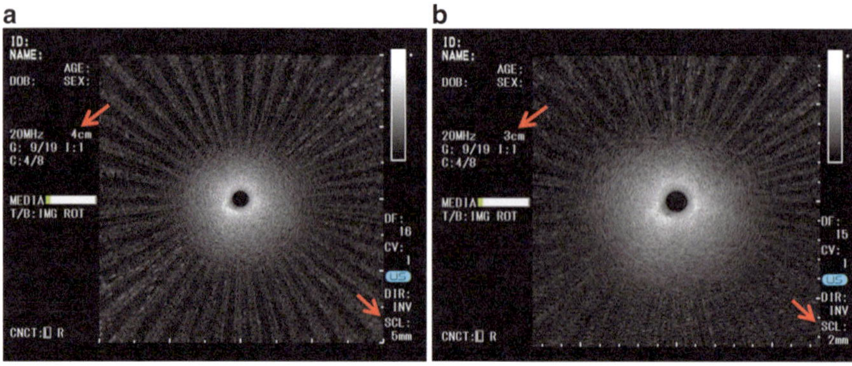

Fig. 17.1 Basic configuration of the ultrasound image for GGO. Changes in configuration of signal images depend on changes in display ranges. (**a**) At a display range of 4 cm (*red arrow*), the scale on the right side corresponds to 5 mm (*red arrow*). (**b**) At a display range of 3 cm (*red arrow*), the scale on the right increases to 2 mm (*red arrow*) and enables visualization of subtle changes in echogenicity. *GGO* ground-glass opacity

the correlation of the R-EBUS mixed-blizzard sign and blizzard sign with high-resolution computed tomography (HRCT) images and pathologic findings of GGO lesions [5]. Of note, this latter study only included lung adenocarcinoma cases that were pathologically confirmed by surgical resection; the GGO cases diagnosed by EBUS-GS as inflammation or organizing pneumonia were excluded because surgical resection was not performed to confirm the diagnoses.

17.2 Basic Configuration of the Endobronchial Ultrasound Processor

The basic settings of the R-EBUS processor for scanning GGO lesions are the same as that for regular R-EBUS for solid lesions: gain value of 9/19, contrast value of 4/8, image quality of 1, and inverse (INV) scanning direction. However, since the R-EBUS findings of GGO are very subtle, the display range (Fig. 17.1) is often set at 3 cm (scale of 2 mm), instead of the usual 4 cm (scale of 5 mm), in order to visualize the changes precisely.

17.3 R-EBUS Findings of GGO

1. Blizzard sign
   A blizzard sign seems to be similar to the snowstorm appearance of normal lung (Fig. 17.2a); however, on closer inspection, it is characterized by hyperechoic and coarse R-EBUS signals that clearly enhance in a wider area within a lesion.

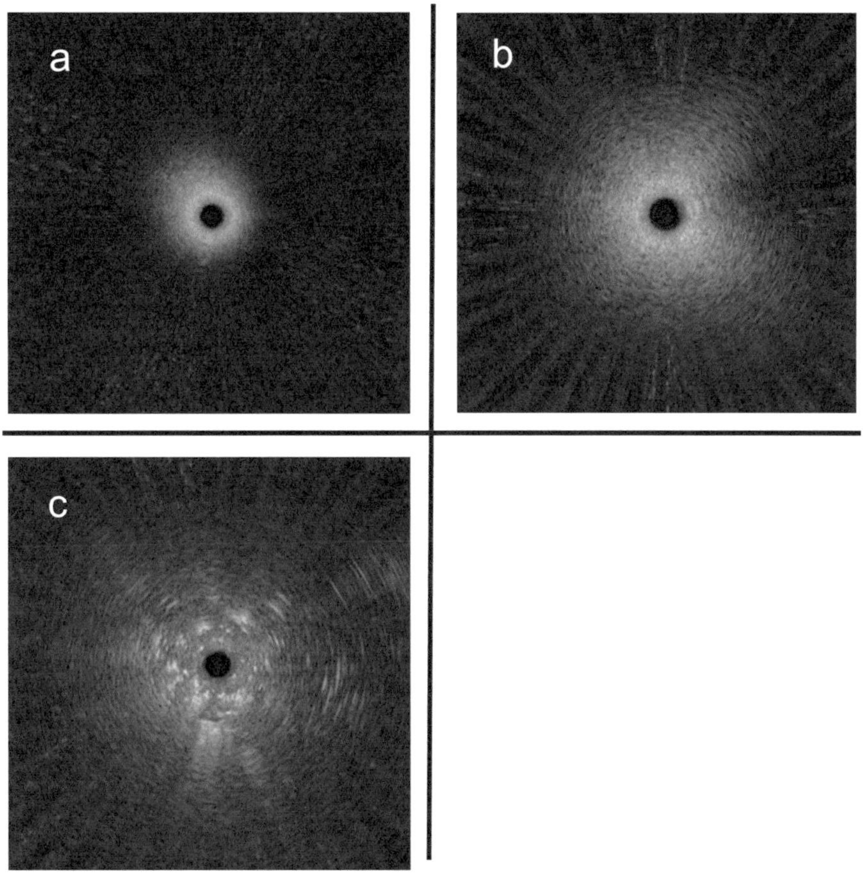

Fig. 17.2 Comparison of different R-EBUS findings. (**a**) A normal lung shows the typical snowstorm appearance; (**b**) A GGO lesion shows blizzard sign; (**c**) A part-solid lesion shows mixed-blizzard sign. Adapted from Izumo et al. [5]. *R-EBUS* radial endobronchial ultrasound, *GGO* ground-glass opacity

Specifically, a blizzard sign is defined as a hyperechoic and coarse R-EBUS signal that extends more than 1 cm away from the center of the ultrasound probe (Fig. 17.2b) [3–5].

2. Mixed blizzard sign
A mixed-blizzard sign is defined as coarse R-EBUS signals that are scattered with hyperechoic dots and lines and mixed with hypoechoic areas [5] (Fig. 17.2c). The typical R-EBUS findings, HRCT findings, and pathologic findings of malignant GGO lesions are shown in Figs. 17.3 and 17.4.

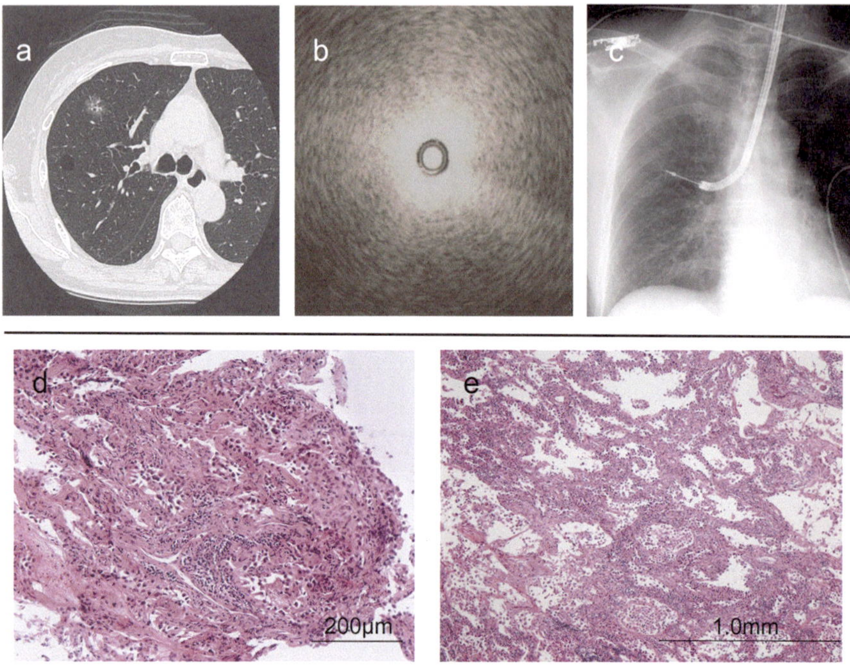

Fig. 17.3 Imaging and histologic correlation of a pure GGO lesion. Axial slice HRCT shows a pure GGO in the right segment 3b (**a**). After confirming blizzard sign on R-EBUS (**b**), EBUS-GS transbronchial biopsy is performed under simultaneous fluoroscopy guidance (**c**) and histopathologic examination (hematoxylin and eosin) reveals adenocarcinoma (**d**). Histopathologic examination of the surgically resected GGO lesion confirms well-differentiated minimally invasive adenocarcinoma (hematoxylin and eosin) (**e**). Adapted from Izumo et al. [5]. *GGO* ground-glass opacity, *HRCT* high-resolution computed tomography, *R-EBUS* radial endobronchial ultrasound, *EBUS-GS* endobronchial ultrasound with a guide sheath

17.4 Targets

From June 2012 to June 2014, 1,134 patients underwent EBUS-GS for peripheral lung lesions. Of them, 187 were found to have GGOs, 116 of which were diagnosed as lung adenocarcinoma by EBUS-GS (Table 17.1); 103 of 116 patients subsequently underwent surgical resection.

17.5 Comparison with HRCT

Table 17.2 shows a comparison of R-EBUS and HRCT findings. Blizzard sign was observed in all cases with pure GGO (9/9). When the R-EBUS findings were correlated with the ratio of GGO on HRCT, it was revealed that lesions with large proportion of GGO (i.e., with less solid component) were likely to show blizzard

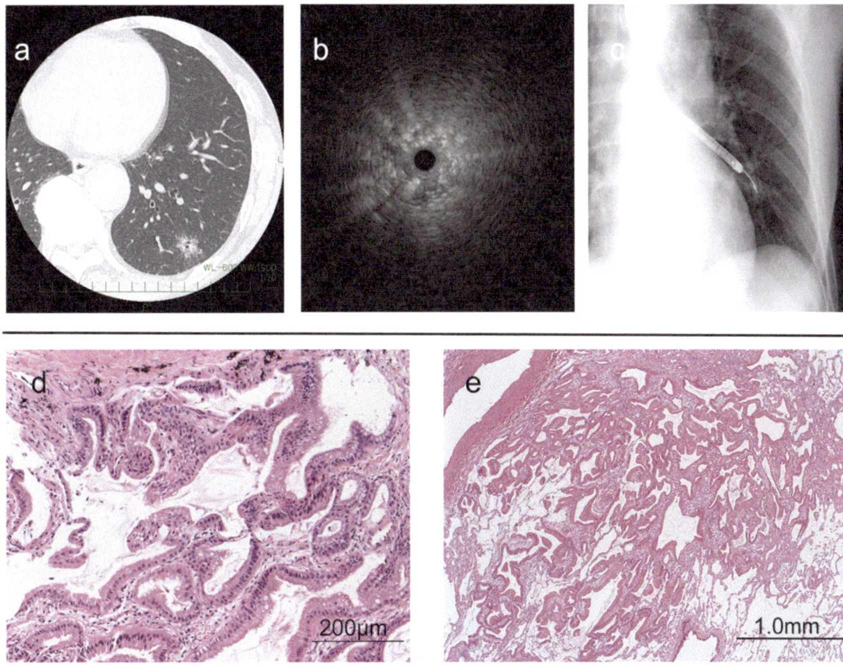

Fig. 17.4 Imaging and histologic correlation of a part-solid GGO lesion. Axial slice HRCT shows a part-solid GGO in the left segment 10a (**a**). After confirming mixed-blizzard sign on R-EBUS (**b**), EBUS-GS transbronchial biopsy is performed under simultaneous fluoroscopy guidance (**c**) and histopathologic examination (hematoxylin and eosin) reveals adenocarcinoma (**d**). Histopathologic examination of the surgically resected GGO lesion confirms well-differentiated invasive lepidic-predominant adenocarcinoma (hematoxylin and eosin) (**e**). Adapted from Izumo et al. [5]. *GGO* ground-glass opacity, *HRCT* high-resolution computed tomography, *R-EBUS* radial endobronchial ultrasound, *EBUS-GS* endobronchial ultrasound with a guide sheath

sign, whereas lesions with smaller proportion of GGO (i.e., with more solid component) were likely to show mixed-blizzard sign. A lesion with a large proportion of GGO on HRCT would be expected to show blizzard sign on R-EBUS. However, R-EBUS findings may vary depending on which part of the lesion the probe is in; this means that in a part-solid GGO lesion, mixed-blizzard sign and/or blizzard sign may be expected on R-EBUS. Therefore, it is important to confirm by HRCT in which part of the GGO lesion the involved bronchus is identified prior to examination [5].

Table 17.1 Baseline characteristics of patients with GGO lung adenocarcinoma ($n=116$)[a]

Variable	No. (%)
Year (range)	69 (44–87)
Gender	
Male	53 (45.7)
Female	63 (54.3)
Lobar location	
Upper	64 (55.2)
Middle or lingula	9 (7.7)
Lower	43 (37.1)
Feature	
Pure GGO	9 (7.8)
Part-solid GGO	107 (92.2)
Lesion size (long axis)	
Median size (range, mm)	23.6 (8.5–56.0)
≤30 mm	88 (75.7)
>30 mm	28 (24.3)
Procedure time (range, min)	23.0 (7.3–50.0)

[a]Adapted from Izumo et al. [5]
GGO ground-glass opacity

Table 17.2 Correlation between HRCT findings and radial EBUS types for GGO lesions diagnosed by EBUS ($n=116$)[a]

HRCT findings		Pure GGO ($n=9$)	Part-solid (>75 % GGO) ($n=7$)	Part-solid (>50–75 % GGO) ($n=29$)	Part-solid (25–50 % GGO) ($n=35$)	Part-solid (<25 % GGO) ($n=36$)
EBUS types	Blizzard sign ($n=44$)	100 (9/9)	85.7 (6/7)	51.7 (15/29)	31.4 (11/35)	8.3 (3/36)
	Mixed blizzard sign ($n=72$)	0.0 (0/9)	14.3 (1/7)	48.3 (14/29)	68.6 (24/35)	91.7 (33/36)

[a]Adapted from Izumo et al. [5]
EBUS endobronchial ultrasound, *EBUS-GS* endobronchial ultrasound with a guide sheath, *HRCT* high-resolution computed tomography

17.6 Comparison with Pathologic Findings

Table 17.3 shows the comparison of R-EBUS findings and pathologic findings ($n=3$). Blizzard sign was observed in lesions in the spectrum of adenocarcinoma in situ to well-differentiated adenocarcinoma, whereas mixed-blizzard sign was considered as reflecting the solid component of a GGO lesion and was observed in lesions in the spectrum of well-differentiated, invasive, lepidic-predominant adenocarcinoma to moderately or poorly differentiated adenocarcinoma.

Table 17.3 Correlation between radial EBUS images and histology of surgically resected GGO ($n = 103$)[a]

Surgical diagnosis	EBUS types	
	Blizzard sign ($n = 39$)	Mixed blizzard sign ($n = 64$)
Adenocarcinoma in situ	1	2
Minimally invasive adenocarcinoma	9	0
Well-differentiated invasive lepidic predominant	18	16
Well-differentiated invasive papillary predominant	8	9
Well-differentiated invasive acinar predominant	2	1
Well-differentiated mucinous (formerly mucinous BAC with invasion)	1	3
Moderately differentiated invasive lepidic predominant	0	1
Moderately differentiated invasive papillary predominant	0	24
Moderately differentiated invasive micropapillary predominant	0	2
Moderately differentiated invasive acinar predominant	0	3
Moderately differentiated mucinous (formerly mucinous BAC with invasion)	0	1
Poorly differentiated invasive solid predominant	0	2

[a]Adapted from Izumo et al. [5]
EBUS endobronchial ultrasound, *GGO* ground-glass opacity, *BAC* bronchoalveolar carcinoma

17.7 Future Perspective

What is the value of diagnostic bronchoscopy for GGO? At some facilities, GGO lesions that have high probability of malignancy are surgically resected, without the need for less invasive histologic confirmation by bronchoscopy. At our facility, bronchoscopy is being developed for therapy of small peripheral pulmonary lesions, including GGOs and beginning lung cancer, by photodynamic therapy, cryotherapy, and radiofrequency ablation. If these modalities of direct and localized therapy prove to be effective, bronchoscopy would have a value in confirming the diagnosis prior to treatment. To this end, we believe that it is important to establish the R-EBUS findings of GGO in order to enable accurate diagnosis by EBUS-GS [5].

References

1. Izumo T, Sasada S, Chavez C, et al. The diagnostic utility of endobronchial ultrasonography with a guide sheath and tomosynthesis images for ground glass opacity pulmonary lesions. J Thorac Dis. 2013;5:745–50.
2. Ikezawa Y, Sukoh N, Shinagawa N, et al. Endobronchial ultrasonography with a guide sheath for pure or mixed ground-glass opacity lesions. Respiration. 2014;88:137–43.

3. Sasada S, Izumo T, Chavez C, et al. Blizzard sign as a specific endobronchial ultrasound image for ground glass opacity: a case report. Respir Med Case Rep. 2014;14:19–21.
4. Chavez C, Sasada S, Izumo T, et al. Image-guided bronchoscopy for histopathologic diagnosis of pure ground glass opacity: a case report. J Thorac Dis. 2014;6:E81–4.
5. Izumo T, Sasada S, Chavez C, et al. Radial endobronchial ultrasound images for ground glass opacity pulmonary lesions. Eur Respir J. 2015;45:1661–8.

Chapter 18
Endobronchial Ultrasound with a Guide Sheath for Peripheral Pulmonary Lesions

Yuji Matsumoto and Takehiro Izumo

Abstract Endobronchial ultrasound with a guide sheath (EBUS-GS) is a useful method that enables localization of a lesion by R-EBUS followed by placement of a guide sheath to allow precise specimen collection. EBUS-GS requires proper basic bronchoscopy skills in order to precisely maneuver the guide sheath to the desired sampling site.

Keywords Endobronchial ultrasound • R-EBUS • Guide sheath • Transbronchial biopsy • Peripheral pulmonary lesion

18.1 Introduction

The diagnostic yield of bronchoscopy for peripheral lung lesions has improved owing to the additional use of radial endobronchial ultrasound (R-EBUS), which has been recommended by the latest guidelines of the American College of Chest Physicians [1]. Placement of a guide sheath (GS) after R-EBUS probe confirmation of the location of a lesion will enable precise collection of specimen from the affected area. In this section, we will present an overview of EBUS-GS.

18.2 Devices

1. *Ultrasound observation device (EU-MEI or EU-ME2, Olympus, Tokyo, Japan)*

Y. Matsumoto
Respiratory Endoscopy Division, Department of Endoscopy, National Cancer Center Hospital, Tokyo, Japan

T. Izumo (✉)
Department of Respiratory Medicine, Japanese Red Cross Medical Center, 4-1-22 Hiroo, Shibuya-ku, Tokyo 150-8935, Japan
e-mail: drtake1118@gmail.com

T. Izumo et al. (eds.), *Respiratory Endoscopy*,
DOI 10.1007/978-981-287-916-5_18

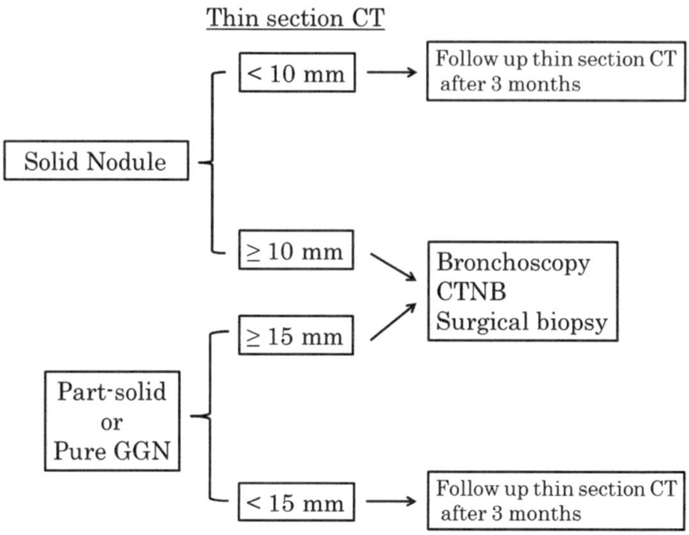

Fig. 18.1 Management algorithm for pulmonary nodules detected on CT scan (This is adapted at the Department of Endoscopy of the National Cancer Center, Japan, and is based on the "Guidelines for the Management of Pulmonary Nodules Detected by Low-dose CT Lung Cancer Screening Version 3" advocated by The Japanese Society of CT Screening [2]). *CT* computed tomography, *CTNB* CT-guided needle biopsy, *GGN* ground glass nodule

2. *Ultrasound probe (UM-S20-17S or UM-S20-20R, Olympus, Tokyo, Japan)*
3. *Disposable guide sheath kit (K-201or K-203, Olympus, Tokyo, Japan)*

18.3 Indications

From January 2012 to December 2013, we performed 1,933 cases of respiratory endoscopic examination at our department; of these, 1,105 cases were peripheral lung lesions that needed fluoroscopy-guided diagnostic bronchoscopy, and most of which were performed with EBUS-GS. The criteria that we used for selecting EBUS-GS as the diagnostic procedure for peripheral lung lesions were almost similar with the guidelines advocated by the Japanese Society of CT Screening (Fig. 18.1) [2].

18.4 Preparation of the Guide Sheath Kit

The disposable GS kit includes one each GS, biopsy forceps, cytology brush, ET stopper, and US stopper. ET stoppers for the biopsy forceps and cytology brush and US stoppers for the ultrasound probe need to be prepared in such a way that the

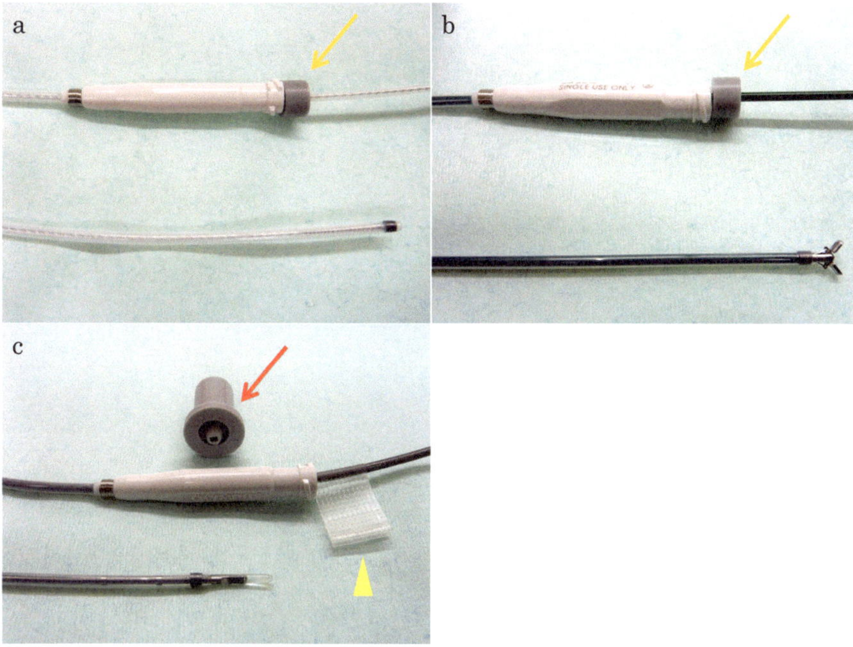

Fig. 18.2 Preparation of a guide sheath kit. Adjust the ET stoppers (*orange arrows*) for the (**a**) cytology brush and (**b**) biopsy forceps so that the distal tip of the GS will accommodate the needed length of each device. For the cytology brush, the distal GS tip should coincide with the distal tip of the plastic sheath covering the brush. For the biopsy forceps, the distal GS tip should coincide with the base of the cup in order to allow protrusion of the distal forceps tip by 2.5–3.0 mm; this would facilitate smooth opening of the cups during biopsy. In setting the (**c**) ultrasound probe, a US stopper (*red arrow*) is provided by the manufacturer; at our department, we prefer to use an adhesive medical tape (*yellow arrowhead*) as a marker that will allow the transducer to protrude out of the GS

distal tip of the GS will accommodate the needed length of each device, as described in detail in Fig. 18.2. Proper preparation will allow smooth R-EBUS scanning and precise biopsy sampling. At our department, we prefer to use an adhesive tape as a stopper for the fragile R-EBUS probe that is prone to breakage.

The ultrasound probe should be connected to the probe driving unit, with the connecting pin pointing upward and the wing downward (Fig. 18.3). If connected the wrong way, the ultrasound probe can sometimes get stuck to the probe driving unit. During examination, the ultrasound probe should be secured in the probe holder to prevent contamination and entry of air bubbles into the surrounding area of the oscillator (Fig. 18.4).

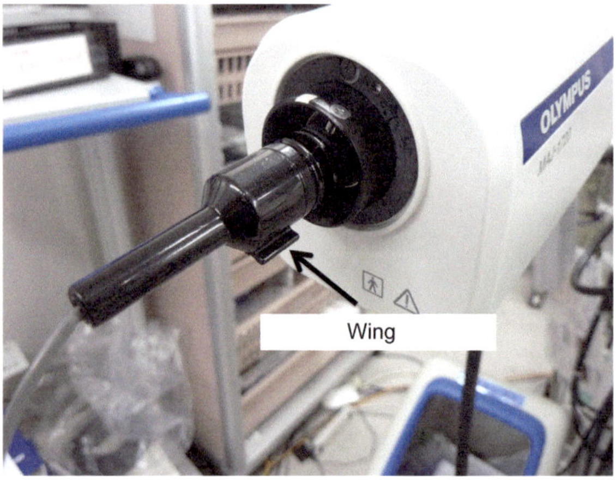

Fig. 18.3 Connecting the ultrasound probe to the probe driving unit. The ultrasound probe should be connected to the probe driving unit with the connecting pin pointing upward and the wing downward

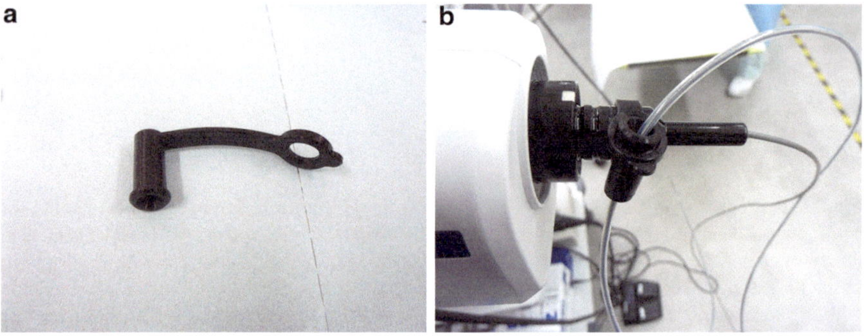

Fig. 18.4 Securing the radial EBUS probe. Using a probe holder (**a**), secure the ultrasound probe (**b**)

18.5 Procedures

18.5.1 Insertion to the Involved Bronchus

Using computed tomography images, confirm the bifurcation of the involved bronchus as far peripheral as possible. Additional use of virtual bronchoscopic navigation system is recommended because selection of a wrong bronchus may prolong examination time and decrease diagnostic yield. Once the bronchial bifurcation is identified, insert the R-EBUS probe with GS toward the target bronchus. The key is to completely suction secretions from the bronchial lumen and bronchoscope working channel and to wedge properly the bronchoscope tip into the involved orifice.

18.5.2 Confirmation of R-EBUS Findings

While observing the positional relationship with the target lesion under X-ray fluoroscopy, insert the R-EBUS probe further to the periphery, and confirm the R-EBUS findings. Once the probe comes to the vicinity of the lesion and is positioned in the center of the display, it will be visualized as a hypoechoic area. When the lesion is visualized, move the R-EBUS back and forth (i.e., toward the periphery and the center) to confirm the range of the lesion and decide where to place the GS. Basically, the GS should be placed 2–3 cm proximal to the site where EBUS visualization is maximal. This is to allow the forceps cup and cytology brush to reach the area of maximal tumor diameter during biopsy. It is also important to note the R-EBUS findings of accompanying blood vessels (Fig. 18.5) and necrotic changes within a lesion, which appear as inhomogeneous hyperechoic areas; these areas should be avoided during specimen collection.

18.5.3 Collecting Specimens

The next step is to place the GS to the target lesion and to collect specimen. At our department, after palpating the lesion using a bronchial brush and with simultaneous X-ray fluoroscopy guidance, we usually prepare a smear sample for rapid on-site cytology evaluation (ROSE). Subsequently, we collect specimen using biopsy forceps while waiting for the results of ROSE; repeat R-EBUS scanning to confirm

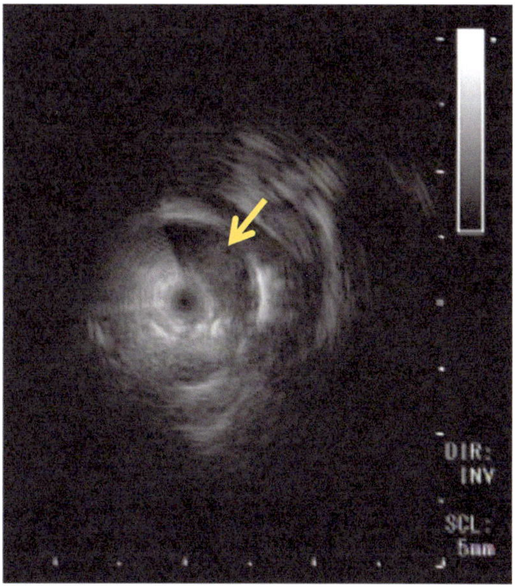

Fig. 18.5 Radial EBUS findings of blood vessels in a peripheral pulmonary lesion. Back-and-forth movement of the probe through the target site shows an anechoic region (*orange arrow*), which corresponds to a blood vessel

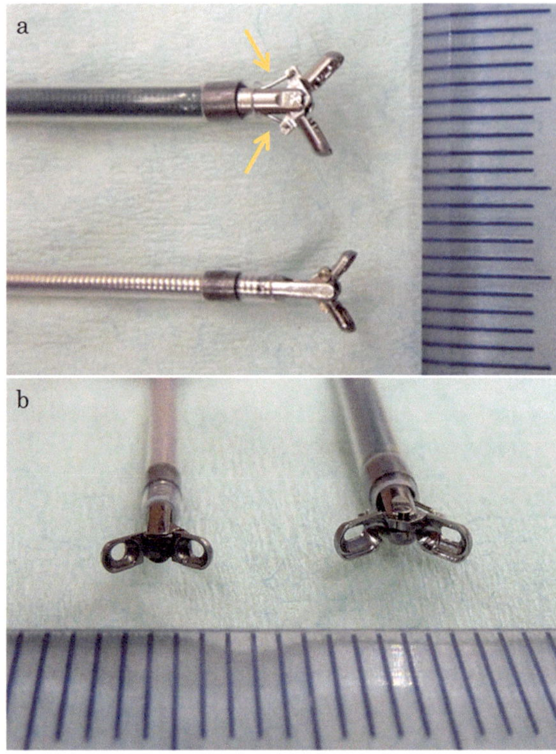

Fig. 18.6 Differences in size of biopsy forceps used for EBUS-GS for peripheral pulmonary lesions. The normal-size forceps (*green handle*; **a**, *upper*; **b**, *right*) has a larger cup and a swing mechanism compared with the small-sized forceps (*silver handle*; **a**, *lower*; **b**, *left*). EBUS-GS, endobronchial ultrasound with a guide sheath

GS placement in the lesion is performed as appropriate. Of note, we always make it a point to secure the bronchoscope and the GS firmly to avoid displacement during sampling, especially when lesions are in the inferior lobe, where diaphragmatic movements during respiration may easily cause displacement of the soft GS. It was reported that diagnostic yield reaches a plateau after more than five specimens are collected [4]; therefore, we recommend performing repeated forceps biopsy until at least five pieces of specimen are collected.

The GS kit comes in two types; K-201 (Olympus, Tokyo, Japan) is supplied with a small-sized biopsy forceps, whereas K-203(Olympus, Tokyo, Japan) comes with normal-sized ones (Fig. 18.6). The small-sized forceps might be prone to yield a small amount of specimen and may lead to diagnostic failure. Our department recommends using normal-sized forceps, especially for peripheral pulmonary lesions that do not invade the mucosa of the involved subsegmental bronchus because the normal-sized forceps has a large cup that allows collection of a larger specimen. In addition, the swing mechanism at the neck supporting its cup enables a stronger force to grip a specimen for easy collection.

However, using the K-203 GS kit necessitates the use of a bronchoscope with a working channel diameter of at least 2.6 mm, which cannot reach more distal subsegmental bronchi, such the superior lobar branches. To address this limitation, our department has started collaborating with a manufacturer to develop a new type of bronchoscope that has a smaller than conventional outer diameter but can accommodate normal-sized biopsy forceps [5].

18.5.4 Removing the GS

After completion of sample collection, the GS should be kept in place for 2 min to tamponade the biopsy site; thereafter, remove the GS smoothly out of the bronchoscope working channel under X-ray fluoroscopy guidance to confirm that its distal tip does not get broken and dislodged in the bronchus.

18.6 R-EBUS Findings and Diagnostic Accuracy

R-EBUS findings are classified into three categories, based on the position of the ultrasound probe relative to the lesion – within, adjacent to, and invisible (Fig. 18.7) – each category has been found to have different diagnostic yields [4, 6]. The results obtained from 296 consecutive cases that underwent EBUS-GS at our department revealed that diagnostic yield was correlated with these categories; a more significant diagnostic accuracy was obtained with better EBUS visualization ($P<0.001$) (Table 18.1). suggesting that the better the cases, from our experience, the significant challenges in performing EBUS-GS have been (1) positioning the probe to the "within" area and (2) increasing the diagnostic accuracy when only "adjacent to" and "invisible" findings can be obtained.

18.7 How to Position the GS to the Optimal Site

When it is difficult to place the GS to the target lesion, use the following methods in combination to reach the optimal target site.

18.7.1 Direct Observation

When the probe is initially found as "invisible" on R-EBUS, it is highly likely that the probe and GS were inserted in a wrong bronchus. When a wrong direction is confirmed under X-ray fluoroscopy, switch back to endoscopic view, go back to the most distal bronchial bifurcation visible, and select a different bronchial branch to approach the target site.

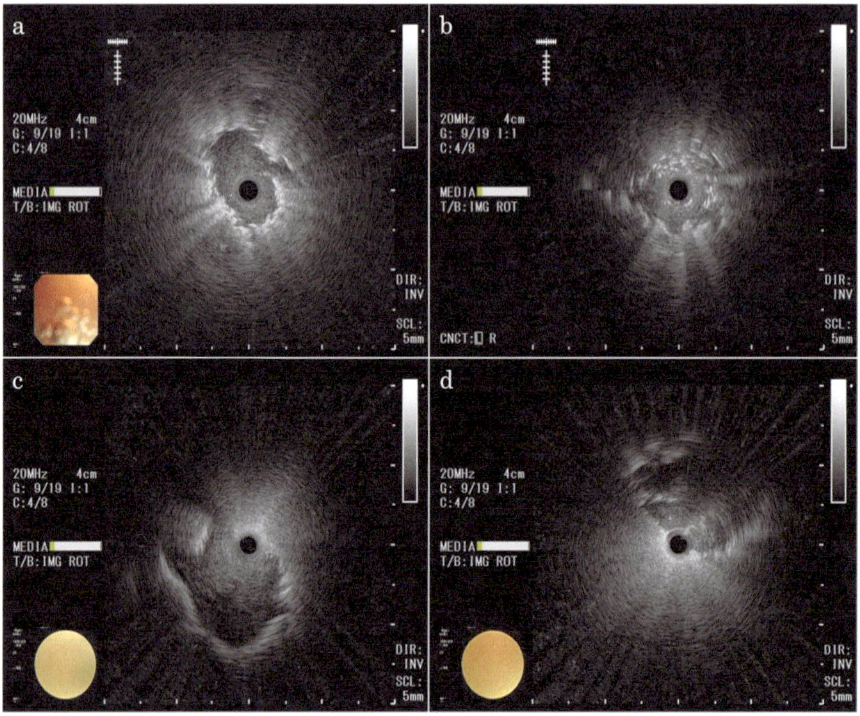

Fig. 18.7 Typical radial EBUS findings of peripheral pulmonary lesions. (**a**, **b**) "Within" pattern shows a heterogeneous, hypoechoic area surrounding the probe circumferentially. (**c**, **d**) "Adjacent to" pattern shows a heterogeneous, hypoechoic area beside the probe, but not surrounding it circumferentially (Adapted from Izumo et al. [3])

Table 18.1 EBUS findings and diagnostic accuracy for patients with peripheral pulmonary lesions ($N=296$)

Obtained EBUS image	Diagnostic no. (%)	P value	Odds ratio (95 %CI)
Within	164 (86.8)	<0.001	7.57 (3.24–18.06)
Adjacent to	55 (69.6)		2.64 (1.10–6.49)
Invisible	13 (46.4)		

EBUS endobronchial ultrasound

18.7.2 R-EBUS

When the probe is found as "adjacent to" a lesion using R-EBUS, confirm the direction of the echoic image enhancement by fine flexion-extension (or up-down) movements of the bronchoscope tip or by slow rotating movements of your operating hand. While firmly maintaining hand position and the direction of the scope, and under X-ray fluoroscopy guidance, pull the scope a bit backward and insert again, until you can insert the probe into the lesion (Fig. 18.8). Try to move the scope

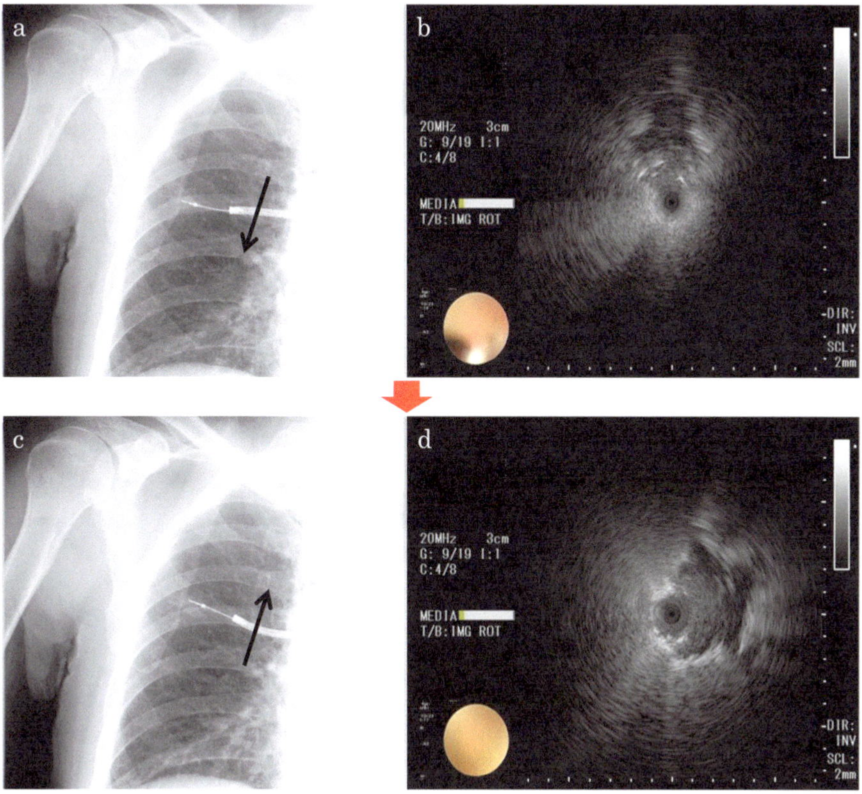

Fig. 18.8 Up-and-down method. By downward movement (*black arrow*) of the bronchoscope, the probe is seen close to the center of the lesion under X-ray fluoroscopy (**a**) but looks far away from the lesion by EBUS (**b**). In contrast, after moving the bronchoscope upward (*black arrow*) while slightly pulling out the probe before reinserting, the probe is seen to shift away from the center of the lesion under X-ray fluoroscopy (**c**) but looks close to it by EBUS (**d**) (Adopted from Izumo et al. [3])

slowly because there is a slight time lag between the actual movement of R-EBUS and the image generated.

18.7.3 X-Ray Fluoroscopy

Similar to the technique described in Sects. 18.7.1 and 18.17.2, the added use of X-ray fluoroscopy will enable a more precise approach. Remove the R-EBUS with GS slowly, and take note of the corresponding site of bronchial bifurcation under X-ray fluoroscopy. From this site, insert the probe toward the periphery, and position it within the lesion (Fig. 18.8a, c).

18.7.4 Introducer

Sometimes, a subsegmental bronchus leading to the target lesion branches off its bifurcation at a sharp and acute angle. Such anatomy often makes it difficult to position the probe with GS even with a combination of the techniques described earlier; in these cases, an introducer will come in handy. Remove the probe from the GS then insert the introducer. Under X-ray fluoroscopy, guide the tip of the introducer along the curved direction of the involved bronchus and lead the GS to the target site. Take note that the anterior and posterior directions would be difficult to distinguish under X-ray fluoroscopy, but observing the bronchoscope direction with right and left rotation will help determine the route that the introducer is heading for. Extra caution is needed because the tip of the introducer is sharp and can easily injure the pleura. At our department, we attempt to reach the target lesion using the introducer for only 1 min or so; if we are not successful, we proceed to the procedure mentioned in Sect. 18.8.

18.7.5 Penetration Using a Biopsy Tool

Even if the correct direction is observed under X-ray fluoroscopy, it is sometimes difficult to visualize the R-EBUS signal of a lesion owing to a resistance, which may be palpated while inserting the probe with GS further. We emphasize the importance of confirming by X-ray fluoroscopy (e.g., oblique view) that this resistance is not near the pleura. If obstruction of the involved subsegmental bronchus is assumed as the cause of this resistance, remove the probe and insert a bronchial brush or biopsy forceps to dilate the obstructed part and guide the GS to the periphery under X-ray fluoroscopy guidance; thereafter, reinsert the R-EBUS probe and confirm whether the target site has been reached.

18.8 Sample Collection from a Noninvolved Bronchus

When collecting a specimen from a lesion that is difficult to reach because of surrounding structure, such as lymph nodes or external compression, transbronchial needle aspiration through a GS (GS-TBNA) is useful [7].

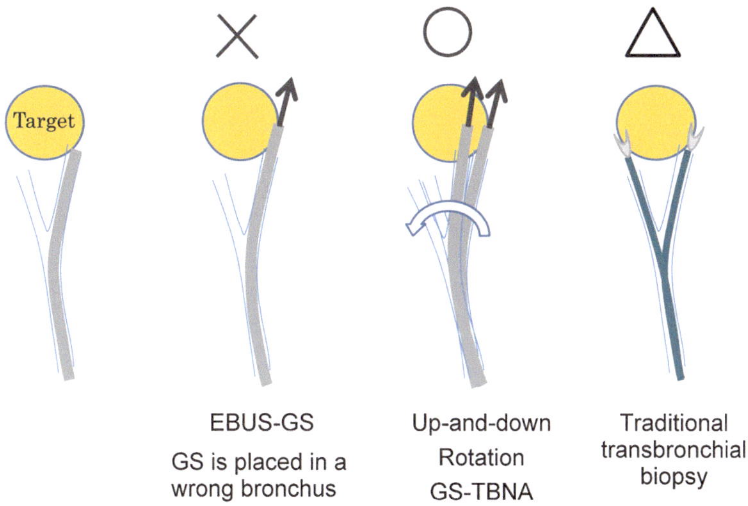

Fig. 18.9 Difference between EBUS-GS and traditional diagnostic bronchoscopy for peripheral pulmonary lesions. Placement of a GS in a wrong bronchus (×) would lead miss sampling of the target site. Fine manipulation movements of the bronchoscope tip and the use of GS-TBNA (*circle*) may overcome this limitation of EBUS-GS. On the other hand, the use of traditional bronchoscopy without GS leads to insertion of biopsy instruments through different bronchial subsegments (*triangle*)

18.9 Pitfalls (Fig. 18.9)

When using EBUS-GS, proper basic bronchoscopy techniques are mandatory. Once the GS is placed, specimen collection can be done at the same site repeatedly. This is an advantage over traditional method without GS, wherein there is high probability of inserting biopsy instruments in a wrong or different bronchus, leading to low diagnostic yield. However, inserting the GS in a wrong bronchus interferes with accurate diagnosis because all specimens collected will be from the same incorrect site where the GS is placed. On the other hand, when using a traditional bronchoscope, a comparatively long distance is needed for the forceps to go through because the most distal subsegmental bronchus that can be reached by the bronchoscope is far from the lesion; in this case, the biopsy instruments may be inserted in different bronchial segments each time. For the latter situation, obtaining more specimens may increase the probability of sampling the correct site and yielding an accurate diagnosis.

It is important to have a vivid image of the rotational direction of the bronchoscope, which can almost be predetermined based on the location of the lesion on axial orientation (Fig. 18.10). Moreover, it is also important from the pathological point of view to process the obtained specimen appropriately.

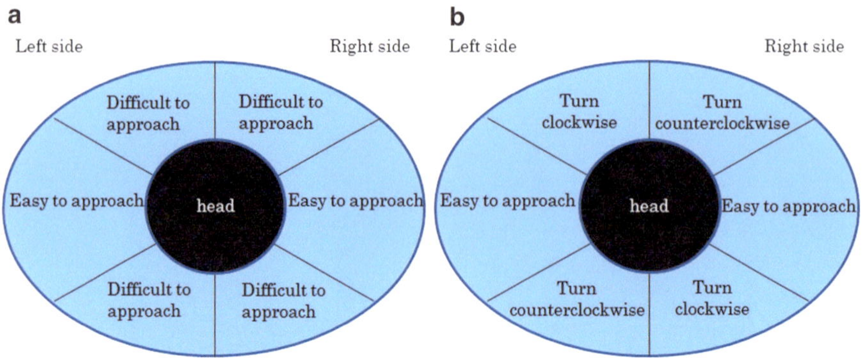

Fig. 18.10 Schematic representation of bronchoscope rotation toward the location of the target lesion

18.10 Conclusions

For proper operation of EBUS-GS, it is necessary for both operators and assistants to understand the procedure well and to establish coordination with each other. As individualized medicine requires us to improve specimen collection, in terms of quality and quantity, it is becoming even more important to master the skills of performing EBUS-GS.

References

1. Rivera MP, Mehta AC, Wahidi MM. Establishing the diagnosis of lung cancer: diagnosis and management of lung cancer, 3rd ed: American College of Chest Physicians evidence-based clinical practice guidelines. Chest. 2013;143:e142S–65.
2. A lung cancer examination by low dose multi-slice CT: a judgment and figure of the pulmonary nodule follow-up http://www.jscts.org/pdf/guideline/gls3rdfig130521.pdf.
3. Izumo T, Sasada S, Matsumoto Y, et al. Radial endobronchial ultrasound and guide sheath for peripheral pulmonary lesions. J Jpn Soc Respir Endosc. 2014;36:392–7.
4. Yamada N, Yamazaki K, Kurimoto N, et al. Factors related to diagnostic yield of transbronchial biopsy using endobronchial ultrasonography with a guide sheath in small peripheral pulmonary lesions. Chest. 2007;132:603–8.
5. Sasada S, Izumo T, Chavez C, et al. A new middle-range diameter bronchoscope with large channel for transbronchial sampling of peripheral pulmonary lesions. Jpn J Clin Oncol. 2014;44:826–34.
6. Tamiya M, Okamoto N, Sasada S, et al. Diagnostic yield of combined bronchoscopy and endobronchial ultrasonography, under LungPoint guidance for small peripheral pulmonary lesions. Respirology. 2013;18:834–9.
7. Takai M, Izumo T, Chavez C, et al. Transbronchial needle aspiration through a guide sheath with endobronchial ultrasonography (GS-TBNA) for peripheral pulmonary lesions. Ann Thorac Cardiovasc Surg. 2014;20:19–25.

Chapter 19
Transbronchial Needle Aspiration Through a Guide Sheath for Peripheral Pulmonary Lesions

Moto Takai and Takehiro Izumo

Abstract In addition to the usual procedure of endobronchial ultrasound with a guide sheath (EBUS-GS), transbronchial needle aspiration through a guide sheath (GS-TBNA) may be performed for peripheral pulmonary lesions. In cases in which the probe is confirmed to be located "adjacent to" a lesion on the EBUS image, a diagnostic yield comparable to that of EBUS probe "within" can be achieved by GS-TBNA.

Keywords EBUS-GS • GS-TBNA • Peripheral pulmonary lesion • Transbronchial biopsy

19.1 Indication

Transbronchial needle aspiration through a guide sheath (GS-TBNA) is an added biopsy technique to transbronchial biopsy (TBB) through a GS during the usual endobronchial ultrasound with a guide sheath (EBUS-GS) procedure for peripheral pulmonary lesions. GS-TBNA is effective for lesions that are assumed to be "adjacent to" a lesion based on the findings on EBUS; for example, the presence of metastatic pulmonary lesions that have spread hematogenously is a good indication.

M. Takai
Department of Pulmonology, Kameda Medical Center, Chiba, Japan

T. Izumo (✉)
Department of Respiratory Medicine, Japanese Red Cross Medical Center, 4-1-22 Hiroo, Shibuya-ku, Tokyo 150-8935, Japan
e-mail: drtake1118@gmail.com

T. Izumo et al. (eds.), *Respiratory Endoscopy*,
DOI 10.1007/978-981-287-916-5_19

19.2 Preparation

Prepare the usual set of equipment and instruments used when performing EBUS-GS for biopsy of peripheral pulmonary lesions. For the GS, use the K-203 kit (Olympus, Tokyo, Japan) so that the sheath of the TBNA apparatus can be accommodated [1]. Specifically, prepare the following:

- Bronchoscope with a working channel diameter of >2.6 mm (e.g., 1 T-260 and LF-TP; Olympus, Tokyo, Japan), so that the sheath of K-203 (Olympus, Tokyo, Japan) can be adapted
- Guide sheath kit with a GS with an outer diameter of 2.55 mm (K-203, Olympus, Tokyo, Japan)
- Metal sheath for TBNA (MAJ-64, Olympus, Tokyo, Japan)
- 21-G aspiration needle without side hole (NA-1C-1, Olympus, Tokyo, Japan)
- T-shaped stopcock and 20-ml syringe

19.3 Actual Procedure

1. The distal tip of the metallic sheath for TBNA is shorter than the forceps and bronchial brush instruments, so it will not reach the distal tip of the GS when inserted. Therefore, the GS needs to be prepared (Fig. 19.1) before starting the procedure in order for it to facilitate smooth TBNA. After preparation, insert the TBNA apparatus into the metallic sheath and connect its proximal end with the T-shaped stopcock with a 20-ml syringe.
2. Observe the endobronchial route as usual and visualize the lesion using radial EBUS (R-EBUS) through a GS.
3. Position the GS in the lesion, as appropriate, and remove the R-EBUS probe. Then, insert the TBNA apparatus with the covering metallic sheath into the GS.
4. An assistant pushes the needle toward the lesion under simultaneous X-ray fluoroscopy guidance.
5. After jabbing the target lesion, the assistant creates a negative pressure through the 20-ml syringe and moves the TBNA apparatus back and forth. Note that instead of the operator, the assistant is the one who performs the needle aspiration, while the operator secures the position of the scope and GS (Fig. 19.2).
6. After about ten times of needle aspiration, close the stopcock while maintaining the negative pressure; otherwise, you might end up pushing the specimen back.
7. Retract the TBNA apparatus into the metallic sheath and remove it from the GS.
8. After puncture, push out the contents of the needle onto a glass slide for cytology. If you find a core specimen, transfer it to a container with formalin and send it for tissue diagnosis. For culture purposes, transfer the samples into a container with normal saline.

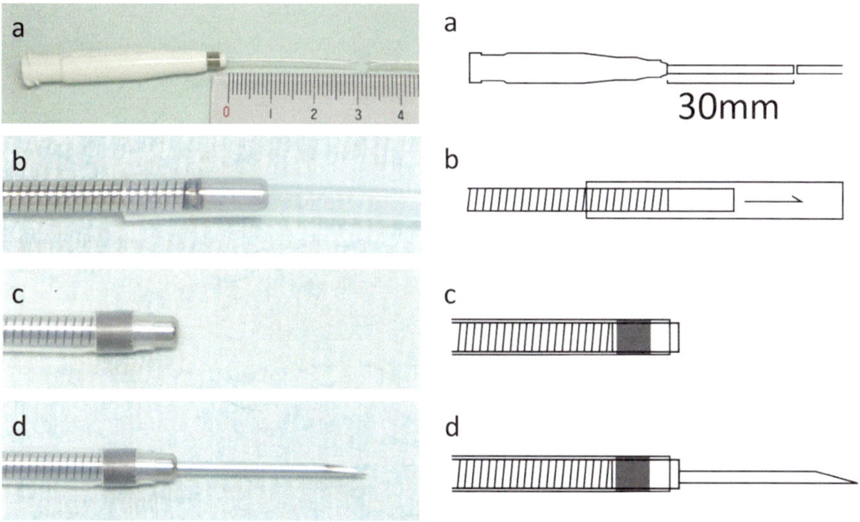

Fig. 19.1 Preparation of the guide sheath. (**a**) Cut the proximal end of the GS by 3 cm and (**b**) insert the metallic sheath from there until its distal tip is confirmed to coincide with that of the GS (**c**); this way, the TBNA apparatus can be pushed out without damaging the GS (**d**). GS, guide sheath; TBNA, transbronchial needle aspiration (Adopted from Takai et al. [1])

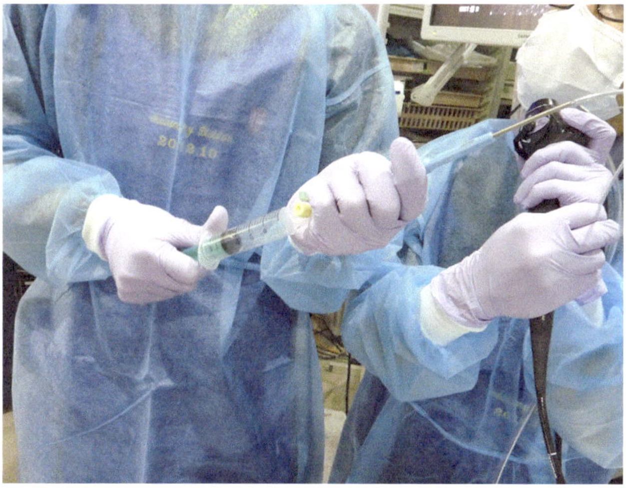

Fig. 19.2 Operation of the needle apparatus and syringe by assistants, as detailed in Sect. 19.3.5

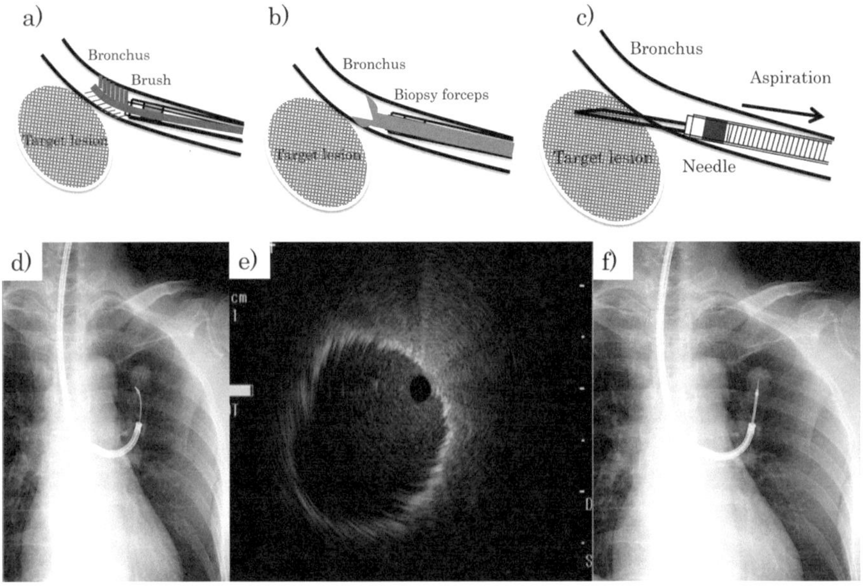

Fig. 19.3 Representative case of GS-TBNA for diagnosis of peripheral pulmonary lesions. (**a**–**c**) Schematic diagram on how GS-TBNA is performed. (**d**) X-ray fluoroscopy image shows that the distal tip of the R-EBUS probe is tangential to the nodular shadow; (**e**) this is confirmed to be "adjacent to" on EBUS scanning. After GS-TBNA, repeat insertion of the probe to the center of the lesion becomes easy, as shown on X-ray fluoroscopy (**f**). GS-TBNA, transbronchial needle aspiration through a guide sheath; R-EBUS, radial endobronchial ultrasound

9. While the assistants process the specimen, the operator reconfirms the position of the lesion using R-EBUS. It is assumed that GS-TBNA would create a tract through the barrier to the lesion and enable easier localization and biopsy (Fig. 19.3) [2]. The goal of this procedure is to improve not only the additional yield of TBNA but also the overall diagnostic accuracy, including that of forceps biopsy and other tools. Ideally, it is desirable to confirm by TBNA first then alternate with R-EBUS scanning until the probe shifts from a position of "adjacent to" the lesion to "within" the lesion.
10. Finally, perform forceps biopsy and bronchial brushing through the GS.

19.4 Limitations and Countermeasures

1. The benefits of GS-TBNA have been demonstrated for solid peripheral pulmonary lesions, but not for ground-glass opacity lesions.
2. In our study, we found one case that developed pneumonia after puncture of a lung abscess. When lung abscess is suspected, empiric antibiotic treatment should be considered immediately after the procedure.

Table 19.1 Diagnostic efficacy of GS-TBNA according to the location of the R-EBUS probe relative to the lesion before biopsy

	Total (N=37)	Within (N=21)	Outside (N=16)	P value
Sensitivity (%)	84.8	89.5	78.6	0.39
Specificity (%)	100	100	100	1.0
Positive predictive value (%)	100	100	100	1.0
Negative predictive value (%)	44.4	50.0	40.0	0.76
Accuracy (%)	86.5	86.4	86.7	0.98

Adopted from Takai et al. [1]

GS-TBNA: transbronchial needle aspiration through a guide sheath

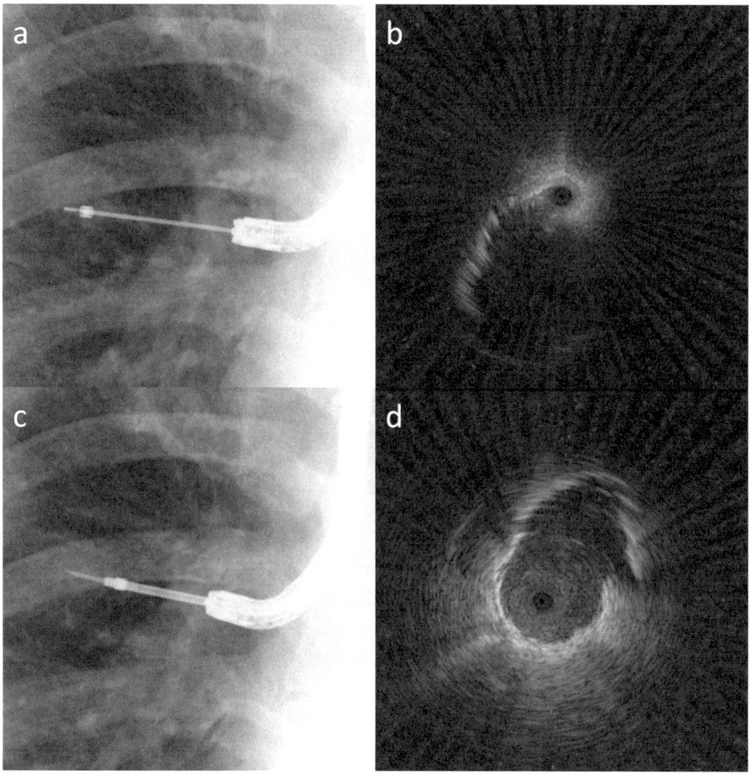

Fig. 19.4 R-EBUS findings before and after GS-TBNA. Upon initial insertion of the R-EBUS probe to the lesion under X-ray fluoroscopy guidance (**a**), EBUS scanning reveals that the probe is "adjacent to" the lesion (**b**). After two GS-TBNA punctures, reinsertion of the R-EBUS probe to the same location (**c**) shows that the probe is now "within" the lesion (**d**). GS-TBNA, transbronchial needle aspiration through a guide sheath; R-EBUS, radial endobronchial ultrasound

19.5 Results

Table 19.1 shows the results of GS-TBNA at our hospital. Adding GS-TBNA to the usual EBUS-GS improved the diagnostic accuracy of "adjacent to" cases to comparable rates as that of "within" cases. It was reported that adding TBNA without using a GS increased the diagnostic accuracy for peripheral pulmonary lesions, compared with transbronchial biopsy using usual EBUS-GS. The diagnostic accuracies for specimens collected by TBNA, regardless of EBUS findings of "adjacent to vs. within," were comparable [3]. Adding TBNA through a GS to conventional methods enabled more thorough and easier repeated TBNA or TBB at the same site [1, 2].

Figure 19.4 shows some representative examples that demonstrate the usefulness of GS-TBNA. Prior to examination, CT bronchus sign was negative and R-EBUS findings were expected to be "adjacent to" the lesion, which was later on the case. After performing two GS-TBNA punctures, repeated R-EBUS scanning showed that the probe could be easily positioned "within" the lesion and enabled smooth forceps biopsy and bronchial brushing. There were no complications after the procedure, and the lesion was successfully diagnosed as adenocarcinoma by bronchoscopy.

References

1. Takai M, Izumo T, Chavez C, Tsuchida T, Sasada S. Transbronchial needle aspiration through a guide sheath with endobronchial ultrasonography (GS-TBNA) for peripheral pulmonary lesions. Ann Thorac Cardiovasc Surg. 2014;20:19–25.
2. Izumo T, Sasada S, Matsumoto Y, et al. Radial endobronchial ultrasound and guide sheath for peripheral pulmonary lesions. J Jpn Soc Respir Endosc. 2014;36:392–7.
3. Chao T-Y, Chien M-T, Lie C-H, Chung Y-H, Wang J-L, Lin M-C. Endobronchial ultrasonography-guided transbronchial needle aspiration increases the diagnostic yield of peripheral pulmonary lesions: a randomized trial. Chest. 2009;136:229–36.

Chapter 20
Virtual Bronchoscopic Navigation for Peripheral Pulmonary Lesions

Yuji Matsumoto and Takehiro Izumo

Abstract Bronchoscopy may be limited in terms of direct endobronchial visualization of farther bronchial subsegments. Therefore, it is necessary to study the computed tomography (CT) images prior to examination in order to count the number of bronchial bifurcations from the trachea before reaching the lesion. It is often difficult to imagine three-dimensional endoscopic images from the two-dimensional images on CT. Virtual bronchoscopic navigation (VBN) system mechanically indicates the route to the target lesion.

Keywords Virtual bronchoscopic navigation • Peripheral pulmonary lesions Transbronchial biopsy • Radial EBUS

20.1 Introduction

Bronchoscopy is limited in terms of field of direct vision. Therefore, when performing diagnostic bronchoscopy for peripheral pulmonary lesions, it is necessary to count the number of bronchial bifurcations from the trachea to the lesion on computed tomography (CT) images prior to examination. The route to a lesion has to be planned carefully, but it is often difficult to imagine the three-dimensional endoscopic view based on two-dimensional CT images. To address this gap, virtual bronchoscopic navigation (VBN) system has emerged and its addition to image-guided bronchoscopy has been recommended by the American College of Chest Physicians [1]. Several VBN systems (Fig. 20.1), such as Bf-Navi and DirectPath by Olympus, are now available, but this chapter will discuss the use of LungPoint (Broncus Ltd.), one of the VBNs that was reported to be beneficial [2].

Y. Matsumoto
Respiratory Endoscopy Division, Department of Endoscopy, National Cancer Center Hospital, Tokyo, Japan

T. Izumo (✉)
Department of Respiratory Medicine, Japanese Red Cross Medical Center, 4-1-22 Hiroo, Shibuya-ku, Tokyo 150-8935, Japan
e-mail: drtake1118@gmail.com

T. Izumo et al. (eds.), *Respiratory Endoscopy*,
DOI 10.1007/978-981-287-916-5_20

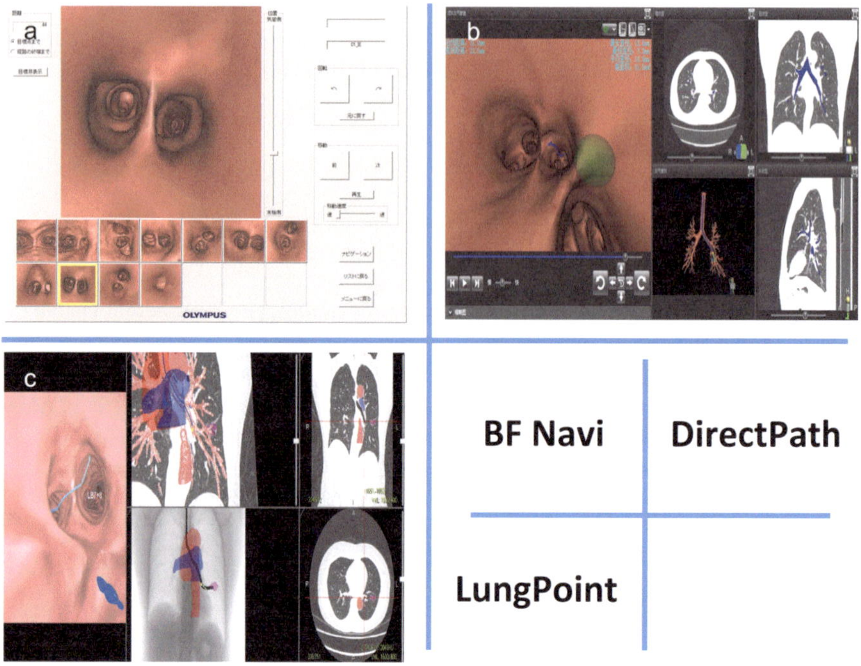

Fig. 20.1 Virtual bronchoscopic navigation systems available

20.2 Requirements

1. LungPoint (Broncus Ltd) (Fig. 20.2)
2. Thin-slice CT images, as recommended by the VBN manufacturer
   - Slice thickness: ≥1.25 mm
   - Interval of reconstruction: >0.625 mm
   - Field of view: bilateral lungs
   - Scanning range: from the apex to the base of the lung

* Note that loading CT images that include information from the entire lung is necessary to visualize bronchial segments precisely.

20.3 How to Operate a VBN

1. Importing images
   Import the CT images into the system. Direct import from the server is possible if connection with picture archiving communication system or other sources, such as CD-ROM and external drives, is available.

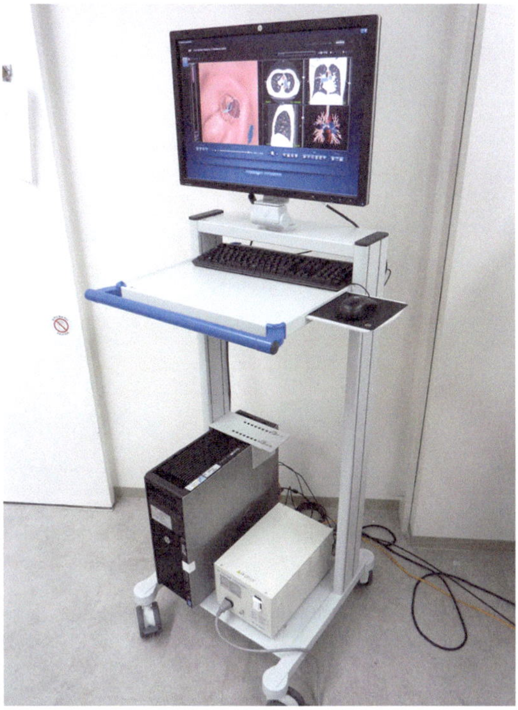

Fig. 20.2 The LungPoint® VBN system

2. Setting the target lesion
   Preset the target lesion on the CT display (Fig. 20.3). Between the two configurations, the outline target better visualizes the lesion compared with the circle target. However, the circle target should be used for lesions that are poorly demarcated from the surrounding structures, such as the chest wall or those having a small attenuation difference with the background lung (e.g., ground-glass opacity, GGO).
3. Display of the virtual endoscopic image
   LungPoint visualizes the airway and major vessels and automatically renders the route to the target lesion. The virtual endoscopic images are displayed on the left side of the screen, with the direction of the endoscope also shown, whereas the axial, coronal, and sagittal images are displayed on the right side of the screen. By default, a three-dimensional diagram of the visualized airway, major vessels, and preset target lesion is displayed on the lower right hand corner, but this may be switched to the virtual endoscopic images as needed (Fig. 20.4).
4. Confirmation of the route
   The center of the route, which may be computed in three different ways, is displayed as a light blue line on the virtual endoscopic image (Fig. 20.5). The bar on the left side of the screen is useful in estimating the distance of the bronchoscope tip to the target lesion, especially when this is difficult to discern on virtual fluoroscopy.

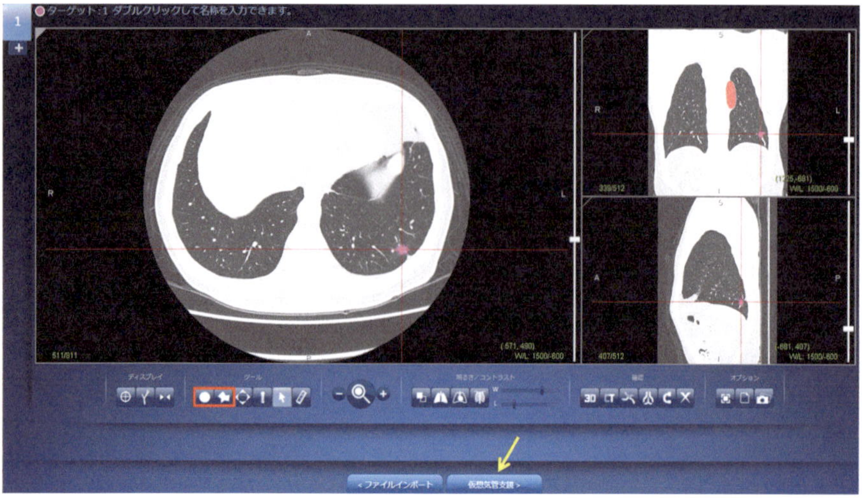

Fig. 20.3 Pre-setting the target lesion. To better visualize the target lesion, use the outline target (*right button* within the *red box*). For lesions that are poorly demarcated from the surrounding structures or for ground glass opacity, use the circle target (*left button* within the *red box*). When using the circle target configuration, the center and the diameter of the circle should be preset. After pre-setting a lesion, click the virtual bronchoscopy button (*yellow arrow*)

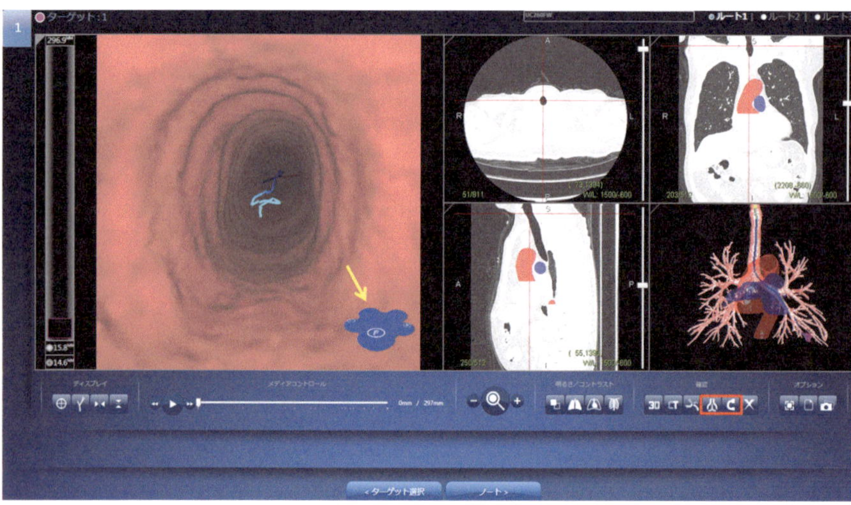

Fig. 20.4 Display of the virtual endoscopic images. On the *left side* of the screen, virtual endoscopic images are displayed, and the direction of the endoscope relative to the body of the patient is also indicated (*yellow arrow*). On the *right side* of the screen, the axial, coronal, and sagittal CT images are displayed. On the *lower right hand corner*, the buttons within the *red box* enable switching from default view (*left button*) to virtual endoscopic view (*right button*). As shown in this photo, the default view shows a three-dimensional image of the airway, major vessels, and preset target lesion

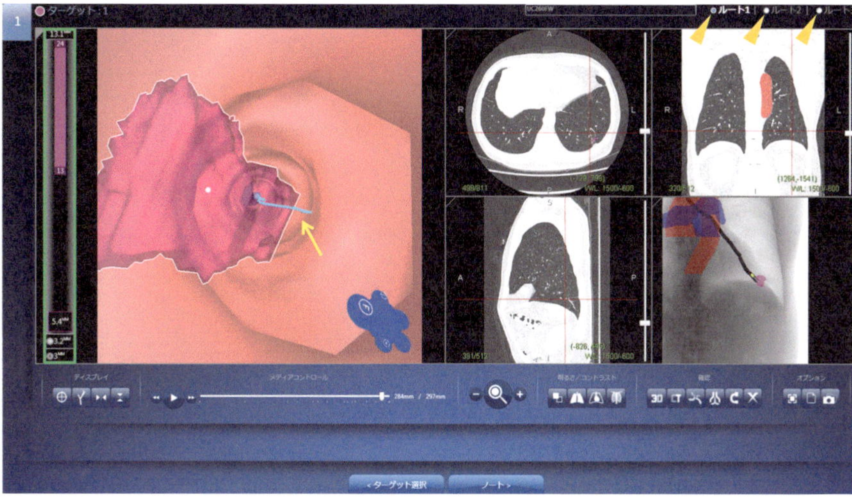

Fig. 20.5 Examples of the image on virtual fluoroscopy. The center of the route is displayed as a light *blue line* on the virtual endoscopic image. The route may be calculated in three different ways (*yellow arrowheads*). The bar (*green frame*) on the left side of the screen indicates the distance of the bronchoscope tip to the target lesion (shaded in *pink*)

The virtual endoscopic image can be turned around using direction keys. Follow the viewpoint just as you do during actual bronchoscopy and proceed to the periphery while confirming the bronchial bifurcations (Fig. 20.6).

20.4 Application for Endobronchial Ultrasound-Guided Transbronchial Needle Aspiration (EBUS-TBNA) (Fig. 20.7)

By using the mediastinal display of the imported CT images, LungPoint may automatically estimate the location of lymph nodes and confirm the positional relationship between the aorta and the main pulmonary artery during EBUS-TBNA.

20.5 Precautions for Use

1. When using the "circle target" configuration
   When using this configuration, attention should be paid to the fact that the shape of the preset target lesion and that of the actual lesion do not coincide. Because there is a possibility that a wrong route could be rendered, it is better to preset a target as small as possible and within the border of the actual lesion.

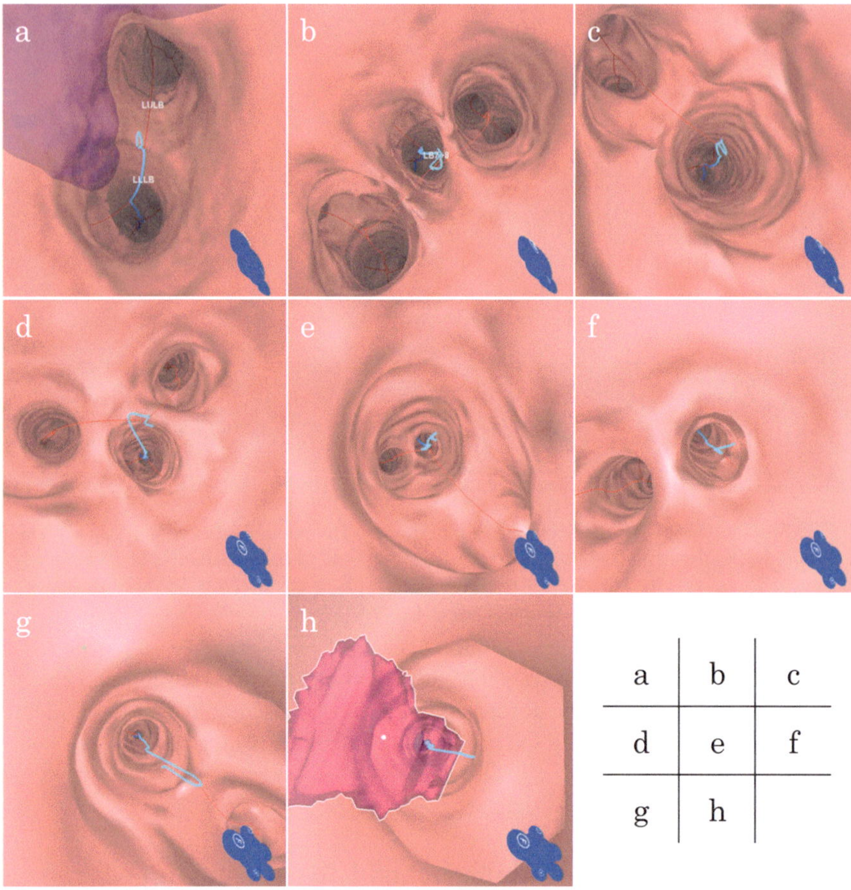

Fig. 20.6 Virtual endoscopic images created by LungPoint®. These images are from the same target lesion in the left segment 9 of the lung, as shown in Figs. 20.2, 20.3, and 20.4. From (**a**–**h**), serial frames at every bronchial bifurcation from the left main bronchus to the target lesion are shown. The route to the target lesion (shaded in *pink*) is indicated by the *light blue line*

2. Narrowing of the involved bronchus (Fig. 20.8)
   LungPoint can usually visualize airways that are more than 3 mm in diameter. It is important to note that stenosed or obstructed airways cannot be visualized and that an erroneous route may be rendered when the system encounters this cutoff. Therefore, it would be preferable to manually confirm by CT if the route indicated by the automatic VBN seems accurate and actually leads to the target lesion.

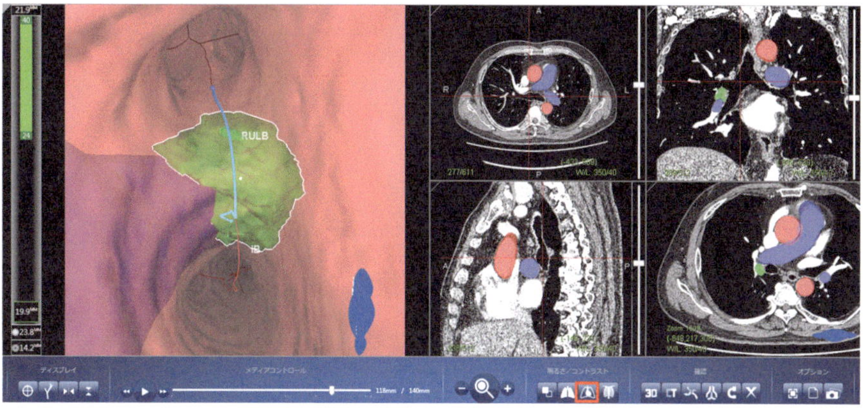

Fig. 20.7 Application for EBUS-TBNA. By switching to mediastinal display (in *red box*) of the imported CT images (*right side* of the screen), lymph nodes may be preset as the target lesion for EBUS-TBNA. In this example, virtual endoscopic images of a right interlobar lymph node (#11) (*green color*) and the main pulmonary artery (*purple color*) are visualized automatically

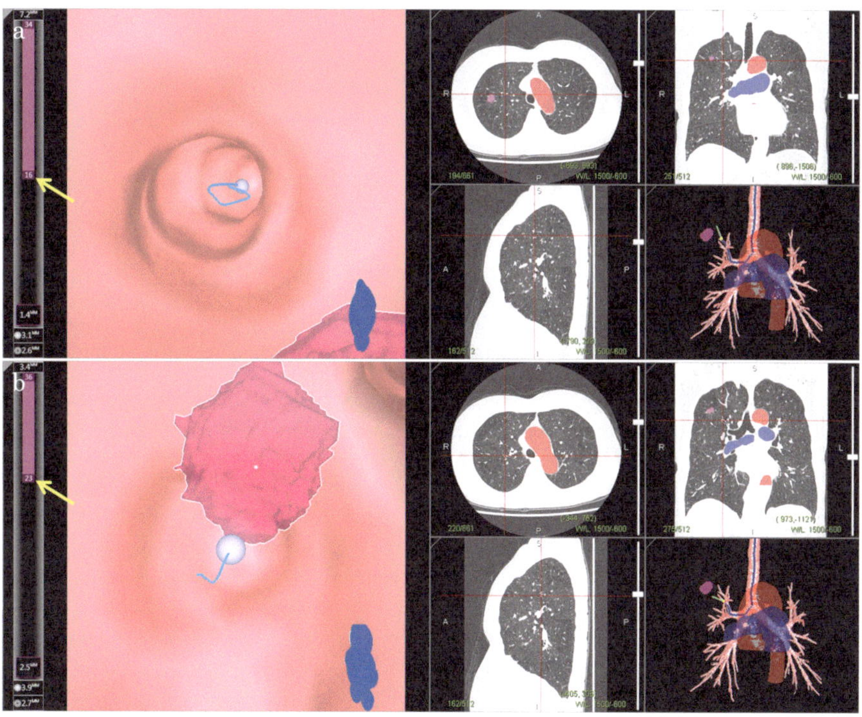

Fig. 20.8 Narrowing of the involved bronchus. The involved bronchus is located in the right segment 1, with surrounding emphysematous changes, thickening of airway walls, and narrowing of the lumen. Both routes created by LungPoint® are disrupted. (**a**) Route 1 indicates a shorter route to the target lesion (*yellow arrow*), compared with (**b**) route 2 which turns out to be the correct route when confirmed manually on CT images

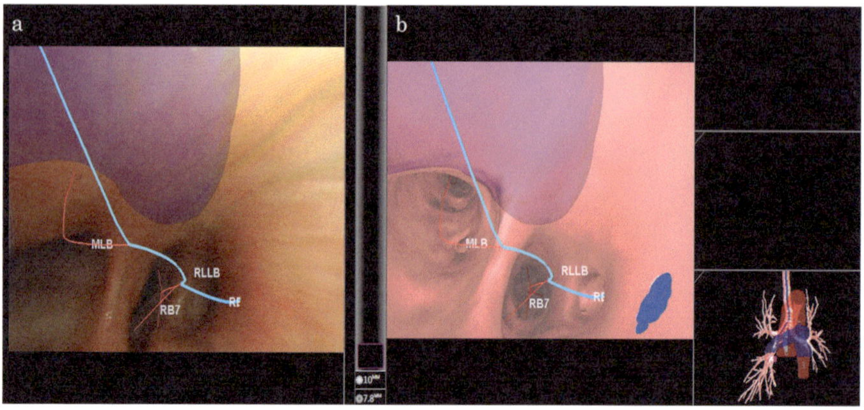

Fig. 20.9 LungPoint VBN SYSTEM®. In the latest model, the synchronization function is available. The actual bronchoscopic image (**a**) and the created virtual bronchoscopic image (**b**) are displayed side by side

20.6 Future Perspectives

The latest model of LungPoint VBN SYSTEM® (Broncus Ltd.) is equipped with synchronization function. Although it is still in the stage of development, further improvement is expected in the future (Fig. 20.9).

References

1. Rivera MP, Mehta AC, Wahidi MM. Establishing the diagnosis of lung cancer: diagnosis and management of lung cancer, 3rd ed: American College of Chest Physicians evidence-based clinical practice guidelines. Chest. 2013;143:e142S–65S.
2. Tamiya M, Okamoto N, Sasada S, et al. Diagnostic yield of combined bronchoscopy and endobronchial ultrasonography, under LungPoint guidance for small peripheral pulmonary lesions. Respirology. 2013;18:834–9.

Chapter 21
Virtual Bronchoscopic Simulation by CT Workstation

Yuji Matsumoto, Takehiro Izumo, and Yasuyuki Mizumori

Abstract An image processing workstation can create virtual bronchoscopic simulation from computed tomography (CT) images, even those taken at another facility. This workstation is versatile and provides benefits that other specialized devices do not have. It can be introduced more easily than a specialized virtual bronchoscopic device because it is widely available and is usually incorporated with multi-detector row CT equipment.

Keywords Virtual bronchoscopic navigation • Virtual bronchoscopic simulation • Peripheral pulmonary lesion • CT workstation • Transbronchial biopsy

21.1 Introduction

Virtual bronchoscopic navigation (VBN) requires installation of specialized devices, such as Bf-Navi (Olympus Ltd) or LungPoint (Broncus Ltd), which may not be readily accessible due to issues on cost and versatility. On the other hand, an image processing workstation is available in almost all facilities that have a multi-detector row computed tomography (CT). In fact, as many as 1,800 facilities in Japan have introduced Ziostation (Ziosoft Ltd), including its several versions [1]. In our clinical practice at our department, we utilize virtual bronchoscopic simulation (VBS) using a workstation. In this section, we will discuss how to create and use VBS [2].

Y. Matsumoto
Respiratory Endoscopy Division, Department of Endoscopy, National Cancer Center Hospital, Tokyo, Japan

T. Izumo (✉)
Department of Respiratory Medicine, Japanese Red Cross Medical Center, 4-1-22 Hiroo, Shibuya-ku, Tokyo 150-8935, Japan
e-mail: drtake1118@gmail.com

Y. Mizumori
Department of Respiratory Medicine, National Hospital Organization Himeji Medical Center, Hyogo, Japan

T. Izumo et al. (eds.), *Respiratory Endoscopy*,
DOI 10.1007/978-981-287-916-5_21

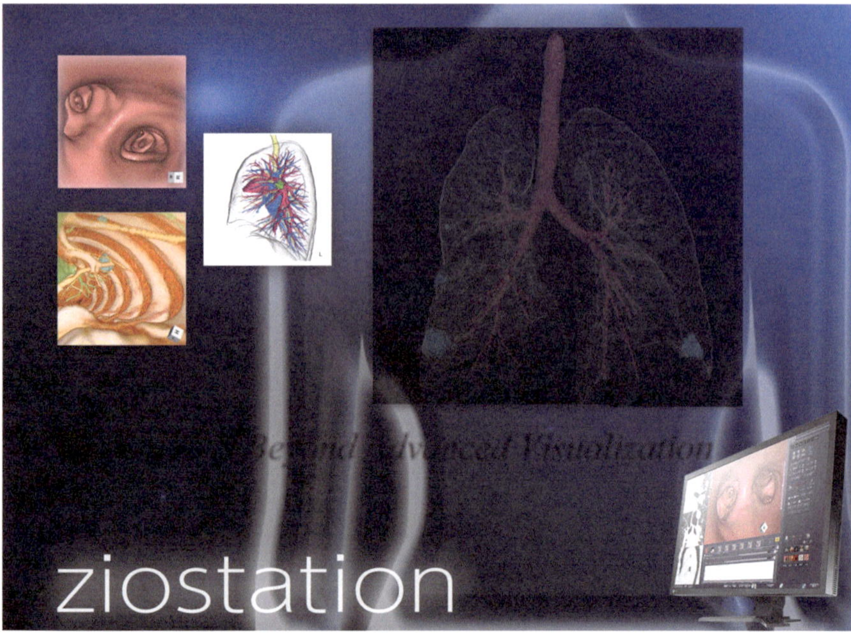

Fig. 21.1 An image processing workstation (Ziostation® or Ziostation2®)

21.2 Requirements

1. An image processing workstation (Fig. 21.1)
2. Thin-slice CT images, as recommended by the manufacturer of the workstation

   – Slice thickness: ≤1 mm
   – Reconstruction function: mediastinal window
   – Field of view: affected lungs
   – Scanning range: from the target lesion to the ipsilateral main bronchus
   ** Note that VBS can still be created even if these requirements are incomplete.*

21.3 How to Create a Virtual Bronchoscopic Image Using Ziostation2

1. Importing the CT images
   Usually, the workstation is connected with the picture archiving and communication system and can directly import CT images from the server.
2. Presetting the target lesion
   Define the target lesion by following the detailed steps and illustrations shown in Fig. 21.2.

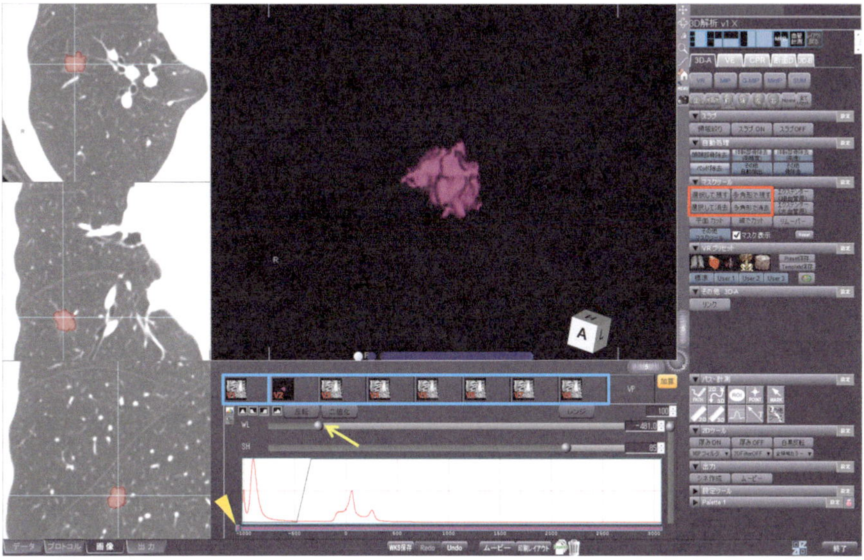

Fig. 21.2 Presetting the target lesion. Click on to the image tags (within the *blue frame*), except for the main V1 tag, and preset the target lesion on the CT display. Select the "create polygonal shape" icon (within the *red frame*) to make an outline of the lesion. Adjust the "window level (WL)" tool bar (*yellow arrow*) to visualize the lesion. Click the visualized lesion using the "select and keep" icon (within the *red frame*) and choose a color (*orange arrowhead*) that you will use to indicate the target lesion. Select the "delete polygonal shape" icon (within the *red frame*) from the mask tools and delete the outline of adjacent chest wall and unnecessary blood vessels. After completion of presetting, click on the main V1 tag (within the *red frame*)

3. Presetting the route
   Trace an accurate bronchial route to the target lesion by following the detailed steps and illustrations shown in Fig. 21.3.
4. Creation of virtual endoscopic images
   Combine the preset target lesion and route to create a VBS motion diagram (Fig. 21.4).

21.4 Differences Between VBS and VBN

In planning the route to a peripheral pulmonary lesion for transbronchial biopsy, both VBS and VBN are useful. A comparison of these systems is shown in Table 21.1.

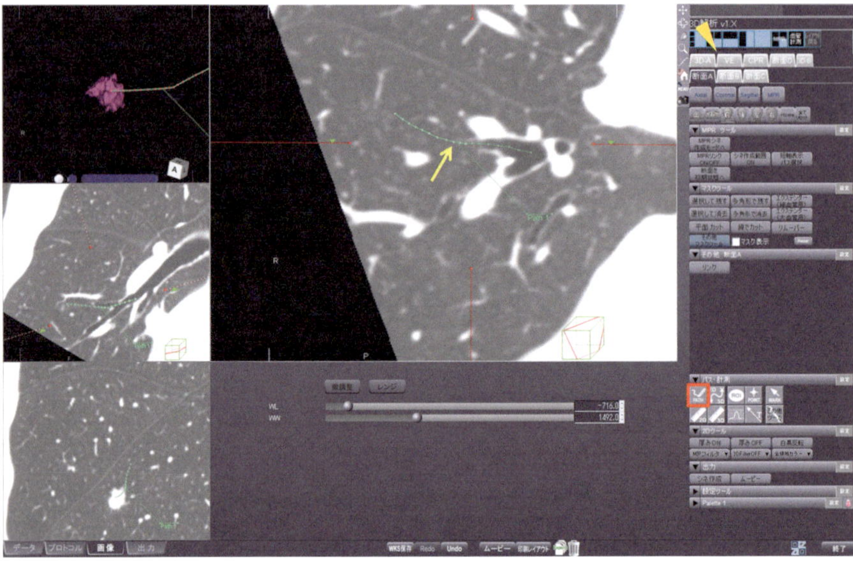

Fig. 21.3 Presetting the route. On the CT display, click the "PATH" icon (within the *red frame*) under the path/measurement tab and a *green dotted line* will pop up (*yellow arrow*). The bronchus involved in the target lesion is defined as the end of the route. From this point, create connecting dots from the periphery to the carina by clicking on intermittent points or at bronchial bifurcations) along the center of the bronchial lumen. The line created by connecting these dots represents the bronchial route from the target lesion to the larger central airways. On the axial CT image, it is difficult to grasp the three-dimensional route of the bronchi. To create a route neatly and quickly, connect the dots using multi-planar reconstruction (MPR) images with intermittent arbitrary references to the axial image when a bronchial lumen becomes straight; this way, contact with the bronchial wall can be avoided. After creating the route, click the VE tab on the right upper corner (*orange arrow*) to switch to the virtual endoscopic image

21.5 Application of VBS

1. Application to bronchus sign-negative cases
   In cases with negative CT bronchus sign [3], VBS may still render an accurate route by following instead the pulmonary artery that flows into the target lesion. In a majority of metastatic pulmonary tumors that are CT bronchus sign negative, the additional use of GS-TBNA (Chap. 19) [please check if you mean GS-TBNA or TBNA only] may increase the diagnostic yield. In such cases, VBS remains applicable by creating a route through the lesion (Fig. 21.5).
2. Application to EBUS-TBNA
   The correct identification of a lymph node for EBUS-TBNA requires good knowledge on anatomic landmarks on the tracheobronchial wall and confirmation of the positional relationship with surrounding vascular structures. This is especially important for lung cancer staging, wherein differentiation of nodal stations based on anatomic landmarks is crucial (Fig. 21.6). However, similar to

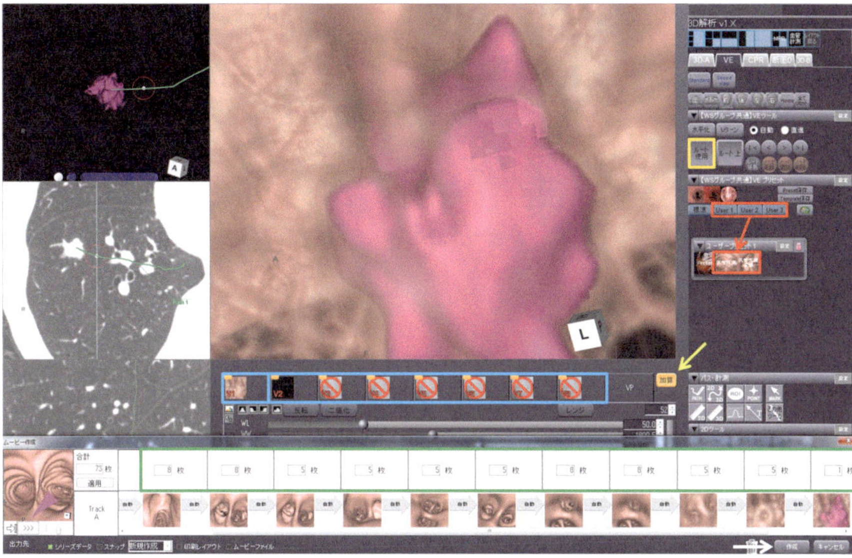

Fig. 21.4 Creation of virtual endoscopic images. Utilizing a user-preset data that were adjusted with the visualization conditions of the virtual bronchoscope (within the *red frame*), add the information from the preset target lesion by clicking on the tab (*yellow arrow*). Click "use the route" button (*orange arrow*) to overlap the preset route. Then, click the "movie" tab (*white arrow*) at the *bottom* to display the movie creation screen. Adjust the orientation according to that expected during actual bronchoscopy and lay out thumbnail images from each bronchial bifurcation up to the end of the route. Upon the completion of the thumbnail layout, input the number of complementation of each image (within the *green frame*). Click the preview button at the *bottom left* to review the created movie picture before clicking on the "create" button on the *bottom right* to render the complete VBS movie picture

Table 21.1 Comparison of virtual bronchoscopy systems

	VBS	VBN
Necessary equipment	Workstation (e.g., Ziostation2®)	Dedicated device (Bf-Navi®, LungPoint®)
Presetting the target lesion	Detailed preset is possible	Only simple preset is possible
Selection of the route	Manual operation	Automatic; manual operation can be added to some devices
Direction of the route	Peripheral to central	Central to peripheral

VBS Virtual bronchoscopic simulation, *VBM* Virtual bronchoscopic navigation

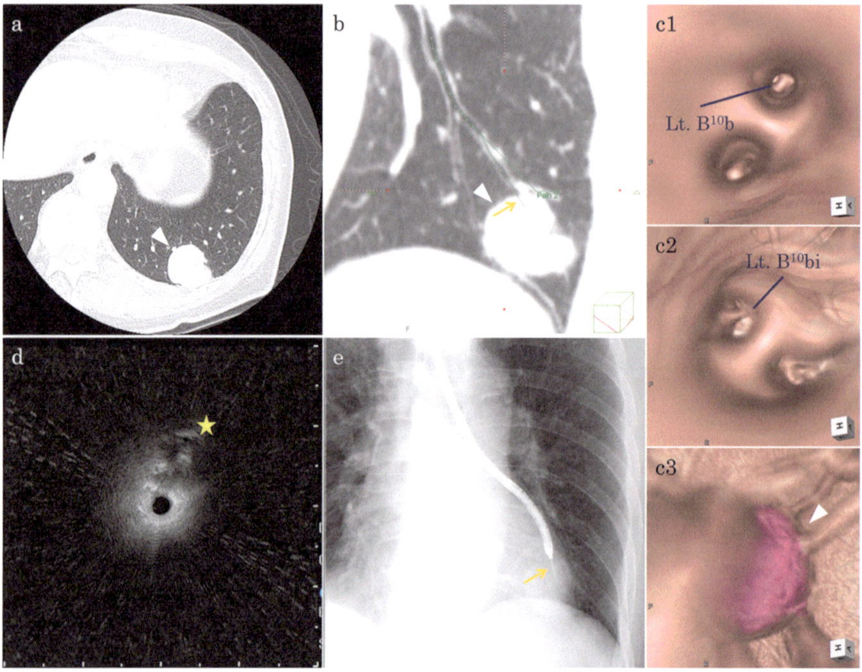

Fig. 21.5 Application of VBS to bronchus sign-negative cases. (**a**) A bronchus sign-negative tumor was observed in the left segment 10 (*arrow head*). (**b**) During presetting of the route, an area in the tumor that was adjacent to the most distal bronchus was marked as the starting point (*yellow arrow*). (**c**) While referring to the created virtual endoscopic images, the R-EBUS probe was inserted, but only an adjacent to pattern (**d**) was possible (*yellow asterisk*). (**e**) TBNA under X-ray fluoroscopy guidance was performed at this site (*yellow arrow*). The patient was diagnosed as metastatic malignant melanoma

peripheral pulmonary lesions, estimation of the three-dimensional structure of mediastinal/hilar structures may be difficult. VBS allows us to create virtual endoscopic images that can easily mark the target lymph nodes and the surrounding vascular structures.

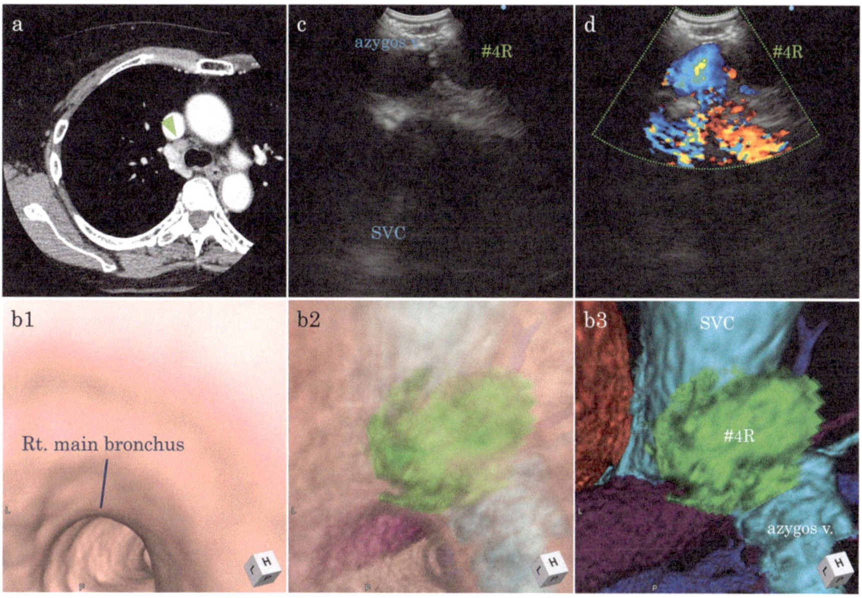

Fig. 21.6 Applications to EBUS-TBNA. (**a**) On CT scan, an enlarged lymph node is seen at station #4R or right lower paratracheal area (*green arrow*). To differentiate from station #10R or right hilar lymph nodes, it is necessary to confirm the positional relationship with the adjacent azygos vein. (**b**) The virtual endoscopic image is marked with the surrounding azygos vein and superior vena cava (*light blue color*), aorta (*red color*), pulmonary artery (*purple color*), and pulmonary vein (*blue color*). By referring to this virtual image during EBUS-TBNA, the position of the target lymph node (*green color*) can be easily grasped. (**c**, **d**) EBUS confirms an enlarged lymph node (#4R) cranial to the junction of the azygos vein with the superior vena cava

References

1. Iwao S, Imaizumi K, Okada T, et al. Virtual bronchoscopy-guided transbronchial biopsy for aiding the diagnosis of peripheral lung cancer. Eur J Rad. 2011;79:155–9.
2. Matsumoto Y, Izumo T, Sasada S, et al. Diagnostic utility of endobronchial ultrasound with a guide sheath under the computed tomography workstation (ziostation) for small peripheral pulmonary lesions. Clin Respir J. 2015. doi:10.1111/crj.12321. [Epub ahead of print].
3. Gaeta M, Pandolfo I, Volta S, et al. Bronchus sign on CT in peripheral carcinoma of the lung: value in predicting results of transbronchial biopsy. AJR Am J Roentgenol. 1991;157:1181–5.

Chapter 22
The Dose and Risk Factors for Radiation Exposure from X-Ray Fluoroscopy During EBUS-GS for Peripheral Pulmonary Lesions

Masahiro Katsurada and Takehiro Izumo

Abstract The dose of radiation exposure from X-ray fluoroscopy during EBUS-GS is much less than we expect; in fact, it was found to be negligibly low, especially for nurses and radiology technicians who usually stand away from the operating table. Wearing a protector can further reduce the dose of radiation exposure to the trunk of the body. However, great care should be taken because the relationship between radiation exposure dose and health hazards is not well clarified yet.

Keywords Bronchoscopy • Radial EBUS • Fluoroscopy • EBUS-GS • Radiation exposure

22.1 Introduction

Bronchoscopic examination can be classified into two methods: fluoroscopy-guided bronchoscopy and non-guided bronchoscopy. Fluoroscopy-guided bronchoscopy includes procedures, such as transbronchial biopsy (TBB), transbronchial lung biopsy (TBLB), and transbronchial needle aspiration (TBNA), whereas non-guided bronchoscopy includes bronchial lavage, bronchoalveolar lavage (BAL), endobronchial ultrasound-guided transbronchial needle aspiration (EBUS-TBNA), bronchial toilette, and endobronchial observation. In Japan, bronchoscopy is often used for diagnostic purposes; therefore, X-ray fluoroscopy is widely used during bronchoscopic procedures. However, almost no data are available regarding radiation exposure dose. In this section, we will discuss the radiation exposure dose during endobronchial ultrasound with a guide sheath (EBUS-GS).

M. Katsurada
Department of Respiratory Medicine, Kobe University Graduate School of Medicine, Kobe, Japan

T. Izumo (✉)
Department of Respiratory Medicine, Japanese Red Cross Medical Center, 4-1-22 Hiroo, Shibuya-ku, Tokyo 150-8935, Japan
e-mail: drtake1118@gmail.com

T. Izumo et al. (eds.), *Respiratory Endoscopy*,
DOI 10.1007/978-981-287-916-5_22

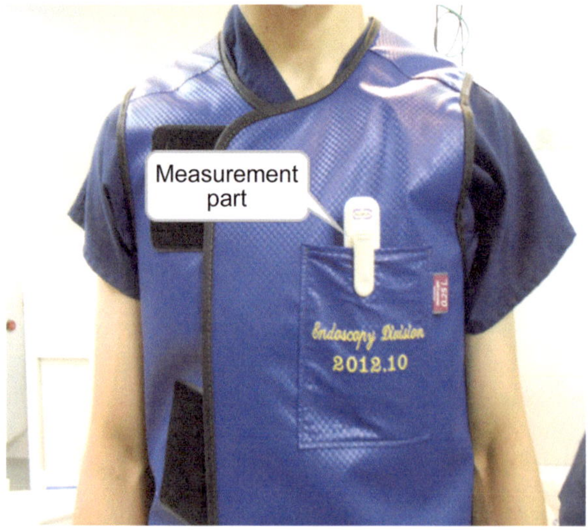

Fig. 22.1 Radiation analyzer

22.1.1 Devices and Measurements

The radiation exposure dose was measured in 132 patients with peripheral pulmonary lesions who underwent EBUS-GS under X-ray fluoroscopy at the Respiratory Endoscopy Division of the National Cancer Center Hospital in Tokyo, Japan from October 2012 to December 2012.

VersiFlex VISTA®(Hitachi, Japan) was used as the fluoroscopy device. Radiation analyzers (MYDOSE mini x, PDM-117®; ALOKA, Japan) were placed inside the pockets (on the chest area in men, on the abdominal area in women) that were located outside the radiation protectors (Fig. 22.1). The targets of the measurements were the medical staff, comprised of operator physicians, assistant physicians, nurses, and radiology technicians. Usually, they are all engaged in bronchoscopic procedures inside the examination room (Fig. 22.2).

22.2 Results

Table 22.1 shows the results of the measurements. The median radiation exposure dose to the operator physicians was low at 12 μSv per exam. The radiation exposure dose to the other medical staff, such as nurses and radiology technicians, was almost negligible low, probably because they stood farther away from the operating table. Logistic regression analysis indicated that increased body mass index (BMI) of the participants and displacement of the radial EBUS (R-EBUS) probe from a lesion were the risk factors for increases in radiation exposure dose [1].

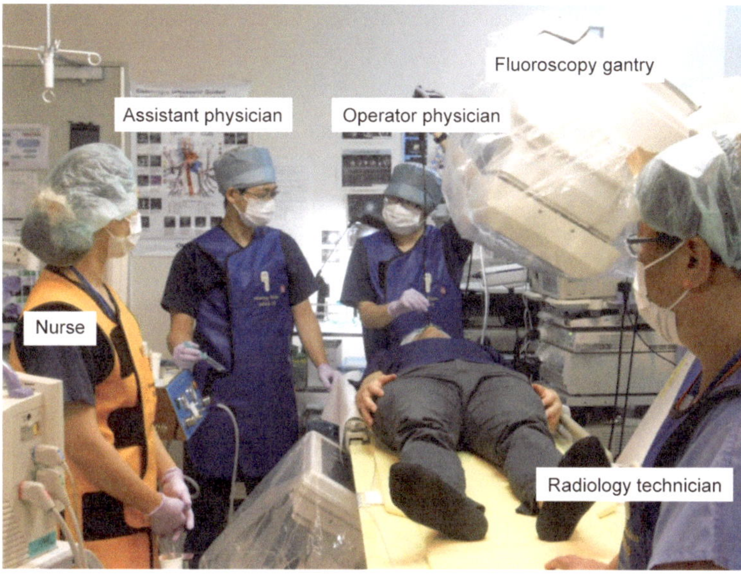

Fig. 22.2 The members of the medical staff as they perform bronchoscopy

Table 22.1 Radiation exposure dose from fluoroscopy during bronchoscopy

	Median (range)	*P* value (vs. operator physician)
Duration of fluoroscopy (min)	7.6 (1.5–23.9)	
Operator physician (μSv/exam)	12 (1–99)	
Assistant physician (μSv/exam)	3 (0–7)	<0.01
Nurse (μSv/exam)	0 (0–9)	<0.01
Radiology technician (μSv/exam)	0 (0–1)	<0.01

Adapted from Ref. [1]

22.3 Discussion

Although some health hazards, such as leukemia and cataract formation, have been reported to arise from radiation exposure, no remarkable health hazard has been reported for radiation exposure dose lower than 100 mSv. On the other hand, there was a report that cataract formation was induced by radiation exposure dose of 100 mSv [2]. Therefore, there remain some uncertainties as to health hazards of radiation exposure. In Japan, the limit of radiation exposure dose to an exposed worker is specified by the Ordinance on Prevention of Ionizing Radiation Hazards, as follows:

1. Not exceeding 100 mSv for 5 years
2. Not exceeding 50 mSv per year

3. For female radiation workers, not exceeding 5 mSv quarterly, in addition to the abovementioned limits
4. For pregnant women
    (a) Not exceeding 1 mSv exposure to internal organs from the diagnosis of pregnancy to childbirth
    (b) Not exceeding 2 mSv exposure to the surface of the abdomen from the diagnosis of pregnancy to childbirth
5. Not exceeding 150 mSv per year for the eye lens
6. Not exceeding 500 mSv per year for the skin

As shown in Table 22.1, the radiation exposure dose to the operator physicians was very low at 12 μSv per exam. At our hospital, each member of the medical staff performs an average of 360 bronchoscopies per year. We estimate that the average annual dose to the staff is low at 4.3 mSv per year. The average annual dose to nurses and radiology technicians is estimated to be almost 0 mSv per year. Moreover, when using a protector made of lead-containing sheet with 0.25 mm of lead equivalence, the actual radiation exposure dose decreases to one-tenth because a high shielding ratio, or an average X-ray transmission rate of 9.2 %, can be obtained [3]. These findings indicate that radiation exposure dose during EBUS-GS under X-ray fluoroscopy is low and safe. Nevertheless, it would still be better to attempt further reductions in radiation exposure dose because there still remain some uncertainties as to the health hazards.

The risk factors for increased radiation exposure dose were greater BMI of patients and improper placement of the R-EBUS probe in the lesion. This could be explained by the fact that greater BMI would require a larger amount of radiation dose to ensure the quality of the X-ray fluoroscopic image; in addition, proper placement of an R-EBUS probe in a lesion would entail the use of X-ray fluoroscopy guidance, and consequent radiation exposure, in many cases. Therefore, we underscore the importance of careful planning of the bronchial route prior to the procedure (i.e., by virtual bronchoscopic navigation system) in order to obtain proper R-EBUS placement as quickly and as safe as possible.

References

1. Katsurada M, Izumo T, Sasada S, et al. The dose and risk factors for radiation exposure to medical staff during endobronchial ultrasonography with a guide sheath for peripheral pulmonary lesions under X-ray fluoroscopy. Jpn J Clin Oncol. 2014;44:257–62.
2. Vano E, Kleiman NJ, Rehani MM, et al. Radiation-associated lens opacities in catheterization personnel: results of a survey and direct assessments. J Vasc Interv Radiol. 2013;24:197–204.
3. JCS joint working group. Guideline for radiation safety in interventional cardiology (JCS 2011) – digest version. Circ J. 2013;77:519–49.

Chapter 23
Endobronchial Ultrasound-Guided Transbronchial Needle Aspiration

Hibiki Udagawa and Takehiro Izumo

Abstract Knowledge on the anatomic relationship between endobronchial view and the position of hilar and mediastinal lymph nodes is an essential requirement for acquiring basic competence in endobronchial ultrasound-guided transbronchial needle aspiration (EBUS-TBNA). Fine rotation movements of the operating hand while maintaining an angle of 3° and doing the aspirations, as if scraping off tissues, may increase the amount of collected samples. Lastly, proper handling of collected specimens is mandatory.

Keywords EBUS-TBNA • Transbronchial needle aspiration • Lung cancer • Lymphoma • Sarcoidosis

23.1 Indications for EBUS-TBNA

1. Lung tumor associated with enlarged hilar and/or mediastinal lymph nodes (for staging)
2. Mediastinal tumors
3. Enlarged hilar and/or mediastinal lymph nodes that may be suspected to be due to lymphoproliferative diseases, such as sarcoidosis and lymphoma
4. Enlarged hilar and/or mediastinal lymph nodes that may be suspected to be due to infectious disease (e.g., tuberculosis)

H. Udagawa
Department of Thoracic Oncology, National Cancer Center Hospital East, Chiba, Japan

T. Izumo (✉)
Department of Respiratory Medicine, Japanese Red Cross Medical Center, 4-1-22 Hiroo, Shibuya-ku, Tokyo 150-8935, Japan
e-mail: drtake1118@gmail.com

T. Izumo et al. (eds.), *Respiratory Endoscopy*,
DOI 10.1007/978-981-287-916-5_23

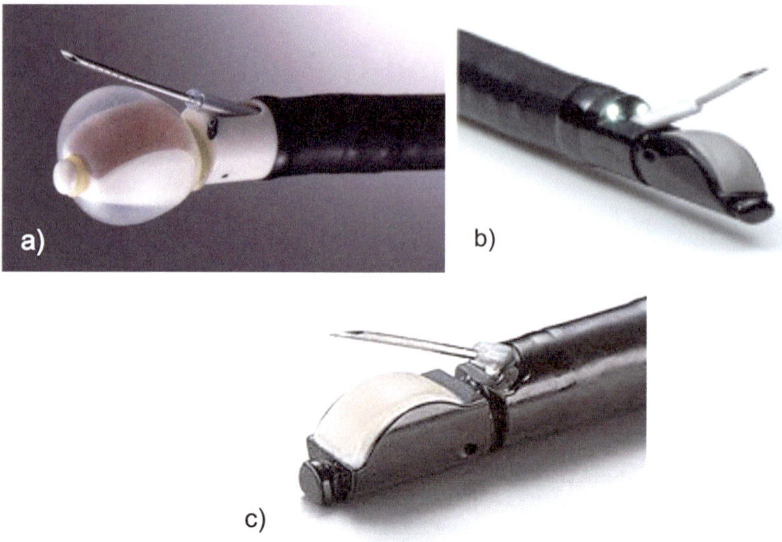

Fig. 23.1 The convex probe endobronchial ultrasound bronchoscope. The different scope models, such as (**a**) BF-UC260FW by Olympus, (**b**) BE-530US by Fuji Film, and (**c**) BE-1970UK by PENTAX

23.2 Preparation of Equipment

1. Bronchoscope with convex probe EBUS (Fig. 23.1)
2. Ultrasound processor (e.g., EU-C2000/EU-ME1/EU-ME2 by Olympus Ltd; ALOKA by Hitachi Ltd)
3. A special needle apparatus for EBUS-TBNA with suction syringe. Examples are ViziShot (Olympus Ltd), SonoTip EBUS PRO (Medi-Globe Ltd), etc.
4. Additional containers, fixing solutions, and the like for obtaining specimen for pathologic analysis, microbiologic culture, and/or molecular studies

23.3 Actual Procedures

In this section, we describe the procedure of EBUS-TBNA with the use of the Olympus EBUS bronchoscope (BF-UC260FW) and needle apparatus (ViziShot).

23.3.1 Insertion of the Bronchoscope

It is important to note that compared with the conventional direct viewing bronchoscope, the convex EBUS bronchoscope has a forward-oblique view (horizontal visible range of 80°; vertical visible range of 30°). For beginners, passing through the larynx and the vocal cords may be difficult and requires mastery of techniques (Fig. 23.2). Therefore, laryngopharyngeal anesthesia becomes even more important than that during conventional bronchoscopy. Table 23.1 shows the anesthesia

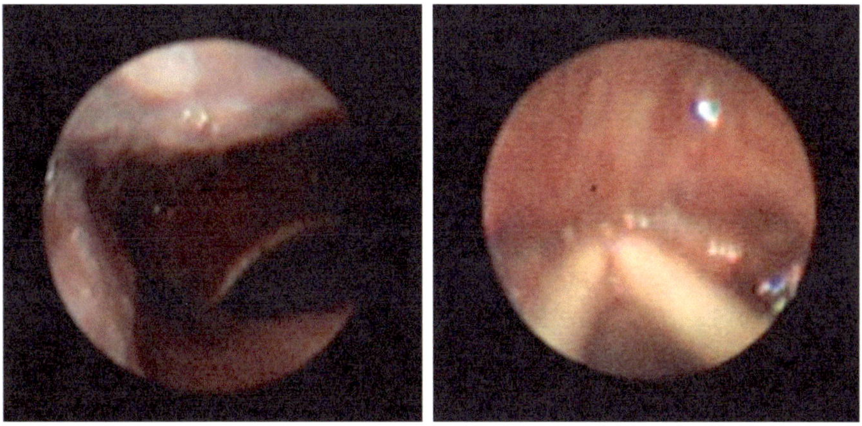

Fig. 23.2 Insert the EBUS scope to the trachea using this view angle of the vocal cords

Table 23.1 Anesthesia and sedation for EBUS-TBNA

Preliminary medication	Pethidine hydrochloride (Opystan®) 35 mg/1 mL is injected intravenously at the following doses:
	Weight >50 kg → 0.5 mL
	Weight ≤50 kg → 0.25 mL
	Age >80 years old → 0.25 mL
	Age ≤80 years old → 0.5 mL
Local anesthesia before bronchoscopy	A total of 5 mL of 4 % lidocaine is applied using a Jackson spray to anesthetize the pharyngeal and laryngeal areas
Sedation before bronchoscopy	Midazolam 10 mg/2 mL (Dormicum®) is diluted in 8 mL of saline to make a 10 mL solution; 2–3 mL of this diluted solution is administered intravenously as follows:
	Weight >50 kg → 3 mL
	Weight ≤50 kg → 2 mL
	Age >80 years old → 2 mL
	Age ≤80 years old → 3 mL
Local anesthesia and sedation during bronchoscopy	If severe coughing occurs, 1–2 mL of 2 % lidocaine is injected through the working channel of the bronchoscope. Additional 1–2 mL of diluted midazolam solution may be administered intravenously

techniques that we employ at our hospital. If bronchoscope insertion is difficult or not feasible, inserting an endotracheal tube before EBUS-TBNA is another option.

23.3.2 Visualizing Lymph Nodes

Inflate the balloon with about 0.3 mL of sterile distilled water or saline solution ad flex the convex EBUS probe tip on the corresponding tracheal or bronchial mucosa to visualize the lymph nodes. Move the bronchoscope slowly, back and forth and from side to side, while scanning to confirm the maximum cross-sectional area of the lymph nodes. Switch to Doppler mode to confirm the location of the large vessels and bronchial arteries, as well as the vascularity within the lymph nodes (Fig. 23.3a). It is often difficult to collect an adequate specimen for diagnosis from lesions without hyperechoic vessels, in which case, tissue necrosis is likely (Fig. 23.3b). Fortunately, the ultrasound processor has been developed and equipped with elastography to enable assessment of tissue hardness by color (Chap. 24) [1].

To stage lung cancer accurately, knowledge on the anatomical position of hilar/mediastinal lymph nodes (Fig. 23.4) and a good understanding of the corresponding location of these lymph nodes on the tracheobronchial lumen (Fig. 23.5) are necessary [2]. The most important points are summarized in Table 23.2.

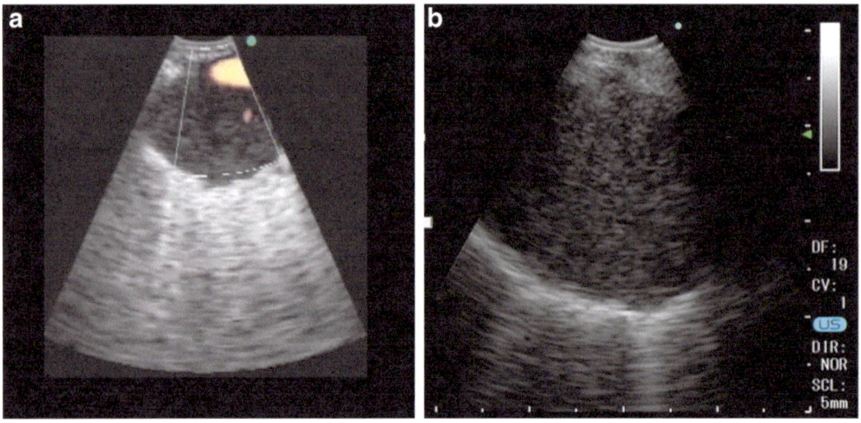

Fig. 23.3 Visualization of a lesion by EBUS. (**a**) Confirmation of blood flow by Doppler mode; (**b**) scattered hyperechoic areas suggest the presence of necrosis

Fig. 23.4 Anatomical location of hilar/mediastinal lymph nodes (Cited from Ref. [2])

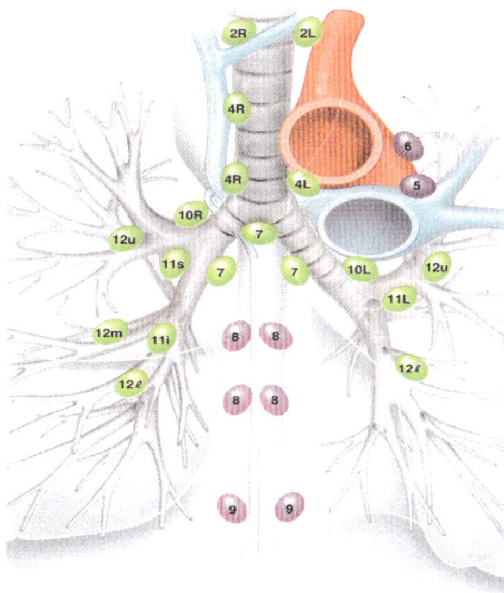

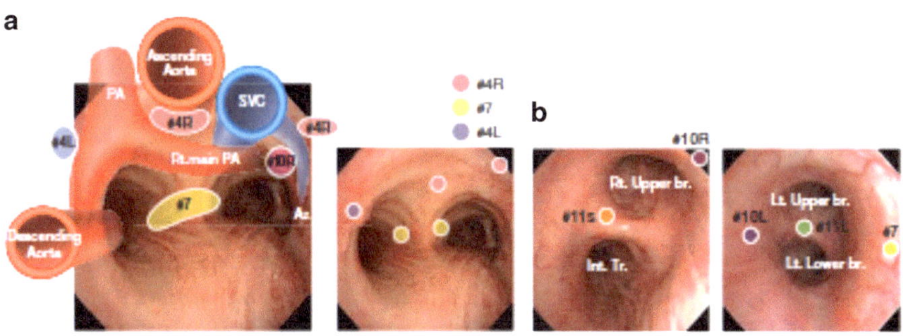

Fig. 23.5 Positional relationship between the endoscopic view and lymph node locations (Cited from Ref. [2])

23.3.3 *Puncture of Lymph Nodes*

After insertion of the needle apparatus in the working channel, take note that the bronchoscope becomes less flexible, and some lymph node stations, such as #4L and #10L, may be difficult to visualize; in this situation, it would be advisable to maximally flex the bronchoscope tip, where the convex EBUS probe is located.

During transbronchial puncture, it is important to avoid the bronchial cartilage and to pass the needle through the intercartilaginous space instead. The bronchial cartilage can be visualized directly on endoscopic view or as a hypoechoic area on EBUS; use these images to adjust the puncture site accordingly (Fig. 23.6). Have an assistant secure the bronchoscope at the corner of the patient's mouth to maintain

Table 23.2 Important landmarks during EBUS-TBNA

The border of the right and left sides	A straight line along the left margin of the trachea
The border of #2R and #4R	The point of where the caudal portion of the brachiocephalic vein crosses the trachea
The border of #4R and #10R	The inferior border of the azygos vein
The border of #2L and #4L	The superior border of the aortic arch
The border of #4L and #10L	The superior border of the pulmonary artery

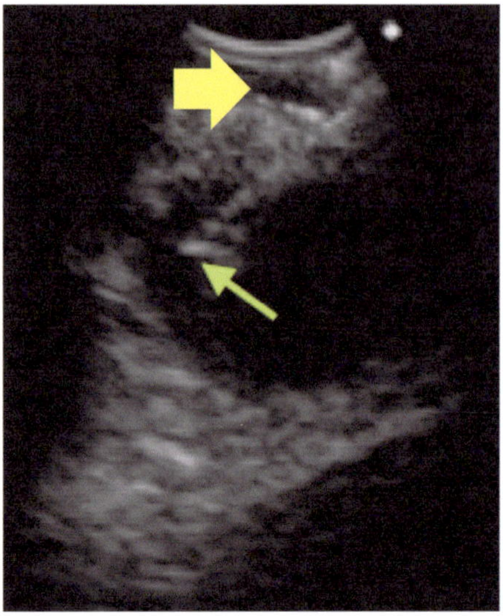

Fig. 23.6 Technique for needle puncture for EBUS-TBNA. Avoid jabbing the needle through a bronchial cartilage (*yellow arrow*), and aim for the intercartilaginous space when inserting the needle (*green arrow*) into a target site

contact of the convex probe with the mucosa (i.e., clear and real-time EBUS image of the target site) while pushing in the needle. At times, it may be necessary for the assistant to push in the bronchoscope, like a piggyback, while the operator inserts the needle.

The stylet of the needle apparatus should be withdrawn slightly before puncture to allow smooth transbronchial penetration of the needle tip. After the puncture, push the stylet through the tip of the needle to remove respiratory epithelium out of the needle lumen before completely removing the stylet and attaching the VacLok Syringe with negative pressure (–20 mL). However, for hypervascular lymph nodes, a smaller negative pressure (–5 or –10 mL) is applied to prevent backflow of blood and allow easier pathologic evaluation of the collected specimen.

During TBNA, confirm the movement of the needle on the ultrasound image display and encompass the widest possible area of the lesion during needle passes of about 20 times. Use fine movements of your operating hand to adjust the EBUS probe as necessary and ensure constant visualization of the needle tip. Simultaneously, watch out for backflow of blood into the VacLok Syringe. To maximize specimen collection, perform TBNA as if you are scraping off portions of the lesion with the beveled needle tip, instead of just passing through the needle into the lesion while applying negative pressure. The amount of collected sample will increase if you move the puncture needle at an angle of about 3° in a fanlike manner.

23.3.4 Processing Specimens

It is mandatory to know the proper way to process the specimen that you collected. Prepare the materials before the procedure and place them together in a designated working area. After this, collect and store the specimens, including core tissue and cytology samples, as appropriate (Fig. 23.7). At our department, we also set aside slide preparations for rapid on-site cytology evaluation.

23.3.5 Needle Apparatus

Usually, the dedicated puncture needle is 22-G apparatus. As of January 2015, two needles have become available in Japan: (1) the 22-G (NA-201SX-4022) and 21-G ViziShot (NA-201SX-4021) needle by Olympus and (2) the 22-G SonoTip EBUS Pro (GUS-45-18-022) with stainless steel by Medi-Globe.

Some studies reported that there was no significant difference in diagnostic yield and tissue sampling rate between 22-G and 21-G needles [3, 4]. We compared the two similar-sized (22G) brands of needles available in Japan (Fig. 23.8) and found out that the diagnostic yield, including cytologic diagnosis, was similar between the two (87.7 % with ViziShot vs. 93.6 % with SonoTip EBUS Pro, $P=0.197$), but tissue sampling rate was significantly higher with the SonoTip EBUS Pro than the ViziShot (61.3 % vs. 74.3 %, $P=0.0035$) [5]. These results were attributed to differences in structure of the needles (Table 23.3).

23.4 Limitations and Countermeasures

1. EBUS-TBNA enables needle puncture of lesions adjacent to the trachea and bronchi. In some cases, endoscopic ultrasound fine-needle aspiration (EUS-FNA) should also be considered.
2. At first, it may be difficult to collect sufficient specimens. As your skills improve, so will the yield for pathologic and molecular diagnoses, such as EGFR mutations and ALK rearrangements.

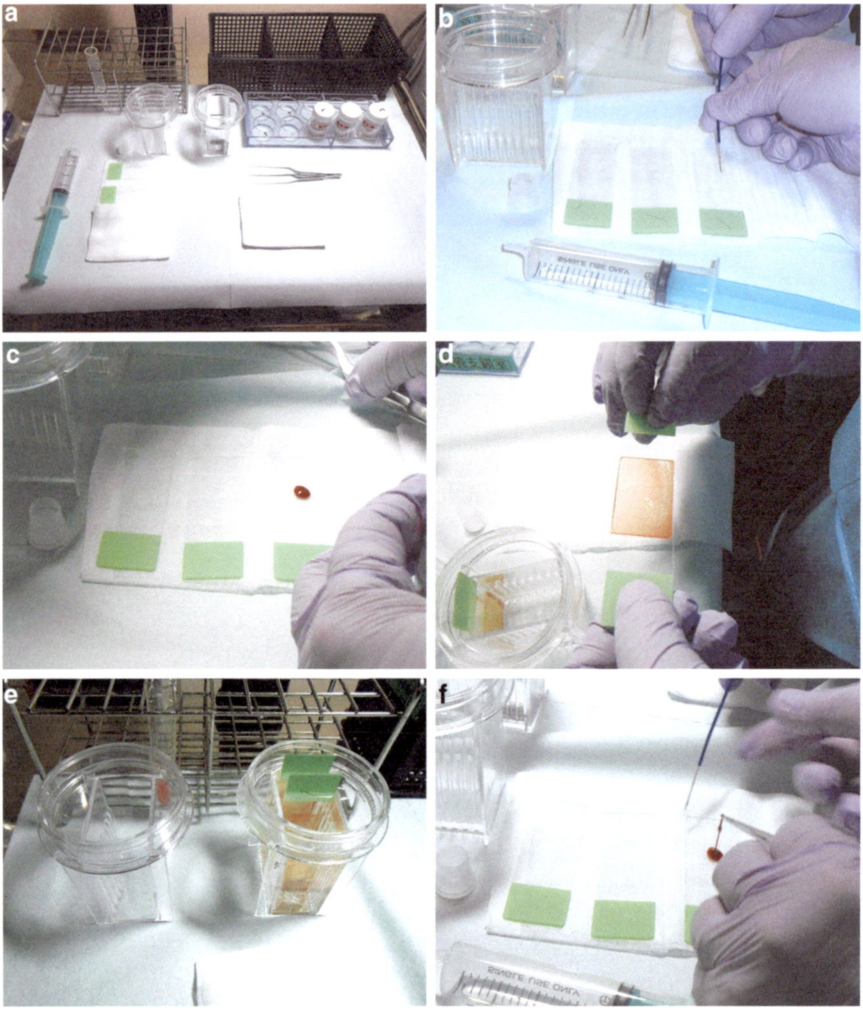

Fig. 23.7 Processing specimens. (**a**) Prepare the materials that you need in one working area. After EBUS-TBNA, remove the needle apparatus from the working channel. (**b**, **c**) Insert the stylet into the needle and slowly push out the collected specimen onto a glass slide. (**d**–**f**) If core tissue is available, gently pick it up with tweezers and transfer it on a filter paper before fixing in formalin. (**g**, **h**) Using another clean glass slide, make a smear from the residual liquid aspirate on the first glass slide; fix one slide in 95% ethyl alcohol, and air-dry the other slide for rapid on-site cytology evaluation. **i** Finally, push out any remaining specimen in the needle apparatus by flushing with 3 mL of saline solution to collect liquid cytology samples for cytology, microbiologic, and/or molecular studies

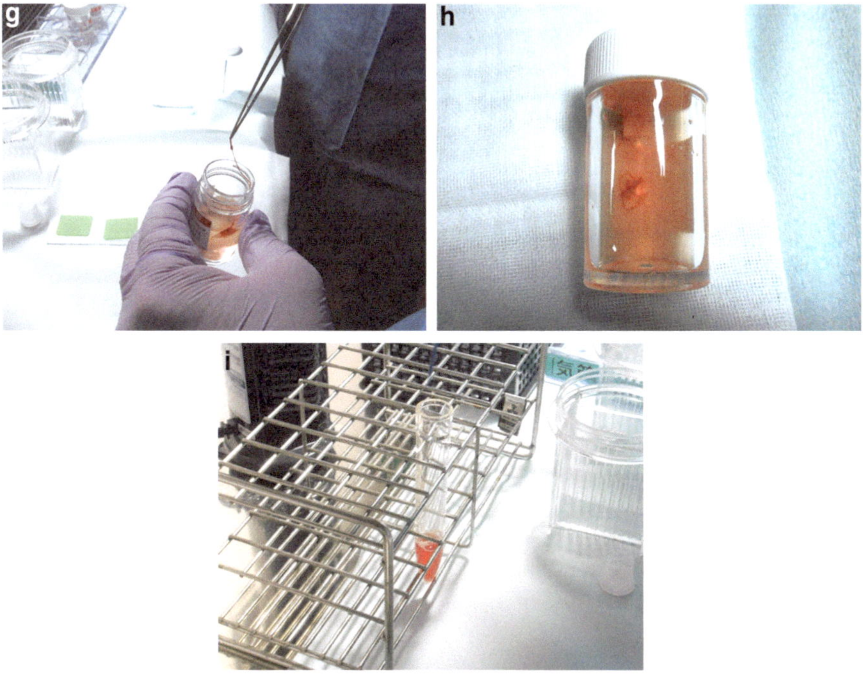

Fig. 23.7 (continued)

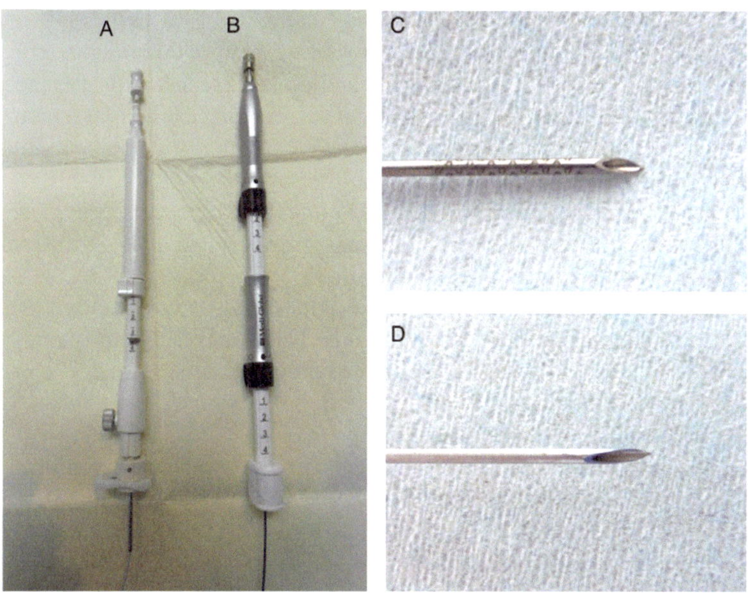

Fig. 23.8 The different types of EBUS-TBNA needle apparatus currently available in Japan. The images show a comparison of the handle and puncturing tip of the (**a**, **c**) ViziShot (NA-201SX-4022, Olympus) and (**b**, **d**) SonoTip EBUS Pro (GUS-45-18-022, Medi-Globe) needles (Adopted from Izumo et al. [5])

Table 23.3 Comparison of EBUS-TBNA needles for tissue collection

Category of histologic specimens	SonoTip EBUS Pro 22-G with stainless steel	ViziShot 22-G	*P* value[a]
A. Diagnostic	74.3 % (159/214)	61.3 % (144/235)	0.0035
B. Nondiagnostic	13.1 % (28/214)	25.5 % (60/235)	
C. No specimen	12.6 % (27/214)	13.2 % (31/235)	

Adapted from Izumo et al. [5]
Data are presented as percentage (number)
EBUS-TBNA, endobronchial ultrasound-guided transbronchial needle aspiration
[a]Using Fisher's exact test, across the sampling yield of diagnostic histologic specimens (A vs. B, C) in each needle group

23.5 Latest Advancements in the EBUS Processor

Since December 2013, Olympus has launched two new ultrasound processors, the EU-ME2 and EU-ME2 PREMIER PLUS, which are equipped with functions, in addition to those already available in the older model. Although the value of these new functions has not been established, they seem to be useful for the evaluation of internal structure and selection of the puncture site. Future research is warranted to clarify these gaps.

1. Elastography (ELST) mode
   ELST mode enables addition of colors according to tissue hardness. Blue color indicates the hardest part of the lesion, followed by green, yellow, and red in the order of hardness (Fig. 23.9). The relative hardness of the tissues is visualized by color, but the pulsations of the surrounding heart and aorta may affect this and need to be taken into account. In addition to the conventional B mode and Doppler mode, ELST is considered useful for selecting a lesion for puncture [1]. More details on these are discussed in Chap. 24.
2. Tissue harmonic echo (THE) mode
   THE mode creates a picture from the harmonic components generated when ultrasound waves are transmitted through biological tissues. With improvements in resolution and reduction of artifacts, few noises appear on the display, and more detailed observation of lymph nodes has become possible. On THE mode, cartilages may be visualized more clearly and facilitate smooth transbronchial needle puncture through an intercartilaginous space.
3. High-flow (H-FLOW) mode
   H-FLOW mode displays blood flow intensity and direction by colors (Fig. 23.10a), without the usual outpouching that is seen on conventional color flow Doppler mode (Fig. 23.10b). This H-FLOW capability allows more precise puncture during EBUS-TBNA, while avoiding blood vessels that are finely and more clearly visualized than those under conventional Doppler mode (Fig. 23.10c).

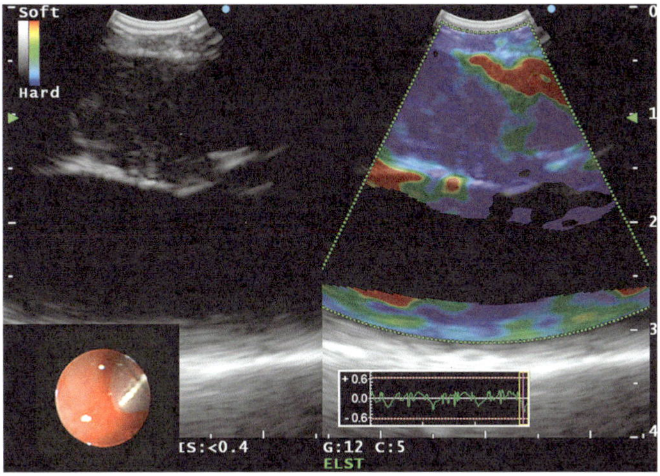

Fig. 23.9 Elastography. The spectrum of hardness, represented by color, is shown in the *upper left hand corner*. The image on the *left* shows B mode scan of a lymph node, whereas the image on the *right* shows a superimposed elastography feature that displays predominantly *blue* color, suspicious for malignancy

4. Pulse wave (PW) Doppler mode
   PW mode displays blood flow rate in the target site on a cross-sectional image. It may be useful for differentiating veins from arteries during EBUS-TBNA, but it might need further assessment.

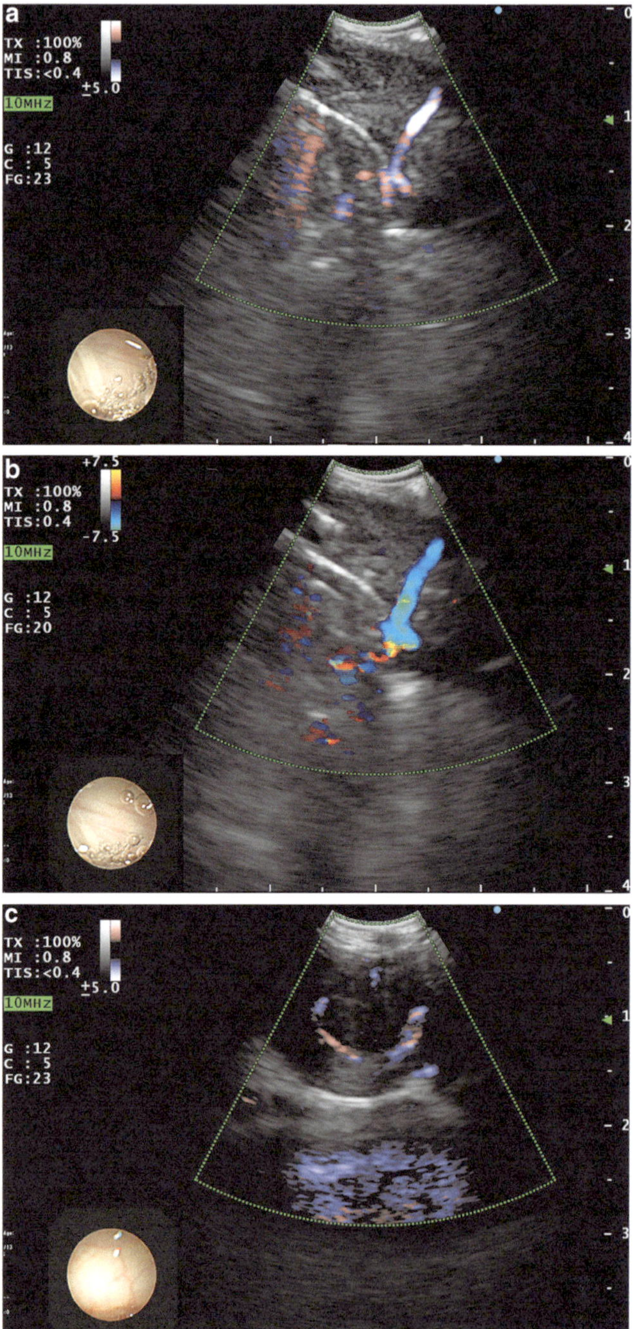

Fig. 23.10 High-flow and color Doppler modes. (**a**) High-flow mode displays thinner and finer outlines of blood vessels, compared with the (**b**) outpouching seen on color Doppler mode. (**c**) On high-flow mode, blood vessels in the lymph nodes are visualized in detail and facilitate safer puncture

References

1. Izumo T, Sasada S, Chavez C, et al. Endobronchial ultrasound elastography in the diagnosis of mediastinal and hilar lymph nodes. Jpn J Clin Oncol. 2014;44:841–5.
2. Nakajima T, Fujiwara T, Izumo T, et al. Handbook for EBUS-TBNA/GS procedures. Olympus medical systems 2013.
3. Oki M, Saka H, Kitagawa C, et al. Randomized study of 21-gauge versus 22-gauge endobronchial ultrasound-guided transbronchial needle aspiration needles for sampling histology specimens. J Bronchology Interv Pulmonol. 2011;18:306–10.
4. Nakajima T, Yasufuku K, Takahashi R, et al. Comparison of 21-gauge and 22-gauge aspiration needle during endobronchial ultrasound-guided transbronchial needle aspiration. Respirology. 2011;16:90–4.
5. Izumo T, Sasada S, Watanabe J, et al. Comparison of two 22 G aspiration needles for histologic sampling during endobronchial ultrasound-guided transbronchial needle aspiration (EBUS-TBNA). Jpn J Clin Oncol. 2014;44:841–5.

Chapter 24
Endobronchial Ultrasound Elastography

Takehiro Izumo

Abstract Endobronchial ultrasound elastography is a new function for assessment of the hardness of a lesion with the use of colors. Blue indicates the hardest portion of a lesion, followed by green, yellow, and red in the order of hardness. Type classification of lesions by color has been reported recently and is expected for future development.

Keywords Endobronchial ultrasound • Elastography • Type classification • Color image

Endobronchial ultrasound-guided transbronchial needle aspiration (EBUS-TBNA) is an excellent method that is known worldwide to visualize the echogenicity of a lesion and collect specimen in real time. It might be best if all suspicious lesions on EBUS can be punctured to collect specimen, but time constraints, possible complications with several punctures, and examiner skills would dictate a need to prioritize the lesions to biopsy. Conventional EBUS procedures have employed the use of B mode and Doppler mode to assess internal structure and blood flow, respectively [1, 2]. In December 2013, a new EBUS processor that is equipped with elastography (EU-ME2 PREMIUM PLUS; Olympus, Tokyo, Japan) was launched.

Elastography mode is a new function that enables addition of colors to lesions according to tissue hardness. Blue indicates the hardest part of a lesion, followed by green, yellow, and red in the order of hardness. EBUS elastography, in addition to the conventional method, is considered useful for selecting a lesion to puncture, and studies about this new technology are in progress worldwide. We reported that classifying elastography findings into three types (Fig. 24.1 and Table 24.1) was very useful for selecting lymph nodes to be punctured [3]. When Type 1 and Type 3 lesions were assigned as nonmalignant and malignant, respectively, the sensitivity, specificity, positive predictive value, negative predictive value, and diagnostic accuracy were as high as 100%, 92.3%, 94.6%, 100%, and 96.7%, respectively

T. Izumo (✉)
Department of Respiratory Medicine, Japanese Red Cross Medical Center,
4-1-22 Hiroo, Shibuya-ku, Tokyo 150-8935, Japan
e-mail: drtake1118@gmail.com

T. Izumo et al. (eds.), *Respiratory Endoscopy*,
DOI 10.1007/978-981-287-916-5_24

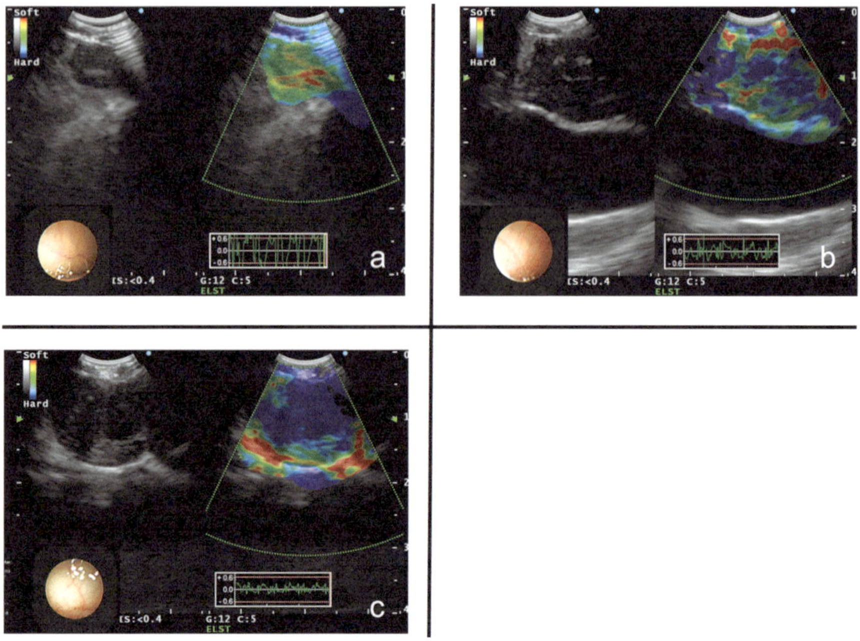

Fig. 24.1 EBUS elastography classification of lymph nodes. The *left* side of the display shows B mode, and the *right* side shows the elastography patterns. (**a**) Type 1 shows predominantly non-blue (*green*, *yellow*, and *red*). (**b**) Type 2 shows part *blue*, part *non-blue* (*green*, *yellow*, and *red*). **c** Type 3 shows predominantly *blue* (Adopted from Izumo et al. [3])

Table 24.1 EBUS elastography classification of LNs

Elastography type	Number of benign LNs/total number (%)	Number of malignant LNs/total number (%)
Type 1 ($n=24$)	24/24 (100)	0/24 (0)
Type 2 ($n=14$)	6/14 (42.9)	8/14 (57.1)
Type 3 ($n=37$)	2/37 (5.4)	35/37 (94.6)

Adopted from Izumo et al. [3]
EBUS endobronchial ultrasound, *LN* lymph node

(Table 24.2). In addition, EBUS elastography types were positively correlated with FDG-PET uptake (Table 24.3). Representative cases are shown in Figs. 24.2, 24.3, and 24.4. Further studies are expected in the future.

Table 24.2 Accuracy of quantitative elastography for the diagnosis of malignant metastasis

	Accuracy (%)	[95 %CI]
Sensitivity	100	[83.8–100]
Specificity	92.3	[73.0–99.0]
Positive predictive value	94.6	[79.8–99.3]
Negative predictive value	100	[78.1–100]
Diagnostic accuracy	96.7	[87.5–99.6]

Adopted from Izumo et al. [3]
This analysis was based on classifying Type 1 as benign and Type 3 as malignant

Table 24.3 Correlation between EBUS elastography types and median values of FDG-PET uptake

	SUVmax	[95 % CI]
Type 1	2.49	[1.08–5.07]
Type 2	4.95	[1.57–8.00]
Type 3	8.5	[6.97–10.03]

Adopted from Izumo et al. [3]
The computed Spearman rank coefficient (r) was 0.54 ($P<0.0001$)
EBUS endobronchial ultrasound, *FDG-PET* fluorodeoxyglucose positron emission tomography, *SUVmax* maximum standardized uptake value

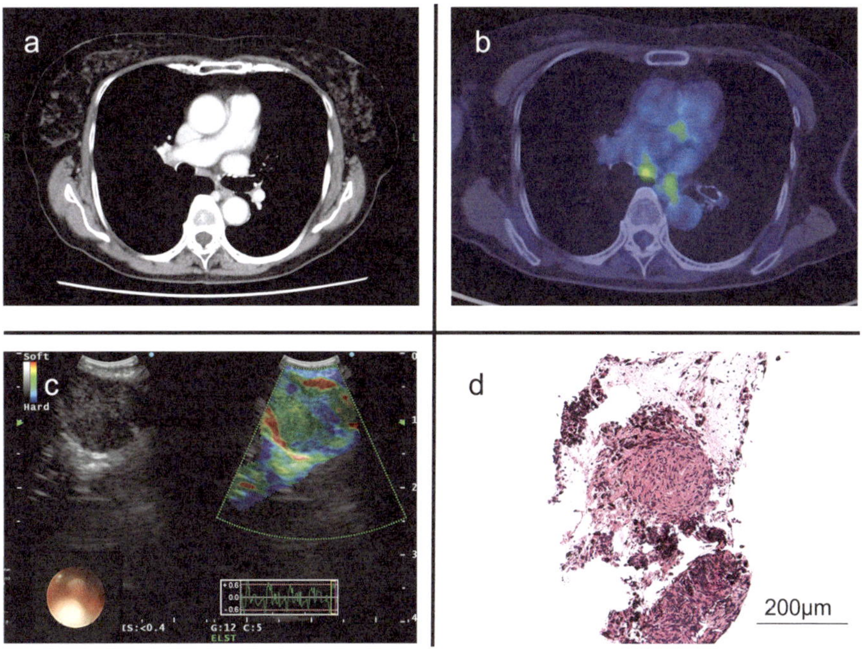

Fig. 24.2 EBUS elastography Type 1 in a case of sarcoidosis. (**a**) Enlargement of subcarinal lymph node (#7) is observed on CT. (**b**) There is significant accumulation on FDG-PET. (**c**) EBUS elastography shows predominantly non-*blue* (*green*, *yellow*, and *red*) pattern. (**d**) Histopathologic examination reveals noncaseating epithelioid cell granuloma, consistent with sarcoidosis (Adopted from Izumo et al. [3]). *EBUS* endobronchial ultrasound, *CT* computed tomography, *FDG-PET* fluorodeoxyglucose positron emission tomography

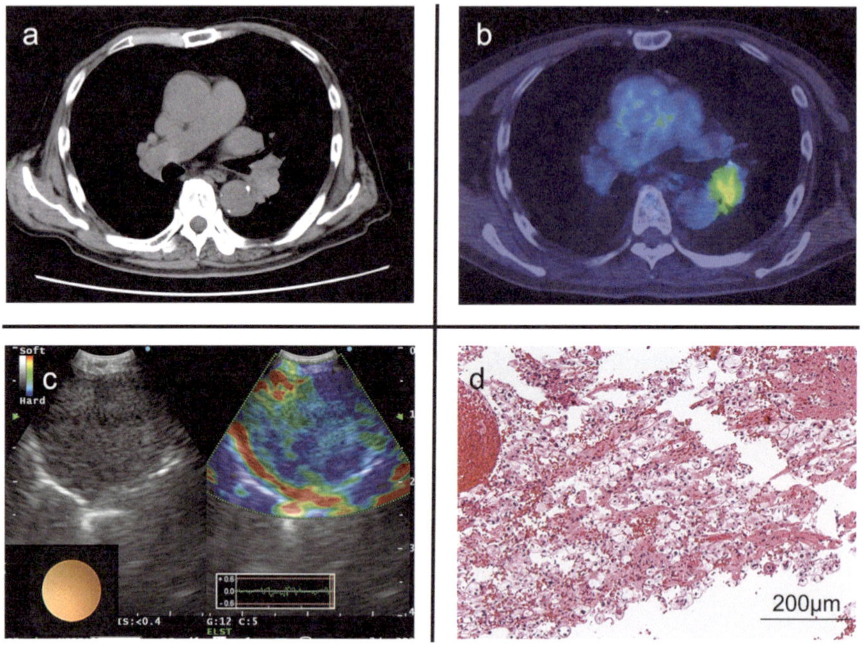

Fig. 24.3 EBUS elastography Type 2 in a case of lymph node metastasis from renal cell carcinoma. (**a**) Enlargement of interlobar lymph node (#11) is observed on CT. (**b**) There is significant accumulation on FDG-PET. (**c**) EBUS elastography shows part *blue* and part non-*blue* (*green*, *yellow*, and *red*) pattern. (**d**) Histopathologic examination confirms lymph node metastasis from renal cell carcinoma (Adopted from Izumo et al. [3]). *EBUS* endobronchial ultrasound, *CT* computed tomography, *FDG-PET* fluorodeoxyglucose positron emission tomography

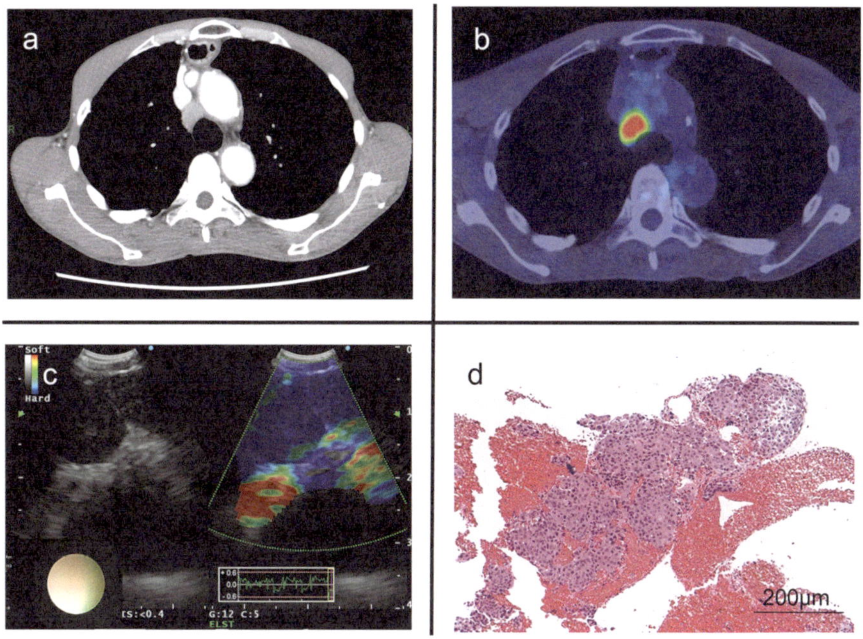

Fig. 24.4 EBUS elastography Type 3 in a case of lymph node metastasis from lung squamous cell carcinoma. (**a**) Enlargement of right lower paratracheal lymph node (#4R) is observed on CT. (**b**) There is significant accumulation on FDG-PET. (**c**) EBUS elastography shows predominantly *blue* pattern. (**d**) Histopathologic examination confirms lymph node metastasis from lung squamous cell carcinoma (Adopted from Izumo et al. [3]). *EBUS* endobronchial ultrasound, *CT* computed tomography, *FDG-PET* fluorodeoxyglucose positron emission tomography

References

1. Fujiwara T, Yasufuku K, Nakajima T, et al. The utility of sonographic features during endobronchial ultrasound-guided transbronchial needle aspiration for lymph node staging in patients with lung cancer: a standard endobronchial ultrasound image classification system. Chest. 2010;138:641–7.
2. Nakajima T, Anayama T, Shingyoji M, et al. Vascular image patterns of lymph nodes for the prediction of metastatic disease during EBUS-TBNA for mediastinal staging of lung cancer. J Thorac Oncol. 2012;7:1009–14.
3. Izumo T, Sasada S, Chavez C, et al. Endobronchial ultrasound elastography in the diagnosis of mediastinal and hilar lymph nodes. Jpn J Clin Oncol. 2014;44:841–5.

Chapter 25
Flex-Rigid Pleuroscopy Under Local Anesthesia

Yukio Watanabe and Shinji Sasada

Abstract The flex-rigid pleuroscope, which has a handle that is similar in design to a standard flexible bronchoscope, is easy to handle and covers a wide field. It is important to perform the procedure in cooperation with a surgeon, while noting that there is a limit. Systematic surveillance during medical thoracoscopy will shorten procedure time and can reduce errors. During pleuroscopy for dry pleural dissemination, identification of the mobility between the parietal and visceral pleura during breathing (sliding sign) by linear probe transthoracic ultrasonography can prevent damage to the lung parenchyma during insertion of the trocar. Full-thickness biopsy is essential in the differential diagnosis of densely thick pleura. Pleuroscopic punch biopsy using insulated-tip diathermic knife (IT knife 2) is a feasible technique for a successful diagnosis of unknown pleural disease. One tip is to hook the short blades of the IT knife 2 into the pleura, then incise while lifting the pleura obliquely.

Keywords Flex-rigid pleuroscopy • Pleural biopsy • Electrocautery • Macroscopic intrathoracic classification • Dry pleural dissemination • Insulated-tip diathermic knife 2

25.1 Procedures and Findings

25.1.1 Introduction

Obtaining an accurate diagnosis of pleural disease is one of the most common problems for a pulmonologist. In fact, 25–40 % of pleural abnormalities remain undiagnosed even after thoracentesis and/or blind pleural biopsy [1, 2]. Medical

---

Y. Watanabe
Division of General Thoracic Surgery, National Cancer Center Hospital, Tokyo, Japan

S. Sasada (✉)
Department of Respiratory Medicine, Tokyo Saiseikai Central Hospital,
1-4-17, Mita, Minato-ku, Tokyo 108-0073, Japan
e-mail: sasastaf@hotmail.co.jp

T. Izumo et al. (eds.), *Respiratory Endoscopy*,
DOI 10.1007/978-981-287-916-5_25

thoracoscopy is an invasive technique that involves examining the pleural space under local anesthesia and which should be used when other simpler methods fail [3, 4]. It yields positive diagnosis in 90 % of pleural effusions [5, 6]. Some doctors use the flexible bronchoscope [7–10], but most prefer a rigid thoracoscope because it allows better observation of the pleural cavity and procurement of larger biopsies [11–13]. The flex-rigid pleuroscope was developed in an attempt to combine the best features of the flexible and rigid instruments [14]. This instrument is easy to handle and covers a wider field because its handle is similar in design to a standard flexible bronchoscope [14–16].

25.1.2 Indications

1. Diagnosis of unexplained pleural effusion
2. Diagnosis of pleural or chest wall tumor
3. Release of adhesions and drainage of empyema
4. Identification of air leak and pleurodesis with sclerosing agent for pneumothorax
5. Detection of lung cancer progression
6. Tissue collection for gene mutation analysis

25.1.3 Contraindications

1. Severe respiratory failure in the contralateral lung
2. Hemostatic dysfunction
3. Severe pleural adhesions
4. Severe hypoxemia
5. Uncontrolled ischemic heart disease and arrhythmia

25.1.4 Devices (Fig. 25.1)

Flex-rigid pleuroscope (LTF-260, Olympus, Tokyo, Japan)
Endoscopy system (light source, image recording device)
Electrocautery equipment
Electrocautery surgical knife (e.g., insulated-tip diathermic knife 2, IT knife 2; Olympus, Tokyo, Japan)
Thoracotomy set
Local injection needle
Flexible trocar and catheter
Alligator biopsy forceps
Coagulation forceps

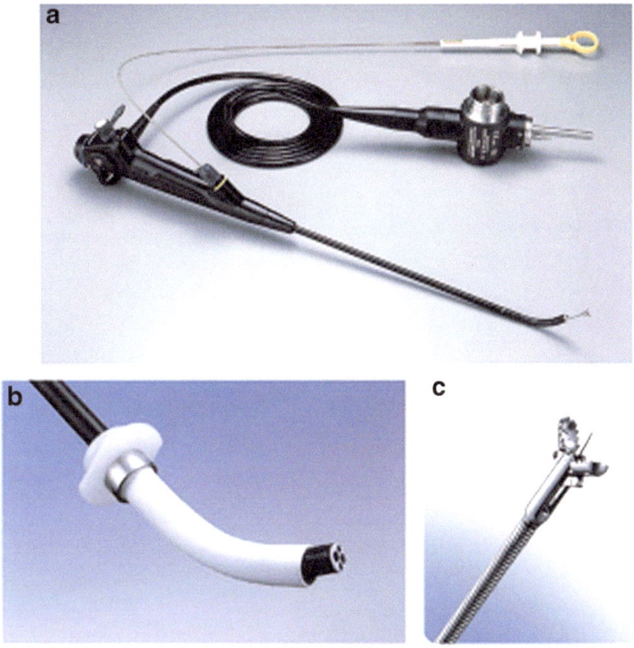

Fig. 25.1 Devices for flex-rigid pleuroscopy under local anesthesia. (**a**) Flex-rigid pleuroscope (LTF-260, Olympus). (**b**) Flexible trocar. (**c**) Alligator biopsy forceps

25.1.5 Preparations and Procedures (Fig. 25.2)

For massive pleural effusion, drain the pleural effusion slowly by use of an indwelling catheter or by repeated thoracentesis, starting from the day before the procedure to prevent re-expansion pulmonary edema.

On the day of the procedure, the patient is placed in the lateral decubitus position, with the diseased side facing upward. The puncture site should be confirmed by checking for pleural effusion and pleural adhesion using chest ultrasound. After administration of local anesthesia with 1 % lidocaine, a 1–2 cm incision is made, followed by blunt dissection through the muscle layers of the chest wall until the parietal pleura is exposed. During this procedure, ensure that adequate anesthesia is delivered to the subcutaneous and muscle layers. Upon reaching the parietal pleura, gently strip it off using a Kocher clamp to avoid injury to the closely apposed visceral pleura. After dissection of the parietal pleura and confirmation of collapse of the affected lung, a disposablc flexible trocar (8 mm inner diameter) is inserted carefully before proceeding with inspection using the flex-rigid pleuroscope.

Upon confirming the location of the pleural lesion, local anesthesia with 1 % lidocaine is administered by subpleural injection needle (4–6 mm, 23–25 G) to reduce a pleural pain before taking biopsies (10–20 times) using alligator forceps (Fig. 25.3). After hemostasis is confirmed on the biopsy site, remove the thoracoscope

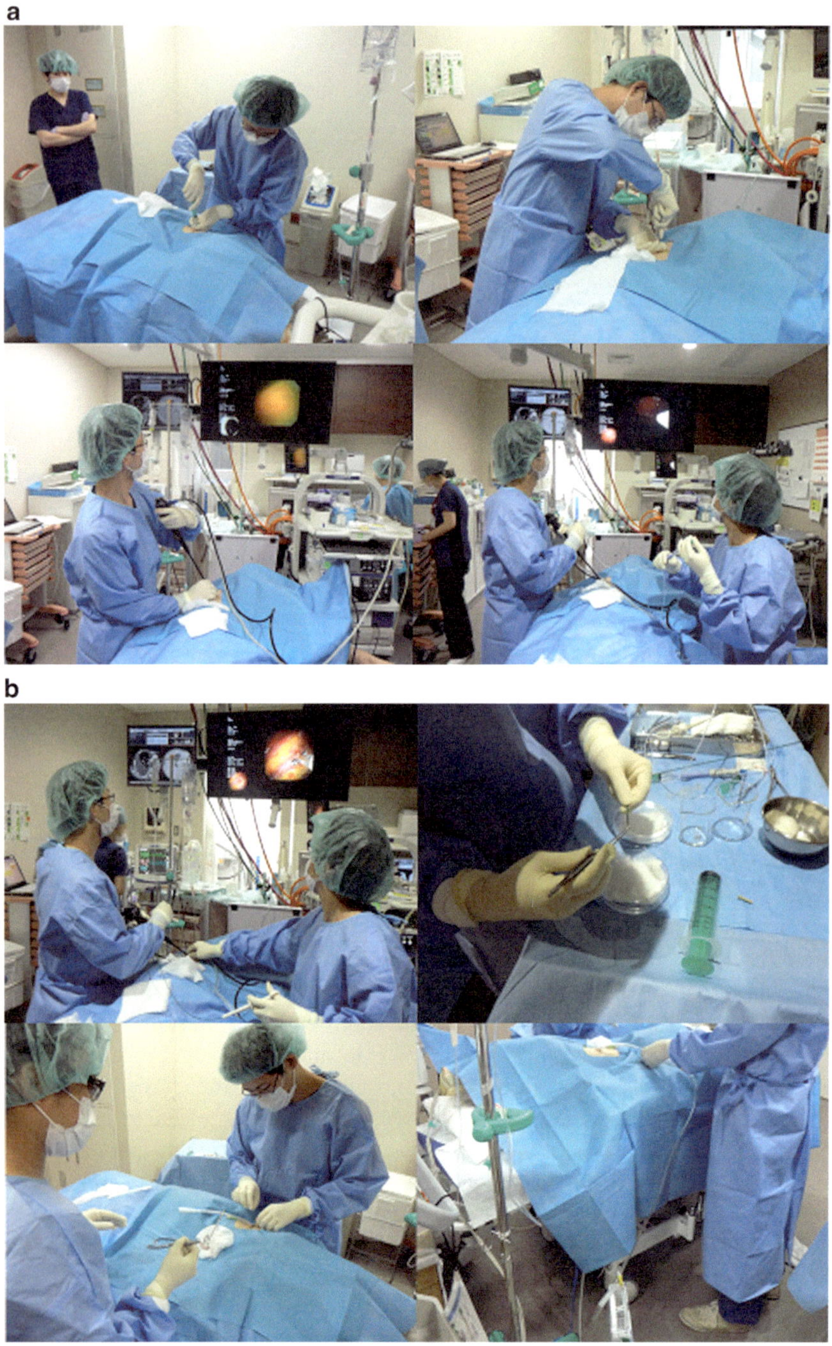

Fig. 25.2 Steps for flex-rigid pleuroscopy under local anesthesia. (**a**) Apply local anesthesia, insert a flexible trocar, inspect the chest cavity, and determine the biopsy site. (**b**) Perform forceps biopsy, collect specimen properly, and insert a chest tube, which will be connected to a water-seal bottle

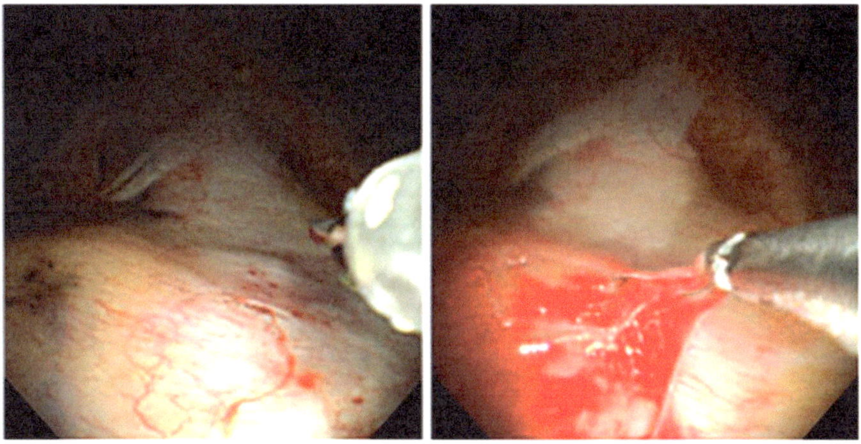

Fig. 25.3 Pleuroscopy findings in nonspecific pleurisy. After injecting lidocaine into the subpleural layer, peel with forceps

and flexible trocar and place a double-lumen chest tube (20–24 Fr), which will be connected to a water-seal bottle for continuous thoracic drainage after the procedure. If there is a large amount of residual pleural effusion, there is no need for immediate application of negative pressure after thoracoscopy closure to avoid re-expansion pulmonary edema.

25.1.6 Limitation of Flex-Rigid Pleuroscopy

1. Mediastinal and apical pleura are difficult to observe, compared with video-assisted thoracoscopic surgery.
2. The presence of extensive fibrin deposition makes inspection of the entire thoracic cavity difficult.
3. Endoscopic hemostasis of arterial bleeding is difficult; that is why cooperation with thoracic surgeons is needed for double setup.
4. The presence of strong pleural adhesions may lead to severe bleeding after peeling for biopsy.

25.1.7 Importance of Thoracoscopic Findings

The main purpose of medical thoracoscopy is to obtain a definitive diagnosis of pleural diseases by visual inspection and biopsy (Figs. 25.3, 25.4, 25.5, 25.6, 25.7, 25.8 and 25.9). The most frequent diseases are cancerous pleurisy from lung cancer, malignant pleural mesothelioma, tuberculous pleurisy, and nonspecific

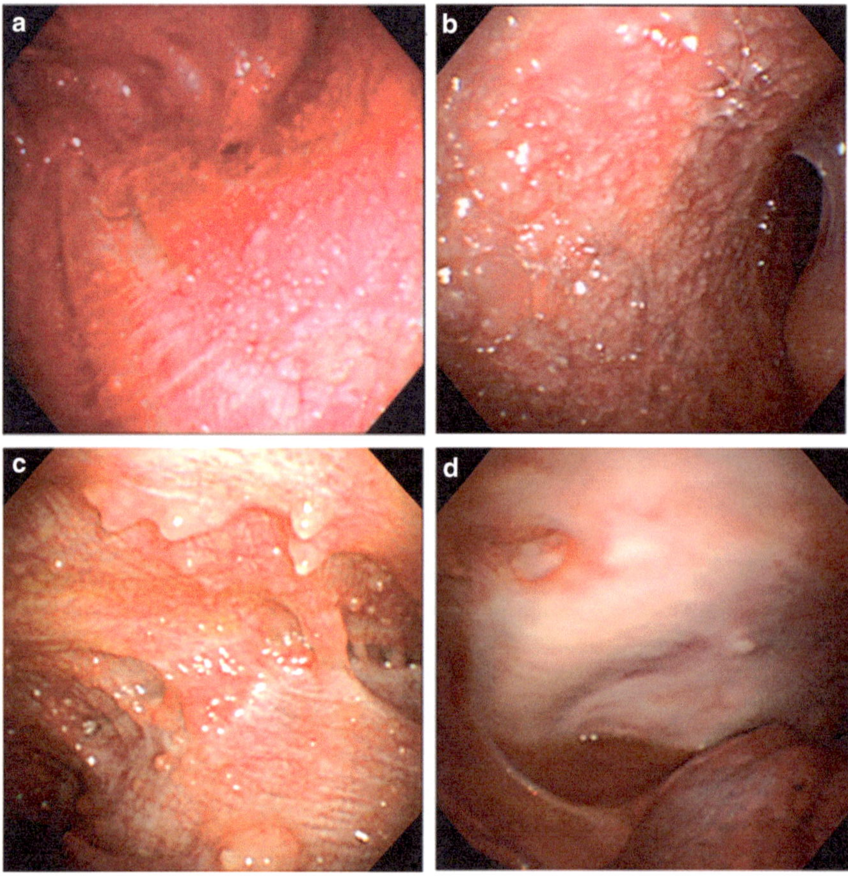

Fig. 25.4 Pleuroscopy findings in tuberculous pleurisy. (**a**) Granular lesions (early phase). (**b**) Nodular lesions. (**c**) Fused nodular lesions. The tip of the cone-shaped nodules is necrotic. (**d**) Dense pleural thickening (advanced phase)

inflammation. Other etiologies are pleural metastasis from other cancer types, malignant lymphoma, empyema, concomitant pneumonia, concomitant pancreatitis, Meigs' syndrome, and collagen diseases. Pleural lesions on thoracoscopy tend to be similar and nonspecific; therefore, these are difficult to clearly classify without biopsy.

It is important to take note that since the local anesthesia under thoracoscopy limits procedure time, quick determination of the pleural biopsy site is required. In the next section, we introduce our system of reporting the thoracoscopic findings that we use in our hospital.

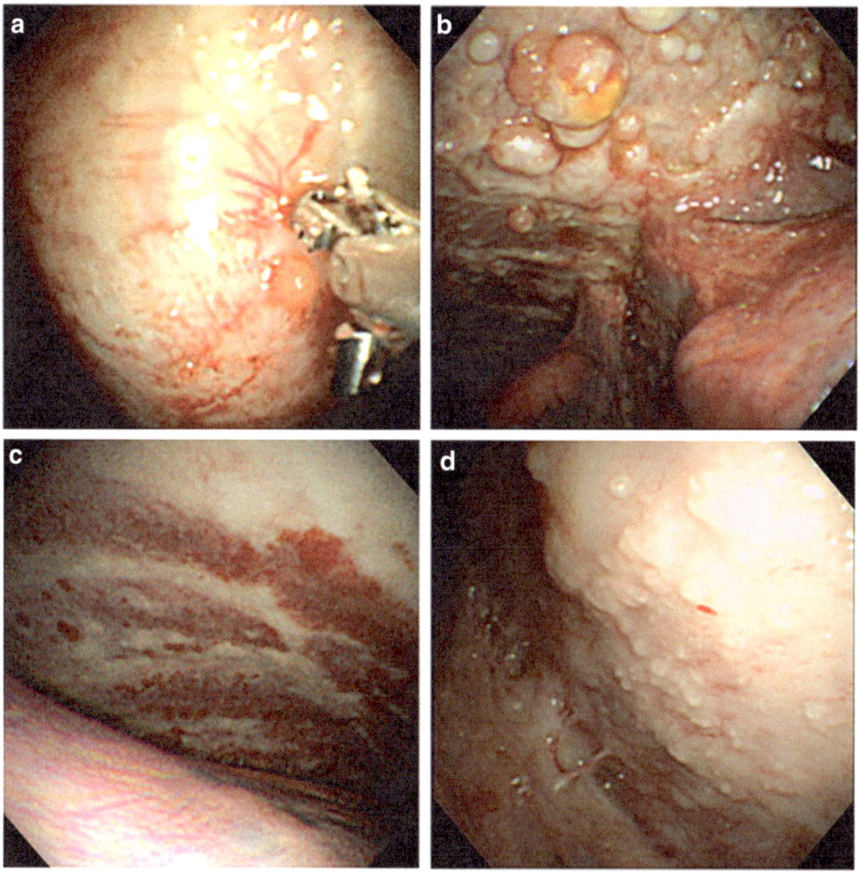

Fig. 25.5 Pleuroscopy findings in lung adenocarcinoma. (**a**) Nodular lesions. (**b**) Multiple mass lesions. (**c**) Wavy whitish pleural thickening (moderate). (**d**) Small nodules with dense pleural thickening (severe)

25.1.8 Classification of Findings that Should Be Noted During Thoracoscopy (Table 25.1)

1. **Polypoid lesions**
   (a) Localization
   (b) Form
   (c) Distribution
   (d) Color
2. **Pleural thickening**
   (a) Grade
   (b) Distribution

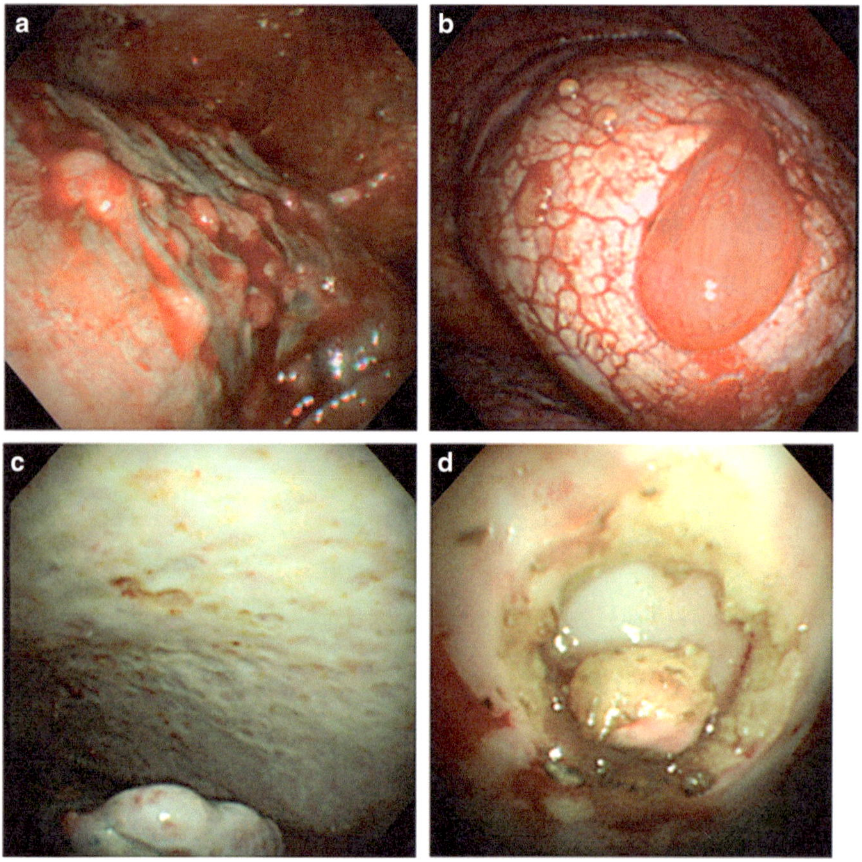

Fig. 25.6 Pleuroscopy findings in metastatic pleural tumor. (**a**) Metastatic thyroid cancer (on the visceral pleura). (**b**) Metastatic peritoneal cancer (cystic lesions). (**c**) Metastatic breast cancer with whitish, densely thickened pleura with cavity. (**d**) Metastatic breast cancer that underwent full-thickness pleural biopsy by IT knife 2

(c) Shape
(d) Color

3. **Others**

(a) Fibrin deposition
(b) Pleurodesis
(c) Hypervascularity
(d) Easy bleeding

Since most pleural lesions consist of polypoid lesions and pleural thickening, it is advisable to take findings of these lesions separately. Systematic taking of abnormal intrathoracic findings will shorten procedure time and can reduce errors.

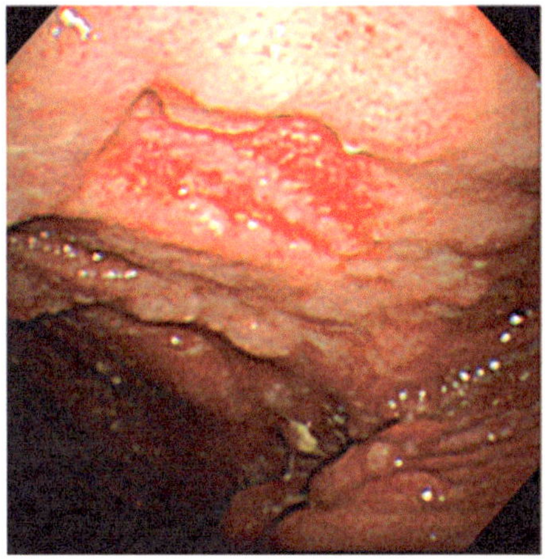

Fig. 25.7 Pleuroscopy findings in malignant lymphoma. Fused whitish, bulging lesions

25.1.9 Pleuroscopic Punch Biopsy by Electrocautery

Malignant pleural mesothelioma is difficult to diagnose by small specimens. The IT knife 2 (Olympus) was specifically designed to electrosurgically treat early gastric carcinoma. It consists of a conventional diathermic needle knife with a ceramic ball at the tip; the outer diameter is 2.2 mm and the length is 4 mm. The IT knife 2 is a disposable tool with a preferred working channel diameter of at least 2.8 mm.

We use the IT knife 2 for thick pleural lesions that are difficult to grasp by flexible forceps (Figs. 25.10 and 25.11) [17]. Local anesthesia is administered almost similar to the method described in Sect. 25, but an additional pleural bulge should be made. Following this, a pinhole is made through the bulge using coagulation forceps. The tip of the IT knife 2 is inserted into the hole, followed by a circular incision through the full thickness of the affected pleura using ENDO-CUT mode electric current at 30–50 W. The incised pleura is then carefully removed by flexible forceps.

25.1.10 Thoracoscopic Findings and Pitfalls in Various Pleural Diseases

Cancerous pleurisy from primary lung cancer is often seen as scattered nodules. Fusion of the pleural lesions may be seen in some cases of malignant pleural mesothelioma (Fig. 25.8), tuberculous pleurisy (Fig. 25.4), or malignant lymphoma (Fig. 25.7). In malignant diseases, pleural thickening may be frequently seen not only in malignant pleural mesothelioma but also in various cases of metastatic cancerous pleurisy. Especially, cancerous pleurisy due to metastatic breast cancer exhibits a high degree of pleural thickening. In our series, full-thickness pleural

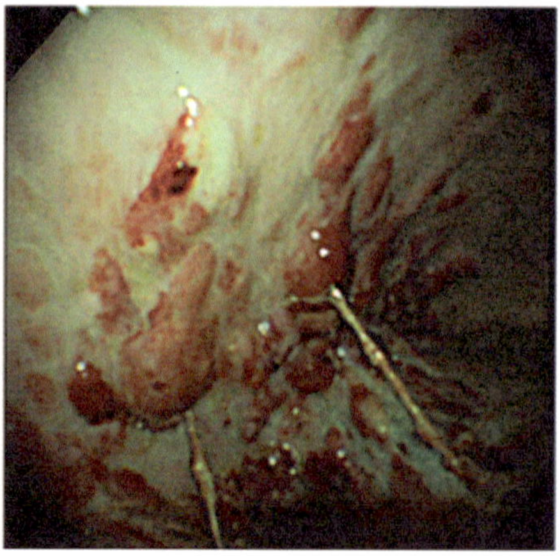

Fig. 25.8 Pleuroscopy findings in malignant pleural mesothelioma (epithelial type). Fused reddish masses accompanied with pleural thickening (moderate)

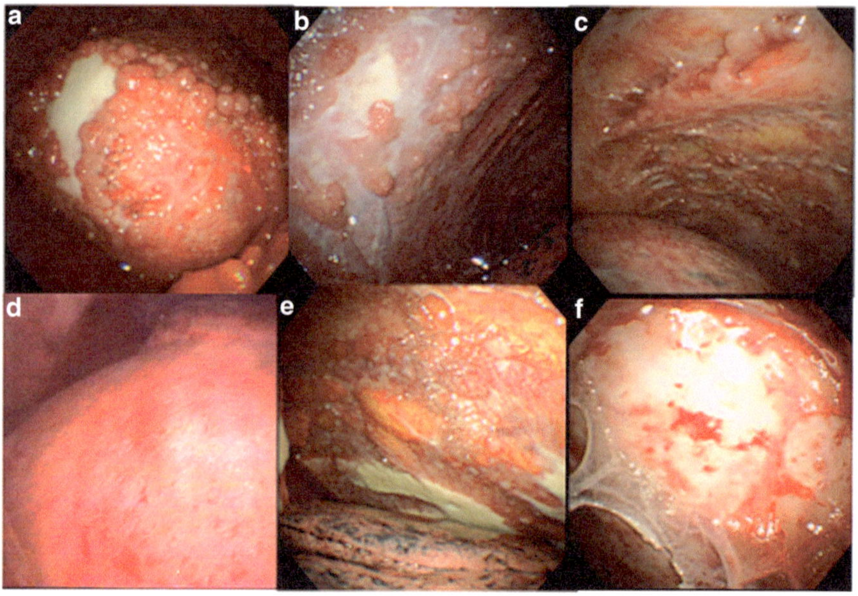

Fig. 25.9 Two types of malignant pleural mesothelioma. (**a–c**) Bulging (nodule, mass) lesions. (**d–f**) Smooth, thickened abnormal lesions. Thickened pleural lesions are difficult to diagnose by forceps biopsy alone; full-thickness biopsy is recommended

biopsy specimen collected by IT knife 2 was useful for determining the diagnosis and for immunohistochemistry analysis [17]. To differentiate from primary lung cancer, breast cancer may sometimes metastasize to the pleura in the form of cavitations on the pleural surface (Fig. 25.6).

When pleural abnormalities present as smooth white pleural thickening without elevated lesions, fibrous pleurisy and desmoplastic malignant pleural mesothelioma

Table 25.1 Reporting of thoracoscopic findings

Polypoid lesion	Present		Absent		
	Localization	Apical	Anterior	Lateral	
		Posterior	Diaphragm	Visceral	
	Form	Granules	Nodules	Polypoid	Mass
	Distribution	Scattered	Fused	Isolated	
	Color	Shiny	Reddish	Whitish	Necrotic
Pleural thickening	Present		Absent		
	Grade	Severe	Moderate	Mild	
	Distribution	Diffuse	Patchy	Localized	
	Shape	Smooth	Wavy	Cavitary	
	Color	Reddish	Whitish	Calcified	
Fibrin deposition	Present		Absent		
Pleurodesis	Present		Absent		
Hypervascularity	Present		Absent		
Easy bleeding	Present		Absent		

Findings that are observed during thoracoscopy are encircled

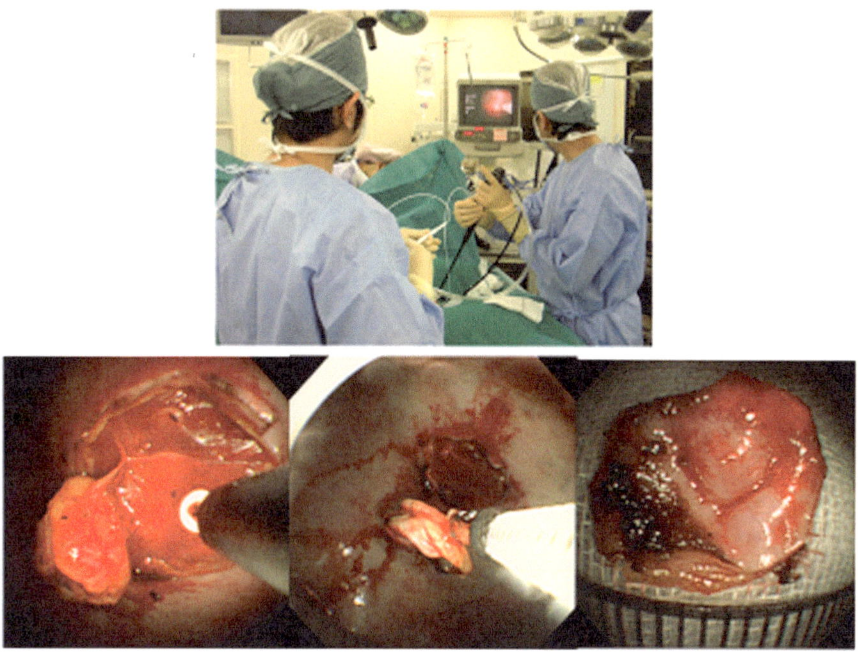

Fig. 25.10 Pleuroscopic punch biopsy by electrocautery (IT knife 2, Olympus)

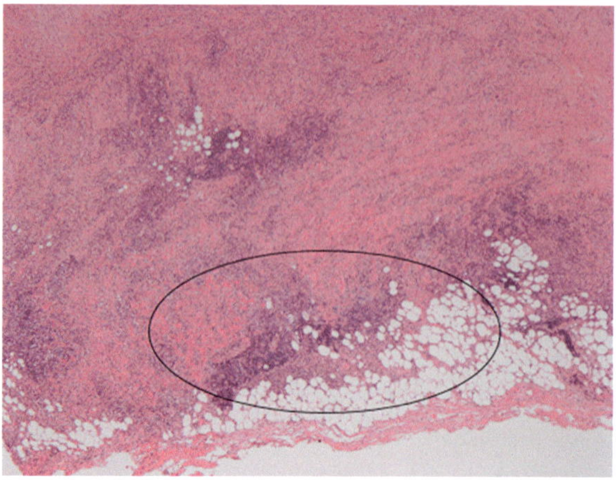

Fig. 25.11 Histopathology findings in sarcomatous mesothelioma (hematoxylin and eosin stain, ×4). Definitive diagnosis was successfully obtained by findings of tumor invasion into the subpleural fat layer (*encircled area*)

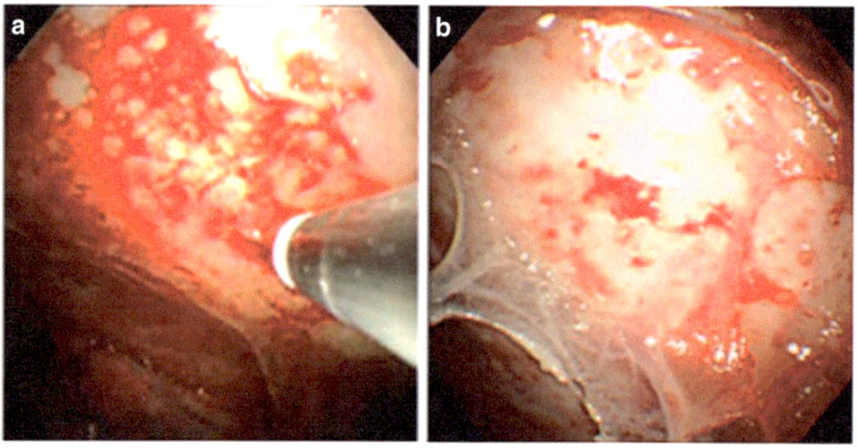

Fig. 25.12 Comparison of thoracoscopic findings. (**a**) Fibrous pleurisy. (**b**) Desmoplastic malignant pleural mesothelioma. These macroscopic findings are quite similar; full-thickness pleural biopsy is necessary for differentiation

must be considered (Fig. 25.12) [18, 19]. Differentiating between these two pathologies is very difficult and biopsy of all pleural layers is recommended [20].

Some cases with cancerous pleurisy present as a nest of fine seeding lesions on the surface of a thickened pleura. Therefore, it is important to examine the pleural surface as close as possible for detailed observation. Narrow band imaging to detect neovascularization can help in the detection of lesions [21]. In re-biopsy cases of EGFR-positive lung adenocarcinoma with prior EGFR-TKI treatment, pleural thickening and scattered nodules with proliferation of blood vessels are often seen (Fig. 25.13).

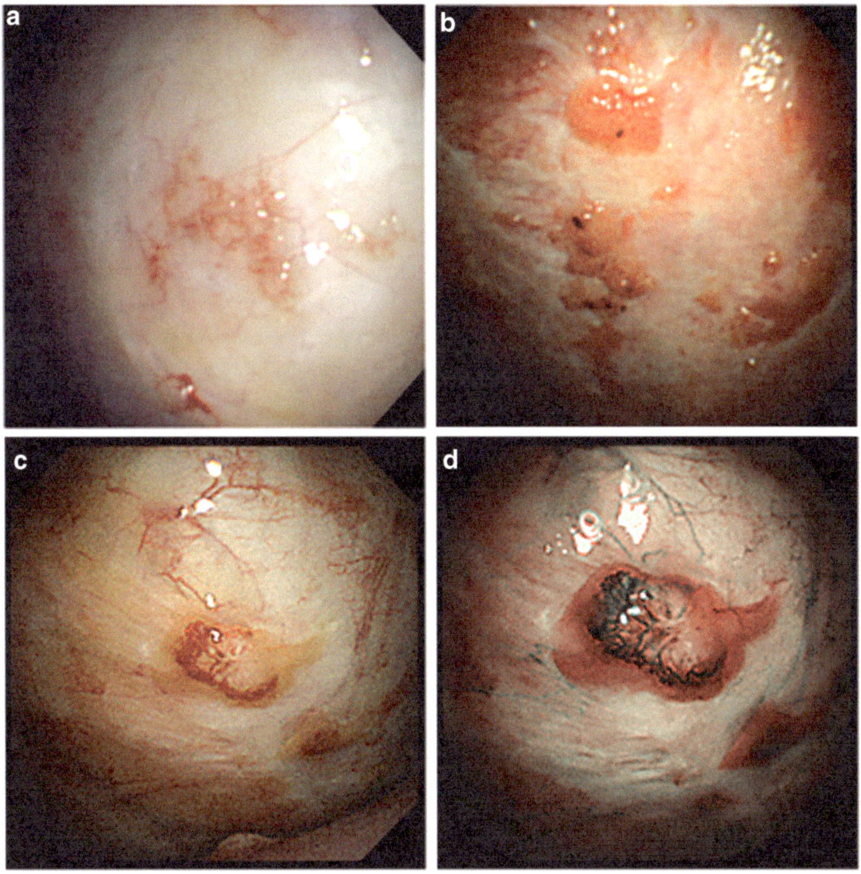

Fig. 25.13 Re-biopsy cases of EGFR mutation-positive (exon 19 deletion) lung adenocarcinoma after therapy with EGFR tyrosine kinase inhibitor. (**a**–**c**) Pleural thickening and scattered nodules with proliferation of blood vessels. (**d**) Narrow band imaging shows neovascularization

25.2 Patients with Dry Pleural Dissemination

25.2.1 Introduction

The British Thoracic Society guidelines on pleural diseases recommend that local anesthesia should generally be undertaken only for patients with radiologically confirmed pleural effusion [22]. Most patients who are suspected to have pleural dissemination with effusion undergo thoracentesis for diagnosis; however, pleural lesions without effusion are sometimes encountered and are referred to as dry pleural dissemination (DPD) [23]. In these patients, thoracentesis cannot be performed and the diagnostic option is limited to thoracoscopy or pleuroscopy. We assessed the diagnostic performance of flex-rigid pleuroscopy under local anesthesia in patients suspected to have DPD based on radiologic findings, in comparison with its performance in patients with pleural dissemination with effusion.

25.2.2 Subjects and Indication

In our series, 56 patients who underwent flex-rigid pleuroscopy from 2011 to 2013 were included [24]. All were suspected to have pleural dissemination and the indication for the procedure was either for diagnosis, staging, or re-biopsy. Forty patients presented with pleural effusion (wet group), whereas 16 patients had asymmetric pleural thickening, pleural nodules, or fissural nodules without pleural effusion on computed tomography (dry group) (Fig. 25.14). In the dry group, history of ipsilateral open lung surgery, extreme pleural thickening, and severe chronic obstructive pulmonary disease were contraindications to pleuroscopy.

25.2.3 Procedures

Lateral decubitus chest radiographs, chest CT scan, and linear-type ultrasonography are used to aid in the selection of an appropriate entry site. Particularly, in the dry group, the mobility between the parietal and visceral pleura during breathing (sliding sign) should be identified to ensure that there are no adhesions that could cause damage to the lung parenchyma during insertion of the trocar.

All procedures are performed in the operating room by one expert pulmonologist and two assistants. A single puncture technique is used. The patient is placed in the lateral decubitus position with the diseased side facing upward. After administration of local anesthesia with 1 % lidocaine, a 1–2 cm incision is performed, followed by blunt dissection through the muscle layers of the chest wall until the parietal pleura is exposed. During this procedure, anesthesia to the subcutaneous and muscle layers should be delivered adequately. Upon reaching the parietal pleura, gently strip it off using a Kocher clamp to avoid injury to the closely apposed visceral pleura. After dissection of the parietal pleura and confirmation of collapse of the affected lung, a disposable flexible trocar (8 mm inner diameter) is inserted carefully before proceeding with inspection of the thoracic cavity with the flex-rigid pleuroscope. Upon confirming the location of the pleural lesion, local anesthesia is administered by subpleural injection of 1 % lidocaine before taking a biopsy using alligator forceps.

The IT knife 2 may be used for thick pleura that is difficult to grasp using standard flexible forceps (SFF). Local anesthesia is administered similar to the method described in the previous paragraph; but this time, a pleural bulge is created. Following this, a pinhole is made through the bulge using coagulation forceps. The tip of the IT knife 2 is inserted into the hole, followed by a circular incision through

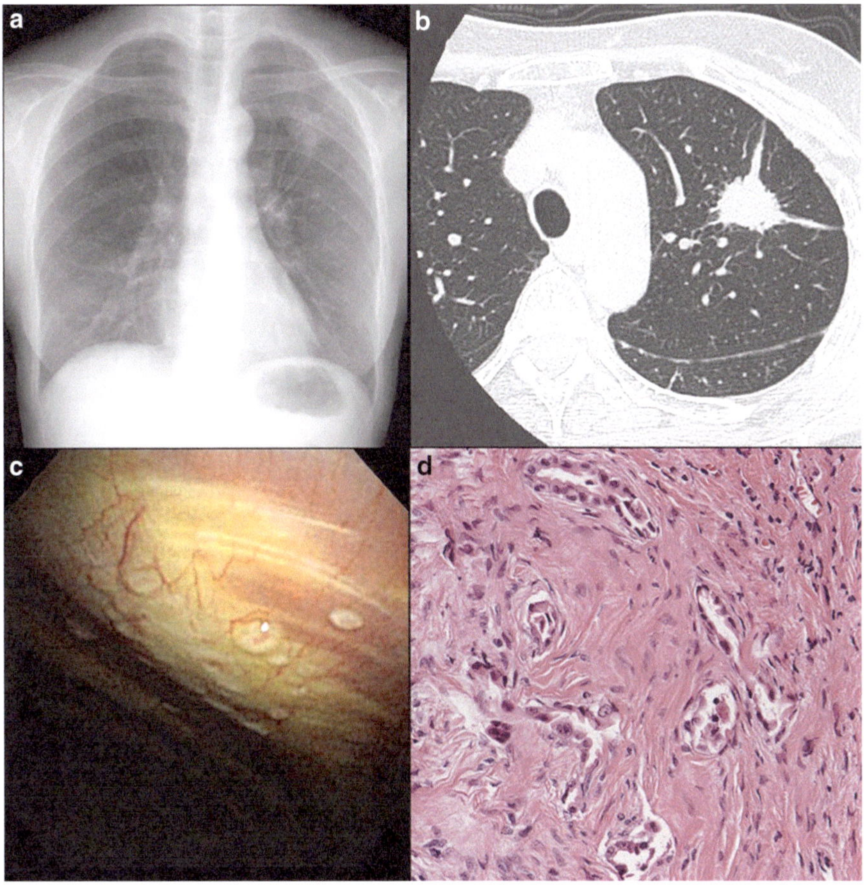

Fig. 25.14 Representative case with dry pleural dissemination. (**a**) Chest X-ray show a mass in the left upper lung field. (**b**) On chest computed tomography, a mass lesion with pleural indentation is seen in the left upper division segment. There is irregular thickening of the interlobar pleura. (**c**) Inspection by flex-rigid pleuroscopy shows small disseminated nodules on the parietal pleura. (**d**) Forceps biopsy specimen shows lung adenocarcinoma (hematoxylin–eosin stain, ×100)

the full thickness of the affected pleura using ENDO-CUT mode electric current at 30–40 W. The incised pleura is then carefully removed with forceps.

25.2.4 Results

The overall diagnostic accuracy in our series was 93.8 % (15/16). Eighty percent of the cases in the dry group were malignant in etiology and included adenocarcinoma from primary lung cancer (83 %) and malignant pleural mesothelioma (MPM) (17 %). One suspected case of MPM was confirmed by pleural re-biopsy under

Table 25.2 Baseline characteristics of patients who underwent pleuroscopy ($n = 56$)

Dry group ($n = 16$)		Wet group ($n = 40$)	p-value
Complications			
Present	2 (13 %)	5 (13 %)	0.66
Absent	14 (87 %)	35 (87 %)	
Operation time (min)			
Mean ± SD	55.3 ± 15.4	58.2 ± 15.9	0.54
Instrument			
SFF	13 (81 %)	27 (68 %)	NS
SFF + IT knife 2	3 (19 %)	13 (32 %)	
Definitive diagnosis			
Success	15 (94 %)	39 (98 %)	0.49
Failure	1 (6 %)	1 (2 %)	

SD standard deviation, *SFF* standard flexible forceps, *IT* insulated tip

general anesthesia. The mean operation duration was 55.3 + 15.4 min. Only two cases had minor complications, including transient hypoxia and mild chest pain. There were no major complications, such as intrathoracic hemorrhage, re-expansion pulmonary edema, or procedure-related death. Drainage by chest tube was continued for a mean duration of 2.31 + 2.26 days; in 69 % (11/16) of the cases, the chest tube was removed on postoperative day 1. The additional use of the IT knife 2 for biopsy was superior to SFF alone in 3 of 16 patients (MPM in two and chronic inflammation in one). In comparison to the wet group (Table 25.2), the dry group did not statistically differ in terms of diagnostic accuracy, operation duration, or complications.

25.2.5 Conclusions

Flex-rigid pleuroscopy under local anesthesia is an efficient and safe diagnostic procedure for radiographic dry pleural dissemination. Because of the higher risk of damaging the lungs during trocar insertion, compared with cases with pleural effusion, ultrasound guidance is important.

25.3 Pleuroscopic Punch Biopsy Using Insulated-Tip Diathermic Knife 2

25.3.1 Introduction

Malignant pleural mesothelioma (MPM) is a mesodermal malignancy of the pleura that is most commonly caused by exposure to asbestos. Desmoplastic malignant mesothelioma (DMM) is a rare subtype of MPM that must be distinguished from chronic fibrous pleuritis for appropriate treatment. However, this can be difficult, particularly on small biopsy samples [25, 26]. Therefore, a biopsy sample of adequate size must be obtained so that an accurate diagnosis can be made. The gastrointestinal electrosurgical knife, an insulated-tip diathermic knife (IT knife), has been demonstrated to be useful for the diagnosis of unknown pleural lesions with thick and smooth abnormalities [19]. From our experience, diagnostic yield from full-thickness pleural biopsy specimens obtained with the IT knife and flexible forceps were 85 % (17 of 20 cases) and 60 % (12 of 20 cases), respectively [17]. IT knife biopsy was superior to flexible forceps biopsy in 8 of 20 patients (malignant pleural mesothelioma in three, nonspecific inflammation in two, metastatic breast cancer in one, and tuberculosis in one). However, the use of IT knife is not always successful in obtaining tissue, especially in extremely dense lesions. IT knife 2 (Olympus, Tokyo, Japan) is a novel electrosurgical device for endoscopic submucosal dissection for early gastrointestinal cancer; it consists of a needle knife with three short blades attached to an insulated ceramic tip (Fig. 25.15) [27]. In this chapter, we describe the utility of pleuroscopic punch biopsy using the IT knife 2 in patients with densely thick pleura.

25.3.2 Pleuroscopic Punch Biopsy Procedures

The procedure is performed under local anesthesia using a flex-rigid pleuroscope (LTF-260, Olympus, Tokyo, Japan) (Figs. 25.16 and 25.17) [28, 29]. The patient is placed in the lateral decubitus position, with the diseased side facing upward. The incision site is anywhere along the fifth to the eight intercostal spaces at the midaxillary line. After administration of local anesthesia with 1 % lidocaine, a 1–2 cm incision is performed, followed by blunt dissection through the muscle layers of the chest wall until the parietal pleura is exposed. During this procedure, deliver anesthesia to the subcutaneous and muscle layers adequately. After dissection of the parietal pleura and confirmation of collapse of the affected lung, an 8-mm flexible trocar is inserted using the single puncture technique.

The flex-rigid pleuroscope is then introduced into the chest cavity for surveillance of the parietal pleura (Fig. 25.17a). If forceps biopsy is difficult because of dense thickening of the pleura, IT knife 2 may be chosen to perform electrosurgical pleural biopsy. Upon confirming the biopsy site, local anesthesia with 1 % lidocaine and epinephrine is injected into the subpleural layer to raise the parietal pleura (Fig. 25.17b). Then, with the use of coagulation forceps or a high-frequency knife, make a pinhole through the bulge (Fig. 25.17c), into which the tip of the IT knife 2 is inserted before performing a circular incision through the full thickness of the affected pleura while applying ENDO-CUT mode electric current at 30–50 W (Fig. 25.17d, e). Finally, the incised piece of pleura is collected by grasping forceps (Fig. 25.17f, g). The median time of a pleuroscopic punch biopsy procedure, from the first pleural injection to specimen removal, is around 20 min; the median largest diameter of the specimen is 10–20 mm. Mild pleural bleeding and chest pain may

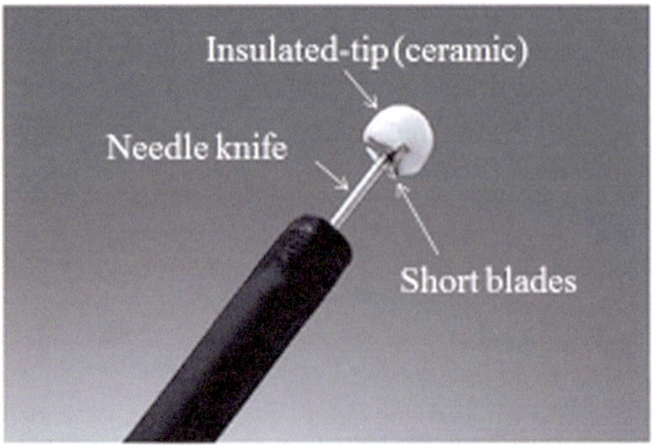

Fig. 25.15 Insulated-tip diathermic knife 2 (Olympus, Tokyo, Japan)

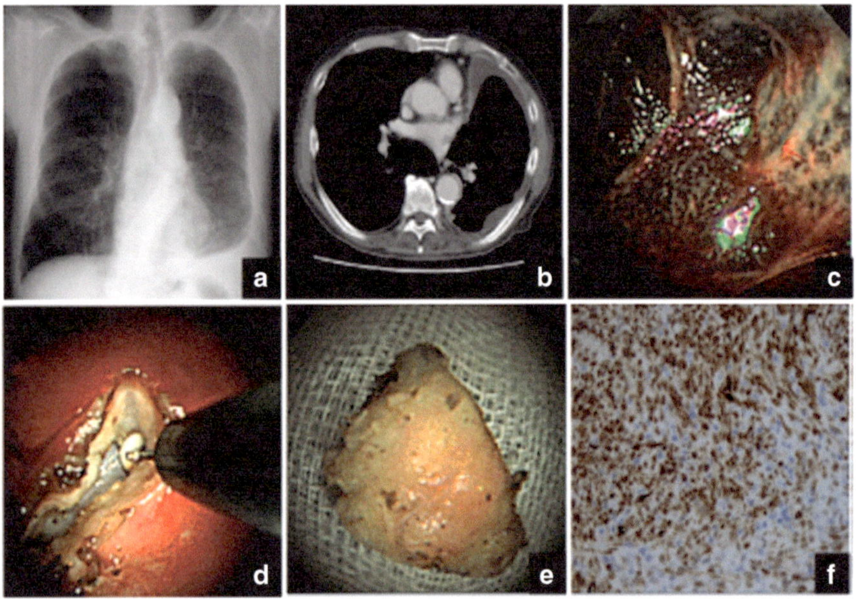

Fig. 25.16 Sarcomatoid malignant pleural mesothelioma confirmed by full-thickness biopsy specimen. (**a**, **b**) Radiologic images indicate encapsulated, left-sided pleural effusion and pleural thickening, with involvement of the mediastinal pleura. (**c**) On pleuroscopy, there are diffuse and dense fibrosis of the pleura, hypervascularization, and extensive fibrous adhesions within the thoracic cavity. (**d**) The tip of the IT knife 2 is inserted below the parietal pleura; the short blades are hooked under the pleura. (**e**) Full-thickness biopsy specimen with a size of 12×8×4 mm is obtained. (**f**) Immunocytochemistry demonstrates strongly positive Wilms tumor susceptibility gene (*WT1*) staining of the nuclear area, findings that are suggestive of malignant mesothelioma (×400)

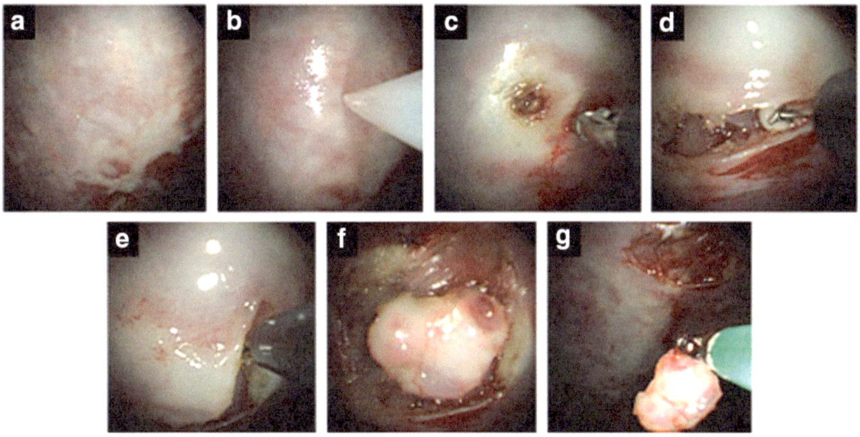

Fig. 25.17 Techniques of pleuroscopic punch biopsy in a case with desmoplastic malignant pleural mesothelioma. (**a**) Whitish and thick pleura is seen on pleuroscopy. (**b**) Subpleural needle injection of lidocaine plus epinephrine solution to create a bulge. (**c**) A pinhole is created through the bulge using coagulation forceps. (**d**) Pleural incision by the IT knife 2; the endothoracic fascia just above the muscle layer should always be kept in view while doing the incision. (**e**) Circumferential pleural incision while applying heat energy. (**f**) The completed circular-shaped incision. (**g**) Peeling by standard flexible forceps

be observed as common complications. In our series, there have been no severe complications experienced during the procedure [17, 19, 28, 29].

25.3.3 Results

A total of 17 patients with undiagnosed thick pleural abnormality who underwent pleuroscopic punch biopsy using IT knife 2 during flex-rigid pleuroscopy under local anesthesia were included in the study from January 2012 to December 2014 (Table 25.3). The patients comprised ten men and seven women, with median age of 68 years (range, 41–79 years). Specimens were separately taken by two devices, IT knife 2 and flexible forceps, from the same patient; the pathologic findings were compared between the two devices. The diagnostic yield with IT knife 2 was significantly higher than that with flexible forceps [94.1% (16/17) vs. 29.4% (5/17); $p=0.0026$; McNemar's test].

Table 25.3 Comparison between IT knife 2 and flexible forceps for pleuroscopic punch biopsy in patients with undiagnosed and thick pleural abnormalities ($n = 17$)

No	Age	Sex	Final diagnosis	Flexible forceps	IT knife 2	Complication
1	41	M	MPM (epithelial)	Failure	Success	None
2	48	F	MPM (biphasic)	Failure	Success	None
3	51	F	MPM (sarcomatous)	Failure	Failure	None
4	51	M	MPM (sarcomatous)	Failure	Success	None
5	54	M	MPM (sarcomatous)	Failure	Success	None
6	63	F	Desmoplastic malignant mesothelioma	Failure	Success	None
7	65	M	Lung cancer (adenocarcinoma)	Failure	Success	Chest pain
8	67	F	Lung cancer (adenocarcinoma)	Success	Success	Success
9	68	M	Lung cancer (adenocarcinoma)	Success	Success	None
10	69	M	Lung cancer (adenocarcinoma)	Success	Success	None
11	70	M	Lung cancer (adenocarcinoma)	Success	Success	None
12	71	F	Lung cancer (adenocarcinoma)	Success	Success	None
13	72	M	Lung cancer (adenocarcinoma)	Failure	Success	None
14	74	M	Lung cancer (adenocarcinoma)	Failure	Success	None
15	75	F	Metastatic breast cancer	Failure	Success	None
16	77	M	Chronic pleuritis	Failure	Success	None
17	79	F	Fibrous pleuritis	Failure	Success	None

Diagnostic yield with IT knife 2 was significantly higher than that with flexible forceps [94.1 % (16/17) vs. 29.4 % (5/17); $p = 0.0026$; McNemar's test]
MPM malignant pleural mesothelioma

25.3.4 Tips

The biggest reason for unsuccessful pleuroscopic punch biopsy is insufficient creation of the pinhole before cutting by IT knife 2. The pinhole should be thoroughly examined inside by bluntly expanding the hole using the IT knife 2 before applying heat current. If the endothoracic fascia or if adipose tissue with outflow of fat droplets is observed, complete penetration of the affected pleura is confirmed. If insufficient, repeat the process of injection and creation of a pinhole. For success, the tip of the IT knife 2 should be slipped just above the endothoracic fascia and hook the short blades to the pleura, then incise with an image of lifting the pleura obliquely (Fig. 25.18). If lifting the pleura is not enough, the patient may feel pain from stimulation of intercostal muscles during heat energy application. These being said, it is most essential to recognize the normal structures of the chest wall during the procedure.

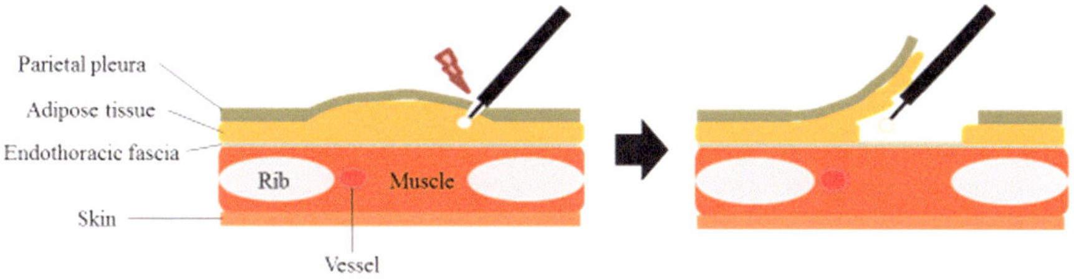

Fig. 25.18 Schematic diagram of pleuroscopic punch biopsy using IT knife 2

25.3.5 Conclusion

Pleuroscopic punch biopsy using IT knife 2 is a feasible technique for successful diagnosis of undiagnosed pleural disease. We have observed that the IT knife 2 can be used to obtain full-thickness samples from densely thick abnormal pleural lesions, including DMM, which are difficult to diagnose with small biopsies using flexible forceps biopsy.

References

1. Poe RH, Israel RH, Utell MJ, et al. Sensitivity, specificity, and predictive values of closed pleural biopsy. Arch Intern Med. 1984;144:325–8.
2. Prakash UBS, Relman H. Comparison of needle biopsy with cytologic analysis for the evaluation of pleural effusion: analysis of 414 cases. Mayo Clin Proc. 1985;60:158–64.
3. McLean AN, Stephen RB, Lawrence GM, Andrew JP. Investigation of pleural effusion: an evaluation of the new Olympus LTF semiflexible thoracofiberscope and comparison with Abram's needle knife. Chest. 1998;114:150–3.
4. Boutin C, Viallat JR, Cargnino P, Farisse P. Thoracoscopy in malignant pleural effusions. Am Rev Respir Dis. 1981;124:588–92.
5. Canto A, Blasco E, Casillas M, et al. Thoracoscopy in the diagnosis of pleural effusion. Thorax. 1977;32:550–4.
6. Weissberg D, Kaufmann M. Diagnostic and therapeutic pleuroscopy. Experience with 27 patients. Chest. 1980;78:732–5.
7. Senno A, Moallem S, Quijano ER, et al. Thoracoscopy with the fiberoptic bronchoscope. A simple method in diagnosing pleuropulmonary diseases. J Thorac Cardiovasc Surg. 1974;67:601–11.
8. Gunnels JJ. Perplexing pleural effusion. Chest. 1978;74:390–3.
9. Ben Isaac FE, Simmons DH. Flexible fiberoptic pleuroscopy: pleural and lung biopsy. Chest. 1975;67:573–6.
10. Kerby GR, Pierce G, Ruth WE. Clinical experience with pleuroscopy utilizing the bronchofiberscope. Ann Otol. 1975;84:602–6.
11. Oldenburg FA, Newhouse MT. Thoracoscopy. A safe, accurate diagnostic procedure using the rigid thoracoscope and local anesthesia. Chest. 1979;75:45–50.
12. Ash SR, Manfredi F. Directed biopsy using a small endoscope. Thoracoscopy and peritoneoscopy simplified. N Engl J Med. 1974;291:1398–9.
13. Boushy SF, North LB, Helgason AH. Thoracoscopy: technique and results in eighteen patients with pleural effusion. Chest. 1974;4:386–9.

14. Ernst A, Hersh CP, Herth F, Thurer R, LoCicero III J, Beamis J, Mathur P. A novel instrument for the evaluation of the pleural space: an experience in 34 patients. Chest. 2002;122:1530–4.
15. Sakuraba M, Masuda K, Hebisawa A, Sagara Y, Komatsu H. Diagnostic value of thoracoscopic pleural biopsy for pleurisy under local anesthesia. ANZ J Surg. 2006;76:722–4.
16. Munavvar M, Khan MAI, Edwards J, Waqaruddin Z, Mills J. The autoclavable semi-rigid thoracoscope: the way forward in pleural diseases? Eur Respir J. 2007;29:571–4.
17. Sasada S, Kawahara K, Kusunoki Y, et al. A new electrocautery pleural biopsy technique using an insulated-tip diathermic knife during semi-rigid pleuroscopy. Surg Endosc. 2009;23:1901–7.
18. Masai K, Sasada S, Izumo T, et al. Pleuroscopic punch biopsy using insulated-tip diathermic knife-2 for the diagnosis of desmoplastic malignant mesothelioma. J Bronchol Interv Pulmonol. 2013;20:345–8.
19. Sasada S, Kawahara K, Iwasaki T, et al. An electrocautery pleural biopsy for the diagnosis of desmoplastic malignant mesothelioma during semi-rigid thoracoscopy. J Thorac Oncol. 2008;3:803–4.
20. Butnor KJ. My approach to the diagnosis of mesothelial lesions. J Clin Pathol. 2006;59:564–74.
21. Ishida A, Ishikawa F, Nakamura M, et al. Narrow band imaging applied to pleuroscopy for the assessment of vascular patterns of the pleura. Respiration. 2009;78:432–9.
22. Rahman NM, Ali NJ, Brown G, et al. Local anaesthetic thoracoscopy: British Thoracic Society Pleural Disease Guideline 2010. Thorax. 2010;65 Suppl 2:ii54–60. 9.
23. Kim YK, Lee HY, Lee KS, et al. Dry pleural dissemination in non-small cell lung cancer: prognostic and diagnostic implications. Radiology. 2011;260:568–74.
24. Watanabe Y, Sasada S, Chavez C, et al. Flex-rigid pleuroscopy under local anesthesia in patients with dry pleural dissemination on radiography. Jpn J Clin Oncol. 2014;44:749–55.
25. Mangano WE, Cagle PT, Churg A, et al. The diagnosis of desmoplastic malignant mesothelioma and its distinction from fibrous pleurisy: a histologic and immunohistochemical analysis of 31 cases including p53. Am J Clin Pathol. 1998;110:191–9. 3.
26. Churg A, Galateau-Salle F. The separation of benign and malignant mesothelial proliferations. Arch Pathol Lab Med. 2012;136:1217–26.
27. Ono H, Kondo H, Gotoda T, et al. Endoscopic mucosal resection for treatment of early gastric cancer. Gut. 2001;48:225–9.
28. Deng CS, Sasada S, Izumo T, et al. Sarcomatoid malignant pleural mesothelioma confirmed by full-thickness biopsy. Chin Med J. 2013;126:3391–2.
29. Masai K, Sasada S, Izumo T, et al. Pleuroscopic punch biopsy using insulated-tip diathermic knife-2 for the diagnosis of desmoplastic malignant mesothelioma. J Bronchol Intervent Pulmonol. 2013;20:345–8.

Chapter 26
Stent Placement Under X-Ray Fluoroscopy

Shinji Sasada

Abstract Airway stenosis may occur in both benign and malignant diseases, but is most often due to lung cancer. Stent placement is carried out properly with the use of the flexible and/or rigid bronchoscopes. Close cooperation of respiratory physician, respiratory surgeon, radiologist, and anesthesiologists is essential.

Keywords Airway stent • Flexible bronchoscope • Rigid bronchoscope

26.1 Introduction

The goal of intervention in patients with airway obstruction is symptom relief. In a prospective study, airway intervention has improved dyspnea in 85 % and quality of life in 65 % [1]. There was also a report that showed control of hemoptysis in 94 % of patients [2]. However, there has been no clear evidence that airway intervention improves survival rate. Patients who received chemoradiation therapy after airway intervention have been reported to have a median survival of 12.1 months [3]. Nevertheless, all patients with central airway obstruction should be recognized high risk; the complication rate 30 days after airway intervention was 19.8 % and the reported mortality rate was 7.8 % [4].

26.2 Types and Causes of Airway Obstruction

Central airway obstruction can be divided into three types (Fig. 26.1):

1. Endoluminal obstruction
2. Extrinsic compression
3. Mixed stenosis

S. Sasada (✉)
Department of Respiratory Medicine, Tokyo Saiseikai Central Hospital,
1-4-17, Mita, Minato-ku, Tokyo 108-0073, Japan
e-mail: sasastaf@hotmail.co.jp

T. Izumo et al. (eds.), *Respiratory Endoscopy*,
DOI 10.1007/978-981-287-916-5_26

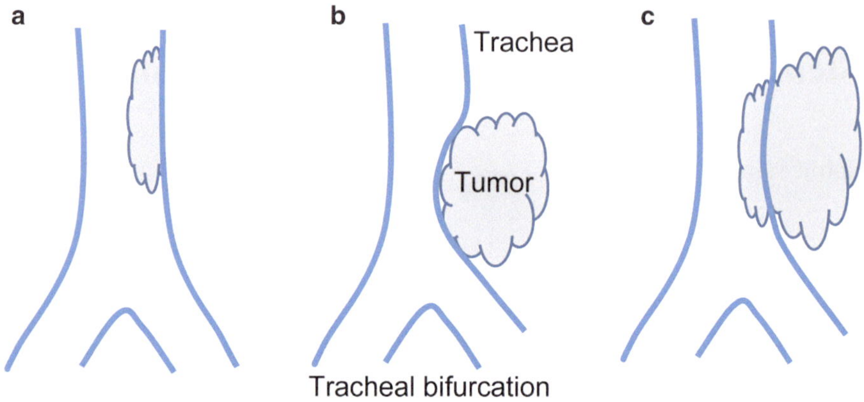

Fig. 26.1 Types of airway obstruction. (**a**) Endoluminal obstruction. (**b**) Extrinsic compression. (**c**) Mixed stenosis

The most common disease that causes central airway obstruction is primary lung cancer (squamous cell carcinoma, adenoid cystic carcinoma, mucoepidermoid carcinoma, carcinoid, etc.), followed by metastatic lung cancer (thyroid cancer, colon cancer, breast cancer, renal cell carcinoma, and malignant melanoma, such as Kaposi's sarcoma) and malignant tumors surrounding the airway (esophageal cancer, laryngeal cancer, and mediastinal tumors, such as malignant lymphoma) [5]. In recent years, the incidence of lung cancer has increased; therefore, the need for pulmonologists who specialize in airway intervention also increases.

26.3 Preparation for Airway Intervention

Prior bronchoscopic inspection of a malignant airway obstruction is important to confirm the area of invasion and the type of tumor. Since it is possible that a large bronchoscope (outer diameter, 6 mm) cannot be inserted beyond the stenosis, a thin bronchoscope (outer diameter, 4 mm) or an ultrathin bronchoscope (outer diameter, 2.8–3.5 mm) should be used. Next, determine whether the needed airway intervention (e.g., balloon, electrocautery, argon plasma coagulation, and stent) according to the extent of a lesion necessitates the use of flexible bronchoscope under local anesthesia or the rigid bronchoscope under general anesthesia.

26.4 Usefulness of the Rigid Bronchoscope (Fig. 26.2)

The greatest benefit of airway dilatation and stenting using a rigid bronchoscope for central airway obstruction is that it enables application of treatment procedures under sufficient and secure airway ventilation. Since airway treatment procedures (tissue coagulation or ablation) with flexible bronchoscopy under local anesthesia

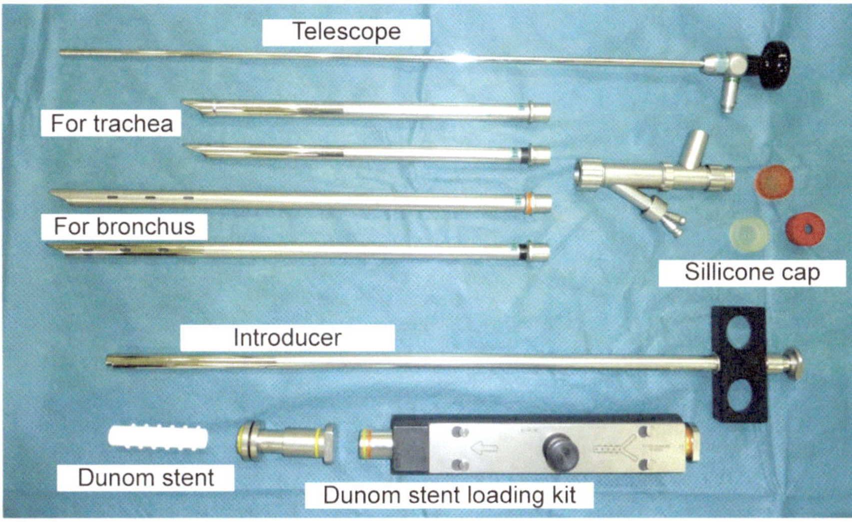

Fig. 26.2 Equipment and setup for rigid bronchoscopy. Rigid bronchoscope set (EFER-DUMON®, Novatech, La Ciotat, France). Rigid bronchoscopy under general anesthesia in the operating room. Cooperation with anesthesiologists is essential

may be distressful for patients, there is a risk for insufficient treatment or severe complications (bronchial damage or suffocation due to airway bleeding). Other advantages of using a rigid bronchoscope are direct hemostasis of a bleeding site and fast relief of airway obstruction by mechanical excision of a larger portion of a tumor with the use of the tip of the rigid bronchoscope (core out).

26.5 Indications for Airway Stenting

1. Progression of airway obstruction that continues to compromise the airway despite other treatment modalities.
2. Unstable airway status.
3. Respiratory symptoms, such as difficulty of breathing, secondary to airway obstruction of 50 %, or more.
4. Estimated survival time is expected to be more than 4 weeks.
5. Lung function is expected to improve after stent placement

26.6 Self-Expandable Metallic Stents

Ultraflex stent has two types, covered and uncovered (Fig. 26.3). The use of covered stent is desired to prevent tumor infiltration into the lumen or to close a tracheo-esophageal fistula. Ultraflex stent® is wound around a delivery catheter in a folded

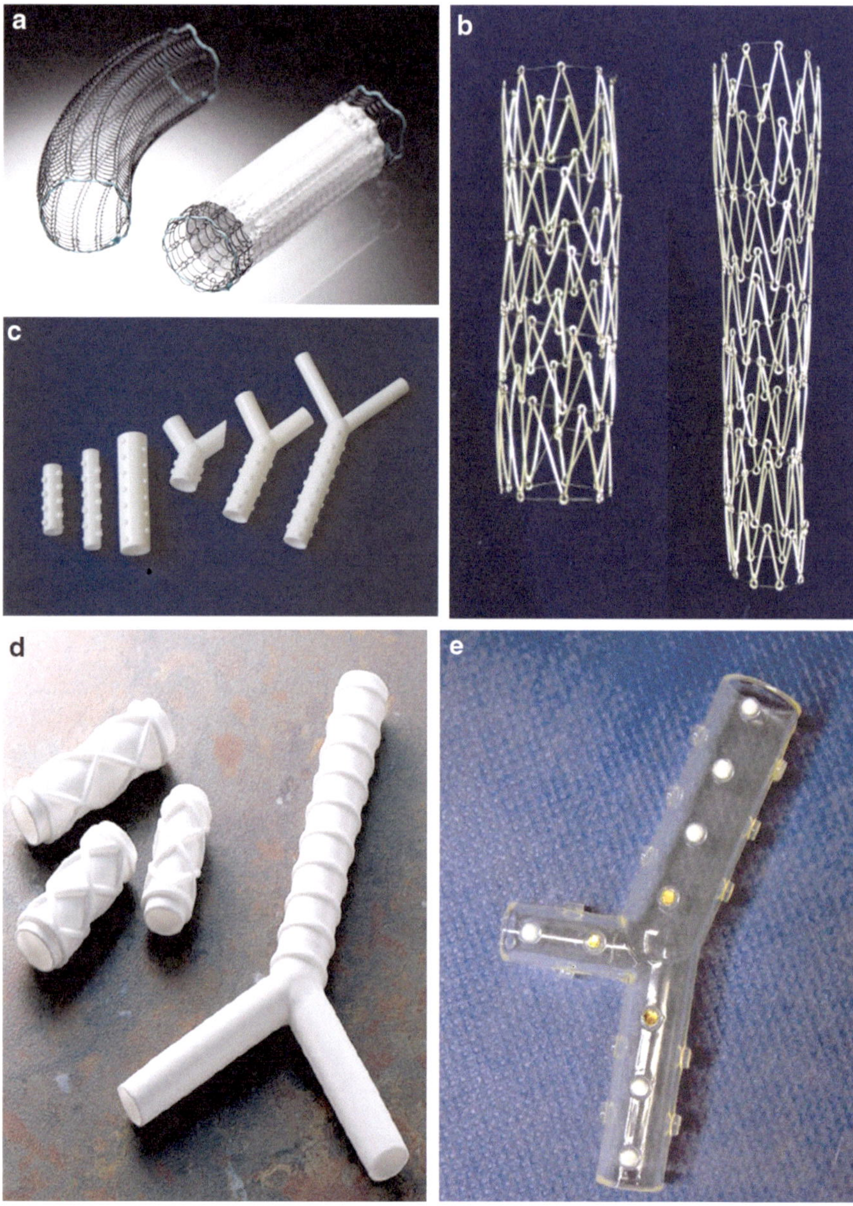

Fig. 26.3 Various types of airway stent. (**a**) Ultraflex stent® (covered or uncovered, Boston Scientific, Natick, Massachusetts, USA). (**b**) Spiral Z stent® (straight or tapered, Medico's Hirata, Osaka, Japan). (**c**) Dumon stent® (straight or Y type, Novatech, La Ciotat, France). (**d**) TM stent® (straight or Y type, Fuji Systems Corp., Tokyo, Japan). (**e**) OKI stent ® (Novatech, La Ciotat, France).

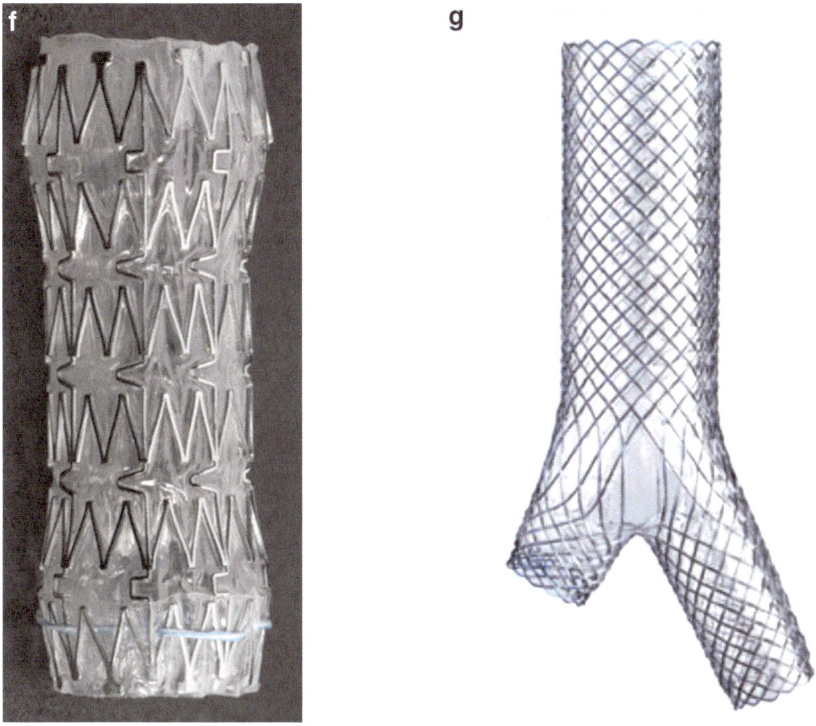

Fig. 26.3 (continued) (**f**) AERO stent® (Alveolus, Inc., NC, USA). (**g**) Leufen Aerstent® (Kapitex Healthcare Ltd., West Yorkshire. England)

state and can be released by pulling a thread. Although its deployment is simple, there is a risk of misplacement when the stent is compressed or deviated at the time of release. When one third of the stent has been released, the appropriate sites for placement can be derived under X-ray fluoroscopy [6].

Spiral Z stent® only has the uncovered type, unlike the Ultraflex stent® (Fig. 26.3). The stent configuration may be straight or with small tapering at the distal end, compared with the proximal end; it is also possible to place a single but long tracheobronchial stent. Precise deployment is easy with the use of the push method. Since the introducer also serves as a dilator, Spiral Z stent® insertion without predilatation may be possible, even if the narrowing is pinhole, if a guide wire can be passed through the stenosis (Fig. 26.4).

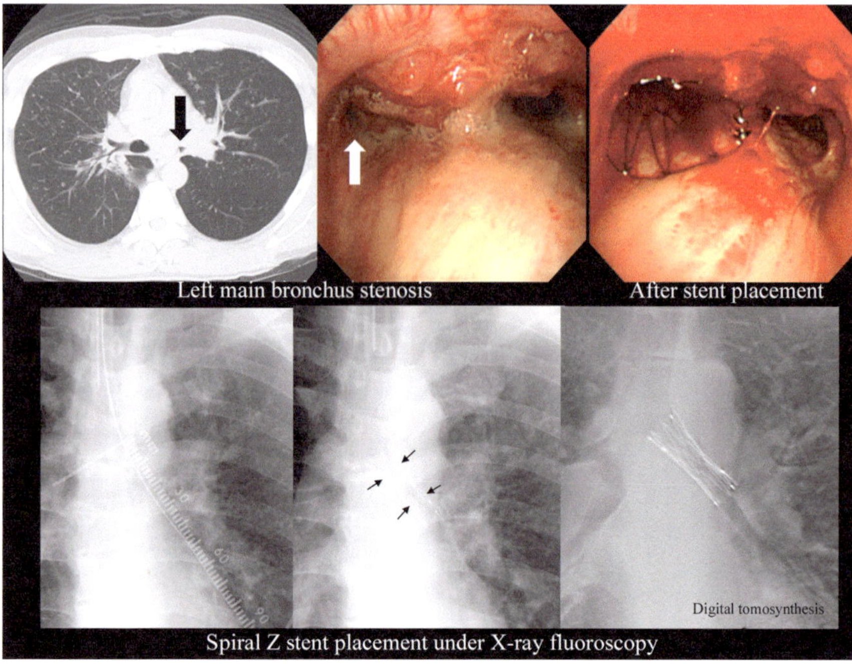

Fig. 26.4 A patient with severe stenosis of the left main bronchus due to lung cancer. There was dramatic improvement of the respiratory condition after spiral Z stent® placement

26.7 Silicone Stent

Silicone stents (Fig. 26.3), such as the Dumon stent® and TM stent®, are used for the purpose of keeping the central airway lumen patent against a tumor-infiltrating stenosis or obstruction. A stent placement kit that is dedicated for use with the rigid bronchoscope is needed. Silicone stents are mixed with barium for visualization under X-ray fluoroscopy and have studs on the surface to prevent migration. Before stent placement, there is a need for pre-dilatation by laser ablation, balloon dilatation, or coring out because the silicone stent is not self-expanding. For tracheal bifurcation stenosis, silicone Y stents are preferred (Fig. 26.5). Deformation Y-type silicone stent (OKI stent®) can be used for stenosis of the right main bronchus to the bifurcation of the intermediate bronchus [7].

26.8 Hybrid Stent

Hybrid stent (AERO stent®) is made of a combination of memory-shaping material, such as nitinol, and another material, such as silicone or artificial blood vessels (Fig. 26.3). Unlike silicone stent, a hybrid stent may be placed without the need for rigid bronchoscope. The greatest feature of this stent is that it can be withdrawn as needed. In recent years, a hybrid Y stent (Leufen Aerstent®) has also become available.

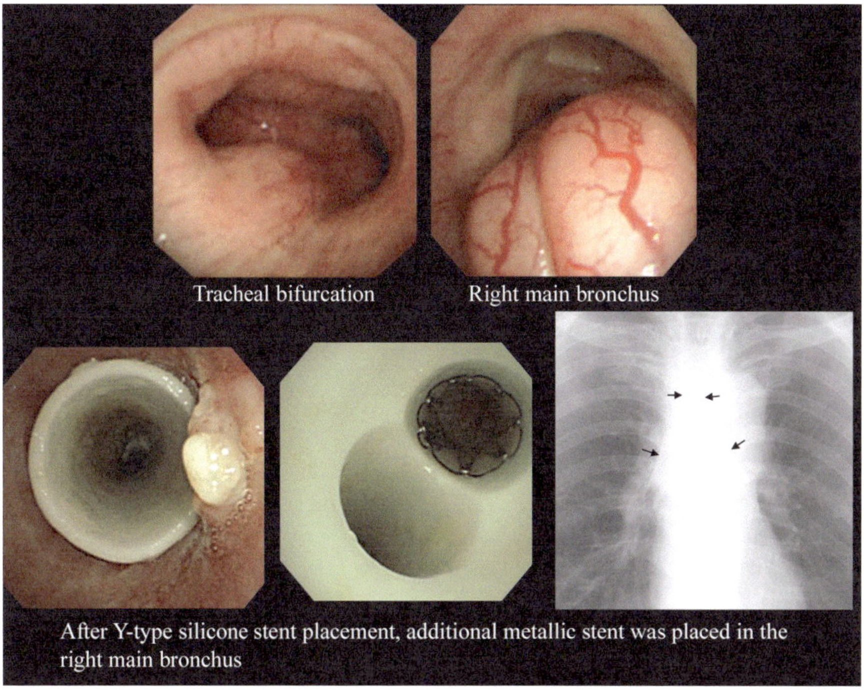

Fig. 26.5 Tracheal bifurcation stenosis due to adenoid cystic carcinoma

References

1. Amjadi K, Voduc N, Cruysberghs Y, et al. Impact of interventional bronchoscopy on quality of life in malignant airway obstruction. Respiration. 2008;76:421–8.
2. Hans CC, Prasetyo D, Wright GM. Endobronchial palliation using Nd:YAG laser is associated with improved survival when combined with multimodal adjuvant treatments. J Thorac Oncol. 2007;2:59–64.
3. Venuta F, Rendina EA, De Giacomo T, et al. Nd-YAG laser resection of lung cancer invading the airway as a bridge to surgery and palliative treatment. Ann Thorac Surg. 2002;74:995–8.
4. Ernst A, Simoff M, Ost D, et al. Prospective risk-adjusted morbidity and mortality outcome analysis after therapeutic bronchoscopy procedures. Results of multi-institutional outcomes database. Chest. 2008;134:514–9.
5. Hadique S, Jain P, Metha AC. Therapeutic bronchoscopy for central airway obstruction. Interventional Bronchoscopy: a clinical guide, respiratory medicine. New York: Springer Science + Business Media; 2013. p. 143–76.
6. Sasada S. Oncologic emergency, airway stenosis. Kokyu. 2014;33:990–7.
7. Oki M, Saka H. New dedicated bifurcated silicone stent placement for stenosis around the primary right carina. Chest. 2013;144:450–5.

Chapter 27
Therapeutic Bronchoscopy for Central Airway Obstruction (Balloon, Argon Plasma Coagulation, High Frequency)

Yukio Watanabe and Shinji Sasada

Abstract Central airway obstruction from the trachea to the segmental bronchi is an indication for therapeutic bronchoscopy. It is important to understand the techniques, advantages, and disadvantages of each procedure. Noting the accompanying serious risk in any treatment modality, the bronchoscopist should always be prepared in managing the worst scenario.

Keywords Airway intervention • Balloon • Argon plasma coagulation • High-frequency devices • Nd-YAG laser

27.1 Indications

Central airway obstruction from the trachea to the segmental bronchi is an indication for therapeutic bronchoscopy. Endoluminal obstruction or mixed stenoses from the following etiologies are indications for ablation, such as argon plasma coagulation (APC), electrocautery, etc.

1. Neoplastic lesions (lung cancer, esophageal cancer, thyroid cancer, and benign tumors, such as hamartomas)
2. Scarring (granulomatous) lesions and stenosis (after intubation, after tracheotomy, after bronchial deformation, endobronchial tuberculosis, after radiation therapy)

Y. Watanabe
Division of General Thoracic Surgery, National Cancer Center Hospital, Tokyo, Japan

S. Sasada (✉)
Department of Respiratory Medicine, Tokyo Saiseikai Central Hospital,
1-4-17, Mita, Minato-ku, Tokyo 108-0073, Japan
e-mail: sasastaf@hotmail.co.jp

T. Izumo et al. (eds.), *Respiratory Endoscopy*,
DOI 10.1007/978-981-287-916-5_27

27.2 Balloon Dilatation

Balloon dilatation for airway stenosis was first reported by Cohen et al. in 1984 [1] and has since been applied to manage stenotic lesions due to various diseases. First, place a marker under X-ray fluoroscopy to identify the site of stenosis while doing flexible bronchoscopy. Then, a guide wire is passed through the channel of the bronchoscope to the area of stenosis. The bronchoscope is then withdrawn while leaving the guide wire in place, as confirmed under X-ray fluoroscopy. After confirming the position of the balloon under fluoroscopic guidance, inflate the balloon using a dedicated device. Care should be taken to adjust the amount of inflation, depending on the degree and location of the stenosis, in order to prevent excessive pressure that may cause rupture of the tracheobronchial mucosa (especially the membranous part). In tracheal stenosis, administration of sufficient oxygen prior to balloon dilation would lessen the expansion time as short as possible. Adding contrast medium into the balloon will enable easy visibility under X-ray fluoroscopy.

27.3 Argon Plasma Coagulation (Fig. 27.1)

APC is a method of applying heat to tissue using argon plasma that is ionized by high-frequency current [2, 3]. Indications are for ablation of tracheobronchial lesions that cause airway compression or obstruction and for coagulation hemostasis of airway bleeding. APC is suitable for a tangentially directed ablation. The

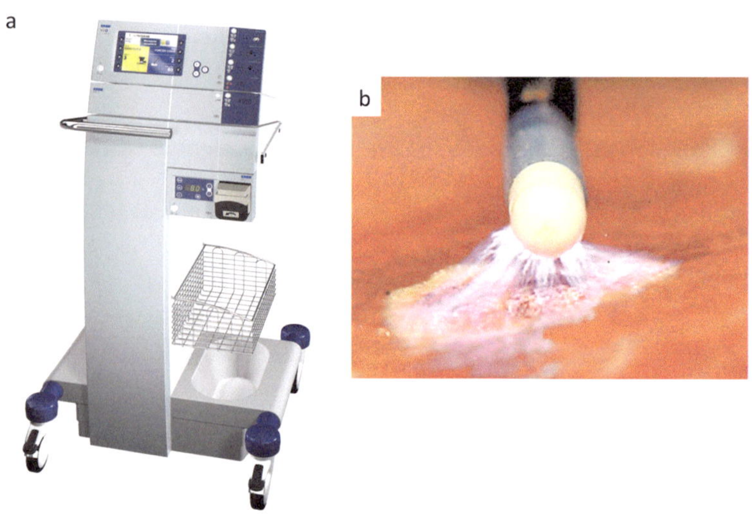

Fig. 27.1 Equipment for APC. (**a**) Electric current generator (VIO300D, Erbe Elektromedizin, Tuebingen, Germany). (**b**) The tip of the APC probe enables ablation in the tangential direction. *APC* argon plasma coagulation

actual procedure is a contact-free heat application at an output 30–50 W, within a 5-mm distance from the lesion, that is, repeated once every few seconds. Oxygen supplementation is reduced to less than 40 % FiO_2 in order to prevent fire or combustible flames. In addition, the APC probe should have a distance of at least 1 cm from the scope tip in order to prevent breakage of the CCD of the videoscope tip. Since the depth of tissue invasion by the ablation is weaker than that of a high-power laser, APC takes more time to achieve ablation.

27.4 High-Frequency Snare (Fig. 27.2)

This device may be applied for resection of a tracheobronchial polypoid tumor (Fig. 27.3) [4]. Check the stalk of the polyp-like tumor by bronchoscopy. Then, hook the tumor stalk with the snare, followed by application of a high-frequency

Fig. 27.2 High-frequency snare

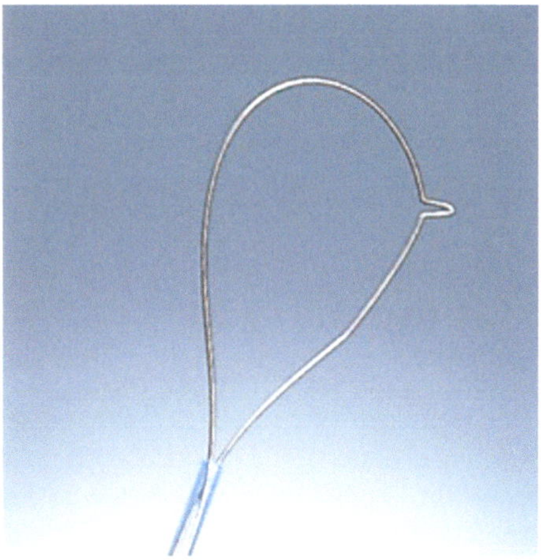

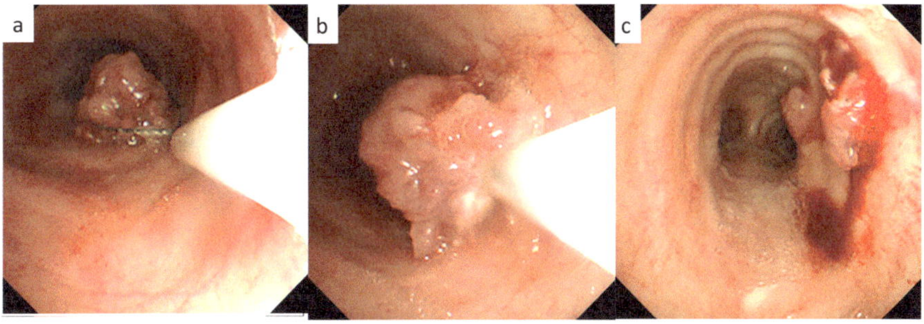

Fig. 27.3 Metastatic lung adenocarcinoma of the trachea treated by high-frequency snare. (**a**) Loop the fully open snare around the tumor base. (**b**) Close the snare while applying thermal energy to incise the tumor base. (**c**) The partial obstruction is reduced after resection

current (30–50 W) to generate heat energy. Avoid prolonged application of the high-frequency current; instead, use short repeated applications every 1–3 s. After dissection, remove the tumor with the use of a grasping forceps or by suctioning with the bronchoscope. A large tumor can be easily removed with basket forceps. It is possible to reduce bleeding after resection by mechanically blocking the tumor blood vessels a few seconds before turning on the power.

27.5 High-Frequency Probe, Coagulation Biopsy Forceps, High-Frequency Knife (Fig. 27.4)

These devices are applied for hemostasis and tumor ablation and to dilate a stenosis. High-frequency probes are used to perform coagulation hemostasis on tumor surfaces. Hot biopsy forceps are used to ablate and resect a tumor. High-frequency knife is used to dilate a stenosis, particularly weblike stenoses after tracheotomy, to dilate mechanically at the tip of the rigid bronchoscope after turn on the break by the high-frequency knife. Even if the tip of these devices is small, the possibility of bronchial wall perforation due to large thermal energy should still be noted. As mentioned in the previous section, avoid prolonged application of the high-frequency current; instead, use short repeated applications every 1–3 s.

27.6 Nd-YAG Laser

This technique often utilizes a noncontact type of probe. Insert the probe into the working channel of the bronchoscope up to a distance of about 5–10 mm beyond the scope tip. Apply laser energy to the lesion while checking the red pilot light. Application of thermal energy begins at intermittent output waves every 0.5–2 s at

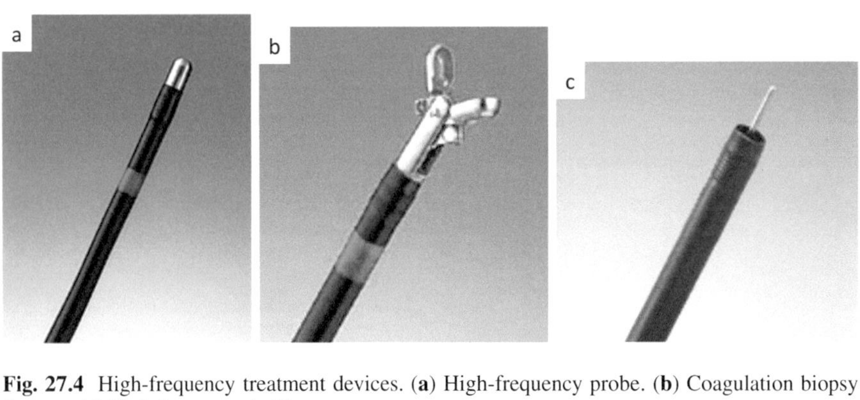

Fig. 27.4 High-frequency treatment devices. (**a**) High-frequency probe. (**b**) Coagulation biopsy forceps. (**c**) High-frequency knife

an average of 20 W (range, 10–40 W). Since the laser beam weakens in tissues with white tone, carbonize the surface initially with an ablation and then proceed with laser irradiation from the lesion edge. The laser depth may be adjusted by irradiation time. It is important to note that deep laser irradiation of the cartilage layer will delay regeneration of the bronchial mucosa and that there is a risk for airway stenosis if two or more cartilages are destroyed. To prevent bronchial perforation, irradiation should be advanced with a low output of 10–20 W while keeping the axis of the bronchus. Since the straight portion of the laser beam is ablated, it is not suitable for treatment of tangential lesions, unlike APC. During laser irradiation, dedicated protection glasses should always be worn to avoid retinal damage by the reflected laser light. Like all other heat application techniques, reduce oxygen supplement to less than 40 % to avoid fire.

References

1. Cohen MD, Weber TR, Rao CC. Balloon dilatation of tracheal and bronchial stenosis. AJR. 1984;14:679–83.
2. Sutedja T, van Boxem TJ, Schramel FM, et al. Endobronchial electrocautery is an excellent alternative for Nd-YAG laser to treat airway tumors. J Bronchol. 1997;4:101–5.
3. Reichle G, Freitag L, Kullmann H-J. Argon plasma coagulation in bronchology: a new method alternative or complementary. J Bronchol. 2000;7:109–17.
4. Pedersen U, Kristensen S, Illum P, et al. Palliative resection with high frequency cutting loop in malignant tracheobronchial disease. J Bronchol. 1994;1:23–5.

Chapter 28
Endoscopic Bronchial Occlusion with Silicone Spigots

Yasuyuki Mizumori and Shinji Sasada

Abstract Endobronchial Watanabe spigot is a cork-shaped silicone bronchial blocker that was originally developed by Watanabe et al. It is easy to insert and remove with the use of flexible bronchoscope and simple grasping forceps. Comprehensive identification of the affected bronchus should be carried out by various methods. In difficult cases, it is important not to give up because various techniques can be employed in inserting the bronchial blocker.

Keywords Endobronchial Watanabe spigot • Silicone • Endoscopic bronchial occlusion • Persistent pulmonary air leak • Intractable pneumothorax

28.1 Introduction

Bronchopleural and alveolopleural fistulas with persistent air leak can cause significant morbidity and increased risk of mortality. These fistulas are usually managed by chest drainage and occasionally by pleurodesis; intractable cases require surgical decortication, direct closure, thoracoplasty, or omental or muscle transposition [1]. However, surgery is often inappropriate for patients with respiratory failure because of the underlying pulmonary pathology. Treatment of prolonged air leak with sclerosing agents, such as fibrin glue, gelatin sponge, and cyanoacrylate, produces only short-term effects [2, 3]. Other endoscopic approaches include insertion of endovascular metallic coil [4, 5], tracheobronchial stent [6], and endobronchial valve [7–9] into the affected airway. The results of these nonsurgical approaches are promising, and the US Food and Drug Administration has approved the humanitarian use of

Y. Mizumori
Department of Respiratory Medicine, National Hospital Organization Himeji Medical Center, Hyogo, Japan

S. Sasada (✉)
Department of Respiratory Medicine, Tokyo Saiseikai Central Hospital, 1-4-17, Mita, Minato-ku, Tokyo 108-0073, Japan
e-mail: sasastaf@hotmail.co.jp

T. Izumo et al. (eds.), *Respiratory Endoscopy*,
DOI 10.1007/978-981-287-916-5_28

bronchial valves to treat selected postsurgical patients with prolonged air leaks [10]. Persistent air leaks sometimes follow a complicated course of severe pneumonia or acute respiratory distress syndrome (ARDS) [8]. In patients with severe respiratory failure, endoscopic approaches may be the only option available after all conventional treatments have failed [11].

28.2 Endobronchial Watanabe Spigot (Fig. 28.1a)

Endobronchial Watanabe spigot (EWS) is a cork-shaped silicone bronchial blocker that was originally developed by Watanabe et al. and reported to be effective in reducing persistent pulmonary air leak by endoscopic bronchial occlusion (EBO) [12, 13]. EWS is available in three sizes based on diameter: 5 mm (S), 6 mm (M), and 7 mm (L). It can be inserted and removed with the use of flexible bronchoscope and simple grasping forceps (Fig. 28.1b). The EWS is inserted through an endotracheal or a tracheostomy tube under sedation to allow spontaneous breathing. Grasping forceps is initially passed through the working channel of a bronchoscope; then, the EWS is held with the forceps and inserted into the affected bronchus (Fig. 28.2).

28.3 Determination of the Affected Bronchi

28.3.1 Balloon Occlusion Test

A chest drainage system is used to assess air leaks. A balloon occlusion test is performed to identify the affected region. After passing a balloon catheter through the working channel of a flexible bronchoscope (Fig. 28.1c), the balloon is inflated to achieve complete occlusion of the lobar, segmental, and subsegmental bronchi (Fig. 28.2). The affected airway is identified if air leak through the chest tube is reduced or stopped 15 s to 1 min after occlusion. When reduction of air leak could not be detected by bronchial occlusion, lung inflation on X-ray fluoroscopy images may be used to identify the affected bronchi.

28.3.2 Chest Computed Tomography Reading

Computed tomography (CT) is useful to identify the responsible bronchus that has continuous communication with the thoracic cavity. It is recommended to refer to a three-dimensional (3D) CT (virtual bronchoscopy) that can be created with 3D workstations (Ziostation, synapse VINCENT, etc.) (Fig. 28.3). From our experience, an extended cyst is less likely a cause of air leakage; rather, a bronchus that leads to the collapsed lesion is more often responsible (Fig. 28.4).

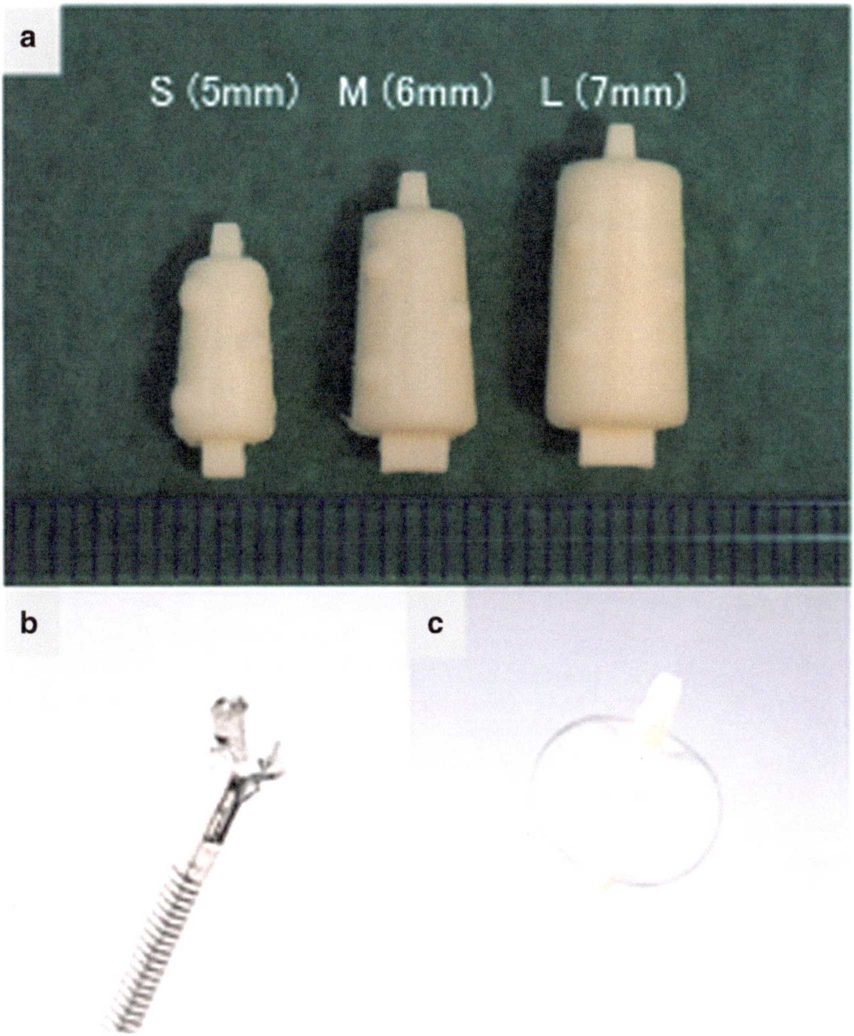

Fig. 28.1 Devices for endoscopic bronchial occlusion. (**a**) Endobronchial Watanabe spigot is a type of silicone bronchial blocker that is available in three sizes based on diameter. (**b**) Grasping forceps. (**c**) Balloon catheter

28.3.3 Bronchography

Inject 5–10 ml of nonionic contrast agent (twofold dilution) forcefully through a bronchoscope and observe for immediate outflow of the contrast into the chest cavity (Fig. 28.5). In other cases, leakage of contrast agent into the chest cavity can be confirmed by gradual visualization of the pleural surface on X-ray fluoroscopy after a few seconds of instillation.

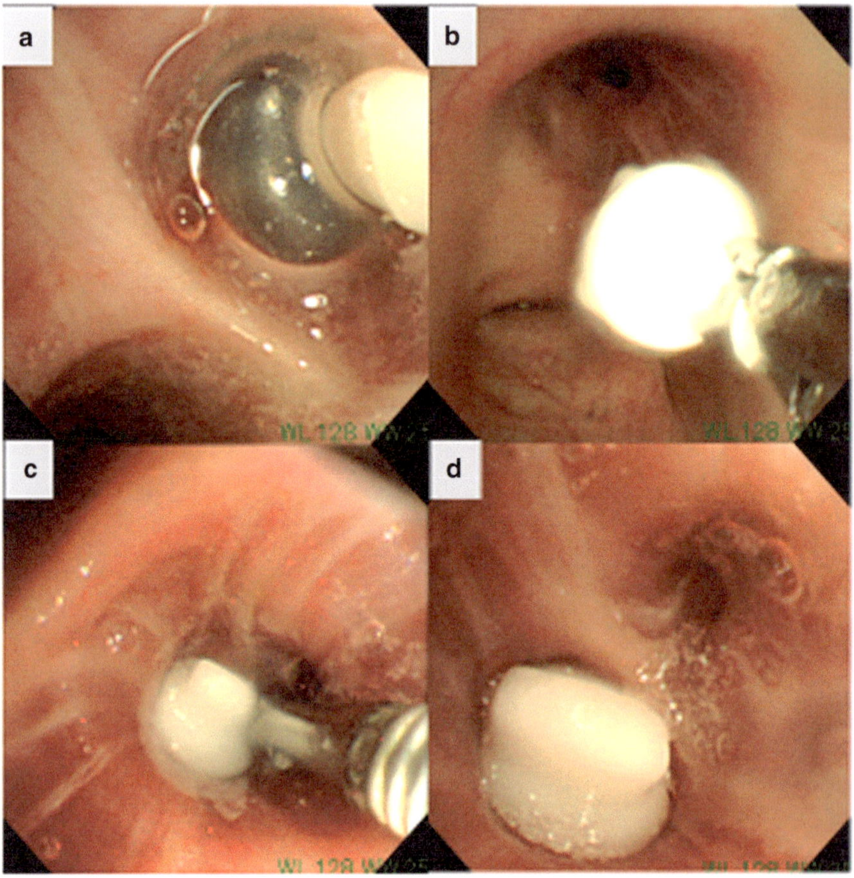

Fig. 28.2 Endoscopic bronchial occlusion by EWS. (**a**) Balloon occlusion test. (**b**–**d**) EWS insertion using grasping forceps. *EWS* Endobronchial Watanabe spigot

28.3.4 Repositioning

Observation of changes in air leakage due to repositioning is useful. Air leakage is reduced when taking a position that is on the bottom.

28.3.5 Intrathoracic Dye Injection

About 10 ml of indigo carmine, diluted twofold in saline, is injected into the thoracic cavity from the drainage tube, followed by additional instillation of approximately 20 ml of saline solution. The bronchus in which reverse flow of dye is observed is indicated as the responsible bronchus. In cases with open

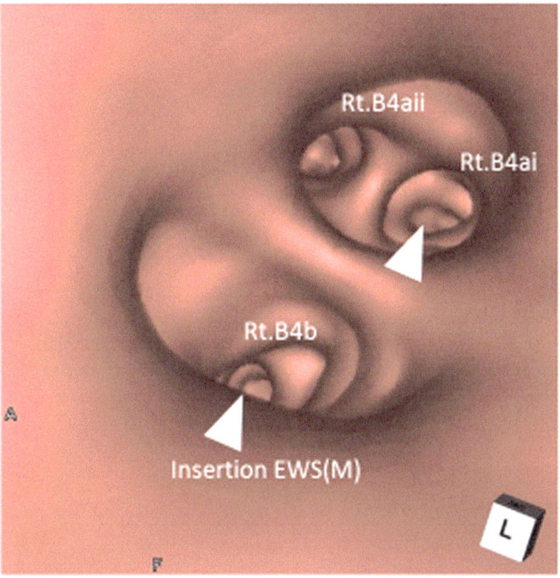

Fig. 28.3 Simulation of Endobronchial Watanabe spigot insertion by virtual bronchoscopy made by a 3D workstation (Ziostation2®, Ziosoft Inc., Tokyo, Japan)

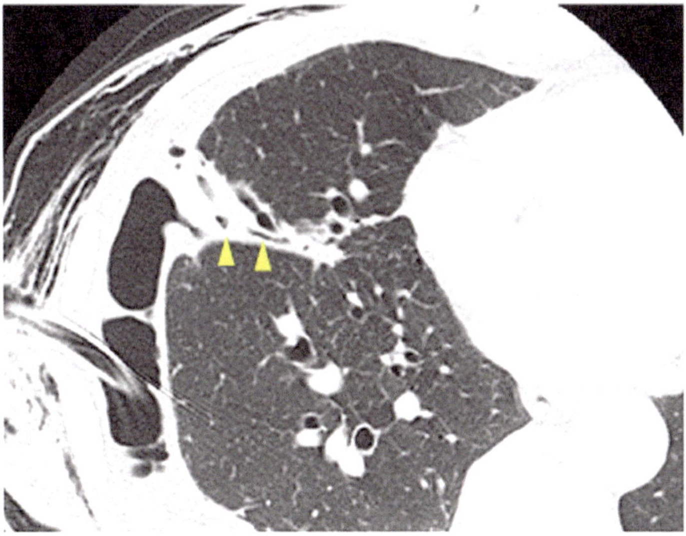

Fig. 28.4 A case of empyema with intractable pneumothorax. The responsible bronchi are identified on thin-slice chest computed tomography (*arrow*)

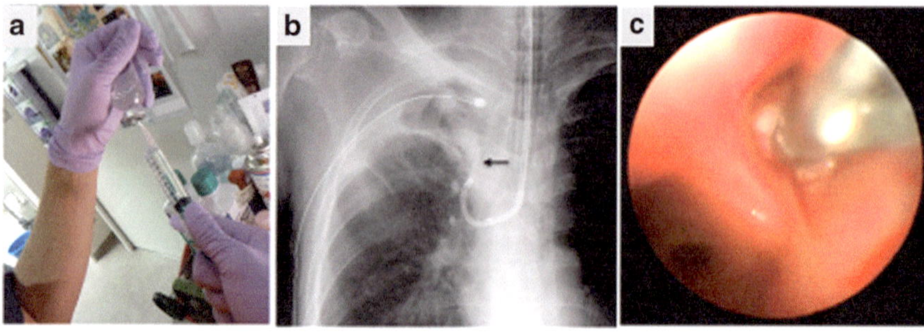

Fig. 28.5 Bronchography. (**a**) Prepare a nonionic contrast agent (twofold dilution). (**b**) Through a bronchoscope, forcefully inject 5–10 ml of the contrast agent into the suspected bronchus (e.g., *right* B1), and observe for outflow into the chest cavity. (**c**) Stop the leakage by inserting an Endobronchial Watanabe spigot to the responsible bronchus (in this case, the *right* B1)

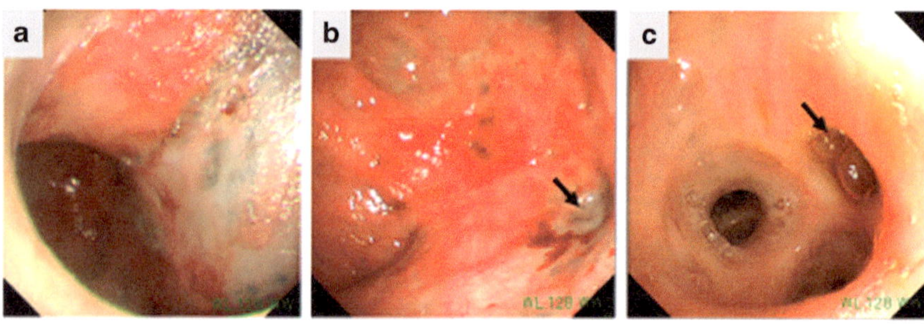

Fig. 28.6 Case of open postsurgical window. (**a**) Bronchoscopic observation through the open window. (**b**) Coat the portion where air leakage is suspected (*black arrow*) with povidone-iodine. (**c**) Identify the bronchus where the povidone-iodine will flow though; in this case, it was the right B6

post-thoracoscopy window, apply povidone-iodine on the surface of the lung where air leakage is suspected then check by bronchoscopy the bronchus where the povidone-iodine flows through (Fig. 28.6).

28.3.6 Thoracic Imaging

Inject a nonionic contrast agent (twofold dilution) into the thoracic cavity from the drainage tube while repositioning under X-ray fluoroscopy, to estimate the site where bubbles appear. When used with balloon test, this method would be more effective because disappearance of bubbles can be seen in real time.

28.4 Techniques of EBO by EWS

The EWS is inserted through an endotracheal or a tracheostomy tube under local anesthesia with moderate sedation to allow spontaneous breathing. In patients with severe respiratory failure requiring mechanical ventilation, the procedure is performed through an inserted tracheostomy tube.

The grasping forceps is initially passed through the working channel of a bronchoscope; then, at the distal end of the scope, the EWS is held with the grasping forceps for insertion and release into the affected airway (Fig. 28.7a). Generally, EWS insertion is difficult. One technique is to align the direction or axis of the EWS with that of the intended bronchus by making an angle with the bronchial wall before insertion (heel kick method, deep heel kick method) (Fig. 28.7b). The distal tip of the EWS may be cut to facilitate insertion (Fig. 28.7c). Curette is also useful. Drill a small hole on the proximal/gripping surface of the EWS and insert the tip of the curette; then, maneuver the EWS into the affected bronchus by rotation and bending (Fig. 28.7d). After EWS insertion, the patient is transferred to the recovery room, where vital signs and oxygen saturation are closely monitored according to the standard hospital practices while waiting for the effects of anesthesia to wean off. Chest radiography is often requested to assess for lung reinflation.

28.5 Efficacy

In our series, 24 patients had persistent pulmonary air leak secondary to pneumothorax ($n = 15$), empyema ($n = 8$), and postsurgical complications ($n = 1$) [14]. After EBO with EWS, the air leaks were completely resolved in 12 patients (50 %) or were reduced in 7 patients (29.2 %); however, 5 patients (20.8 %) showed no improvement. Of the 24 patients in our series, four had underlying infection (tuberculosis, $n = 2$; pneumonia, $n = 1$; empyema, $n = 1$); three of these patients were successfully treated despite concurrent ARDS with severe respiratory failure requiring mechanical ventilation (Fig. 28.8).

Twenty-three patients required chest tube as part of their clinical management, but these were removed after EBO in 15 patients (65.2 %). The median time from chest tube insertion to EBO was 31 days (range, 9–157 days); the median time from EWS insertion to chest tube removal was 18 days (range, 8–90 days).

28.6 Complications and Prevention

In our series, the most frequent EWS-related complication was migration of the spigot [14]. To prevent migration, EWS should be inserted up to the maximum possible distance, and coughing should be minimized with appropriate medications.

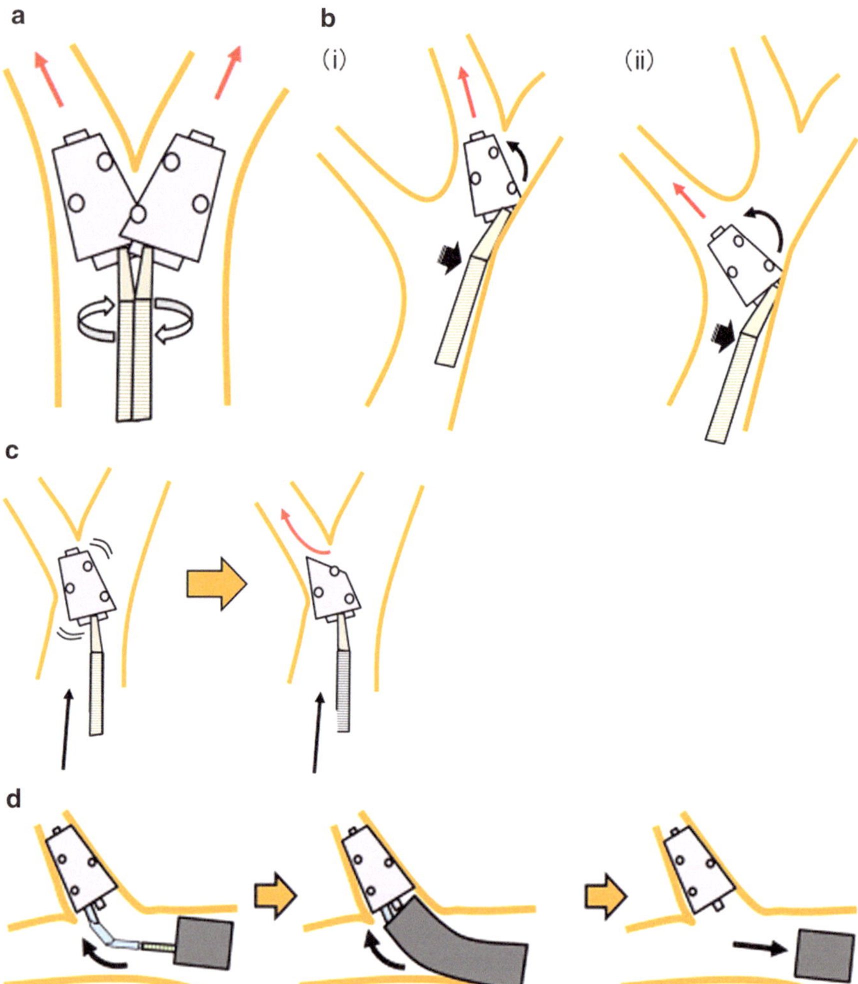

Fig. 28.7 Techniques of EWS insertion. (**a**) Grip the EWS at an angle. Change the direction of the tip as necessary by rotation. (**b**) Align the direction or axis of the EWS with that of the intended bronchus by making an angle with the bronchial wall before insertion. Heel kick method (*left*, acute angle); deep heel kick method (*right*, obtuse angle). (**c**) Obliquely cut the EWS to facilitate insertion. (**d**) EWS insertion using a curette. *EWS* Endobronchial Watanabe spigot

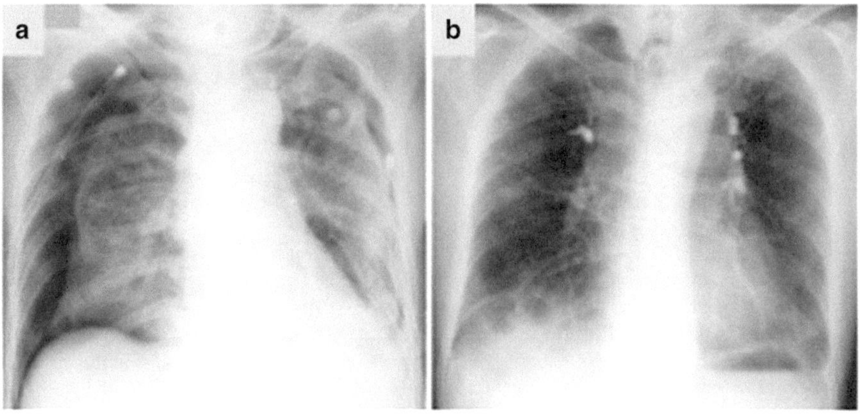

Fig. 28.8 Case of bilateral intractable pneumothorax caused by acute respiratory distress syndrome. (**a**) A representative chest radiograph shows bilateral pneumothorax. (**b**) Chest radiograph at 3 months after placement of six EWS shows reduced pneumothorax

The EWS may be cut obliquely to half its length to facilitate maximum insertion; this reduction in length does not appear to affect the proper functioning of the device. Medium-sized EWS (6 mm diameter) was the most frequently used in this study. If the inserted EWS was smaller or larger than the diameter of the affected bronchus, it was removed and a different size was selected to ensure the optimal fit. In addition, in some cases of EWS migration, factor XIII with fibrinogen was endobronchially administered to seal the orifice of the affected bronchus after EBO.

One patient developed atelectasis, a known complication of bronchial occlusion, and severe respiratory failure after insertion of eight EWSs, which were immediately removed. We found no evidence to support the choice between permanent versus temporary EWS insertion; however, late-phase lung infection will influence this decision. In our series, the case of pulmonary abscess was successfully managed by EWS removal. Although critical infections were not observed in patients with permanent EWSs during the follow-up period, we recommend temporary placement (3 months to 1 year) to prevent late-phase complications.

References

1. Puskas JD, Mathinsen DJ, Grillo HC, Wain JC, Wright CD, Moncure AC. Treatment strategies for bronchopleural fistula. J Thorac Cardiovasc Surg. 1995;109:989–96.
2. Sakai T, Komuro Y. Gelatin-filling therapy for drainage bronchus. J Jpn Soc Bronchol. 1984;6:323–8.
3. Sippel JM, Chesnutt MS. Bronchoscopic therapy for bronchopleural fistula. J Bronchol. 1998;5:61–9.
4. Ponn RB, D'Agostino RS, Stern H, Westcott JL. Treatment of peripheral bronchopleural fistulas with endobronchial occlusion coils. Ann Thorac Surg. 1993;56:1343–7.

5. Sivrikoz CM, Kaya T, Tulay CM, Ak I, Bilir A, Doner E. Effective approach for the treatment of bronchopleural fistula: application of endovascular metallic ring-shaped coil in combination with fibrin glue. Ann Thorac Surg. 2007;83:2199–201.
6. Singh SS, Pyragius MD, Shah PJ, Stubberfield J, Jurisevic CA, Chaloob S. Management of a large bronchopleural fistula using a tracheobronchial stent. Heart Lung Circ. 2007;16:57–9.
7. Fann JI, Berry GJ, Burdon TA. The use of endobronchial valve device to eliminate air leak. Respir Med. 2006;100:1402–6.
8. Travaline JM, McKenna RJ, Giacomo TD, et al. Treatment of persistent pulmonary air leaks using endobronchial valves. Chest. 2009;136:355–60.
9. Wan IYP, Toma TP, Geddles DM, et al. Bronchoscopic lung volume reduction for end-stage emphysema. Report on the first 98 patients. Chest. 2006;129:518–26.
10. Wood DE, Cerfolio RJ, Gonzalez X, Springmeyer SC. Bronchoscopic management of prolonged air leak. Clin Chest Med. 2010;31:127–33.
11. Abu-Hijleh M, Blundin M. Emergency use of an endobronchial one-way valve in the management of severe air leak and massive subcutaneous emphysema. Lung. 2010;188:253–7.
12. Watanabe Y, Matsuo K, Tamaoki A, Hiraki S, Moriyama S. Bronchial embolization using an endobronchial Watanabe spigot for intractable pneumothorax and bronchial fistula. J Jpn Soc Bronchol. 2001;23:510–5.
13. Watanabe Y, Matsuo K, Tamaoki A, Kamoto R, Hiraki S. Bronchial occlusion with endobronchial Watanabe spigot. J Bronchol. 2003;10:264–7.
14. Sasada S, Tamura K, Chang YS, et al. Clinical evaluation of endoscopic bronchial occlusion with silicone spigots for the management of persistent pulmonary air leaks. Intern Med. 2011;50:557–61.

Chapter 29
Photodynamic Therapy for Lung Cancer

Takaaki Tsuchida and Takehiro Izumo

Abstract Photodynamic therapy (PDT) causes a photodynamic reaction by a low-power laser irradiation tumor affinity light-sensitive material, the energy conversion of when the transition to the excited state a result, the antitumor effect by producing the active oxygen. Be familiar with handling of equipment and use the right probe for a particular device. Check whether the laser equipment is operating correctly prior to administration of the photosensitizer. Sequential electronic scope cannot be used. PDT for advanced lung cancer is currently an off-label treatment modality, at least in Japan. The dose of laser irradiation has not been established, but it has been proven to be superior to ablation therapy. PDT for peripheral-type lung cancer is currently an off-label treatment, so its performance needs ethics committee review and should be in the context of a clinical trial. The laser irradiation dose for such purpose has not been established.

Keywords Photodynamic therapy • Photosensitizer • Central-type lung cancer • Advanced lung cancer • Guide sheath • Peripheral lung cancer

29.1 Photodynamic Therapy for Central-Type Lung Cancer

29.1.1 Indications

1. Stage 0 or Stage I lung cancer (Fig. 29.1).
2. Entire tumor can be observed.
3. A tumor that is located on the central side of a subsegmental bronchus.
4. The patient does not have porphyria.

T. Tsuchida (✉)
Department of Endoscopy, Respiratory Endoscopy Division,
National Cancer Center Hospital, 5-1-1, Tsukiji, Chou-ku, Tokyo 104-0045, Japan
e-mail: ttsuchid@ncc.go.jp

T. Izumo
Department of Respiratory Medicine, Japanese Red Cross Medical Center,
4-1-22 Hiroo, Shibuya-ku, Tokyo 150-8935, Japan

T. Izumo et al. (eds.), *Respiratory Endoscopy*,
DOI 10.1007/978-981-287-916-5_29

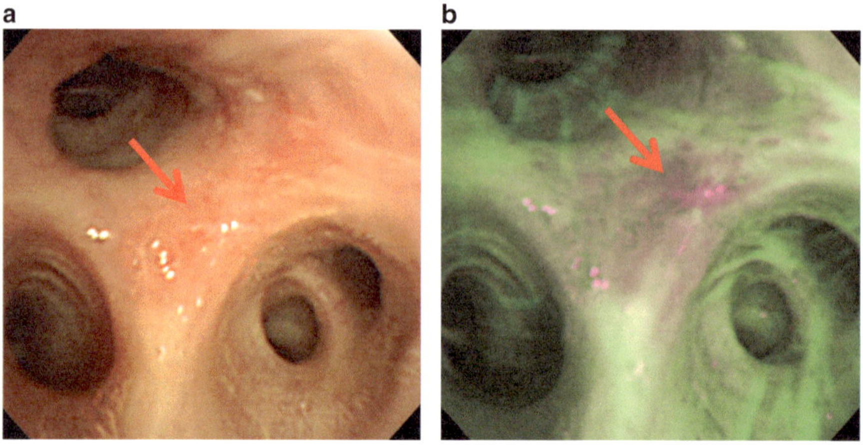

Fig. 29.1 (**a**) There is mild thickening and redness on the mucosa of the left upper lobe bronchus (*arrow*). This was diagnosed as squamous cell carcinoma after biopsy. (**b**) On autofluorescence imaging during bronchoscopy, fluorescence (*arrow*) is seen on the same site

29.1.2 Preparation

- Laser equipment for photodynamic therapy (PDT).
- Laser probes: Be sure to provide a dedicated probe for the laser equipment (Fig. 29.2a, b).
- Bronchoscope or simultaneous type electronic scope through which probe insertion is possible (Fig. 29.2c, d).
- When a bronchoscope is used, a dedicated filter to be attached to the eyepiece is required.
- Photosensitizer

Necessary preparations for light shielding of patients (sunglasses, hat, large mask, clothes to avoid exposure of the skin, and gloves)

29.1.3 Procedure

1. Check whether the laser device is working properly prior to administering the photosensitizer.
2. The photosensitizer is administered intravenously prior to laser irradiation. If talaporfin sodium will be used, injection of the drug should be 4–6 h prior to laser irradiation and the dose is 40 mg/m^2 (Fig. 29.3).
3. Immediately before intravenous injection, the patient is shielded below 500 lx and is asked to wear sunglasses.
4. The patient is kept away from sunlight exposure until the start of treatment.

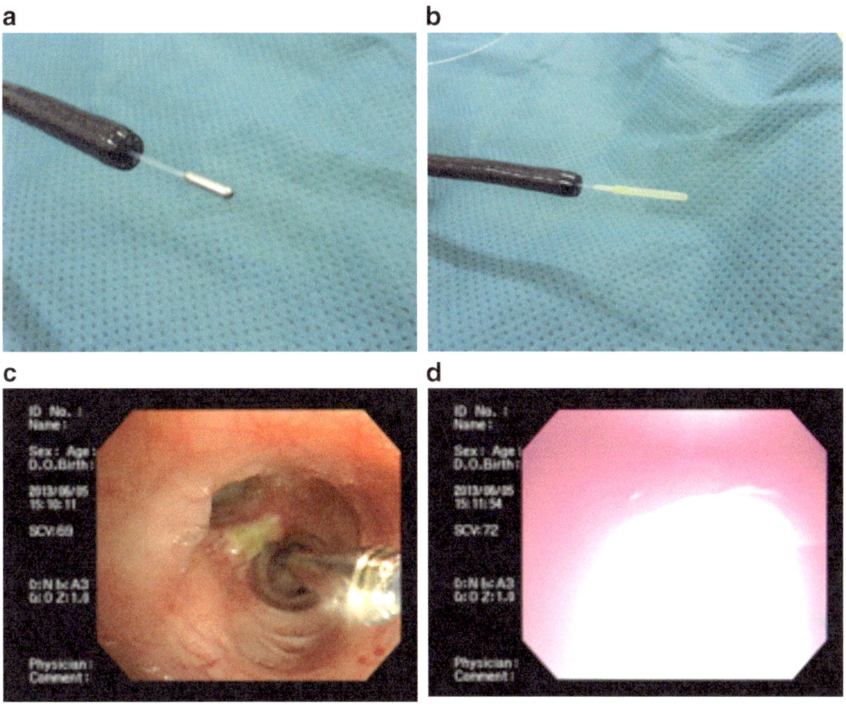

Fig. 29.2 (**a**) Irradiation probe for photodynamic therapy. (**b**) Direct probe. (**c**) Side elevation probe. (**d**) Sequential type electronic scope. (**e**) Screen is white out during laser irradiation

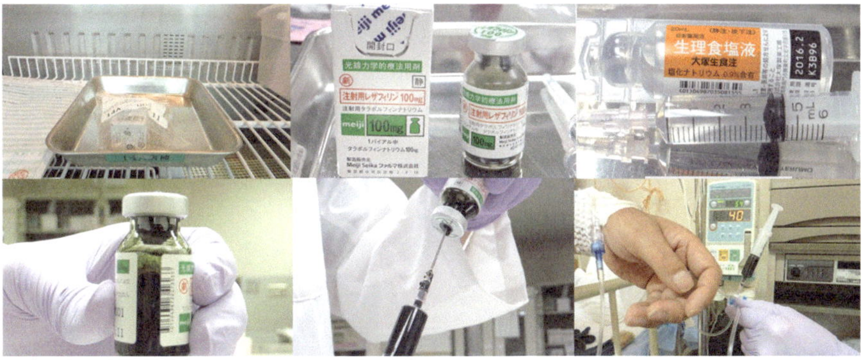

Fig. 29.3 Actual talaporfin sodium administration

5. During local anesthesia, start the laser equipment and perform an output test. The following is the procedure if you use the PD laser®:
   (a) Switch on the PD laser® then put the power switch on the back (Fig. 29.4).
   (b) Wait until warm-up is complete (Fig. 29.5).

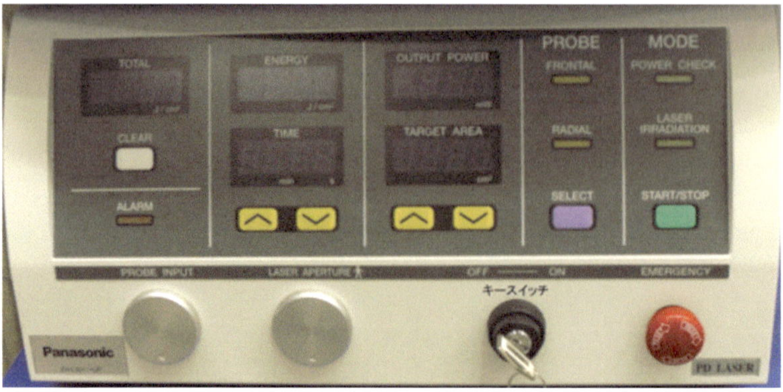

Fig. 29.4 The front panel of PD laser®

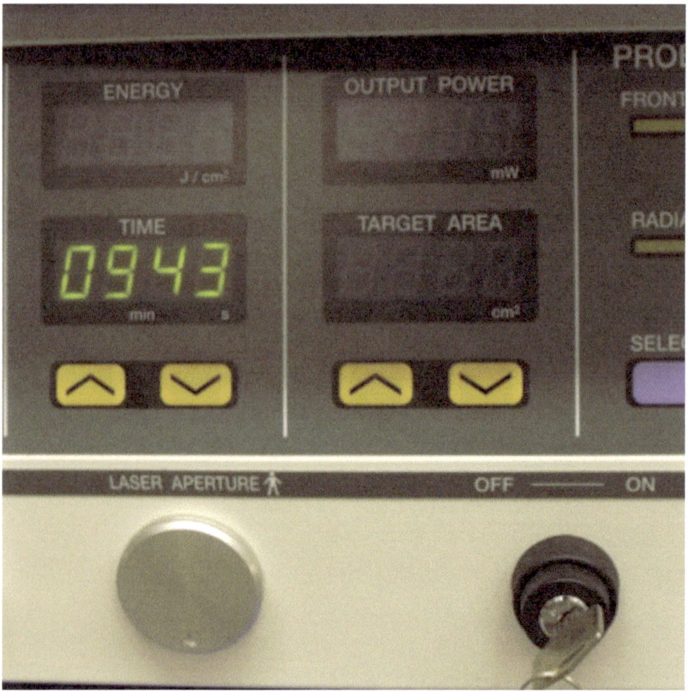

Fig. 29.5 Display during warm-up

(c) When the output test mode is ready, mount the laser probe to the laser equipment body.

(d) For the output test, insert the laser probe to the adapter while pressing the white button (stopper) of the adapter (Fig. 29.6).

(e) Put the adapter with the inserted laser probe to the PD laser® body (Fig. 29.7).

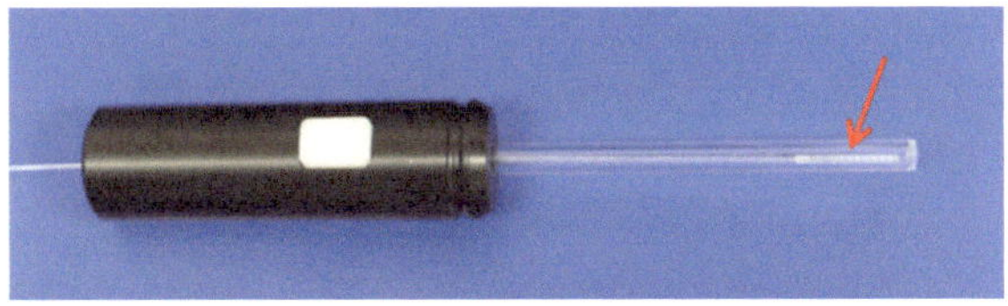

Fig. 29.6 Laser probe that is installed on the output test adapter

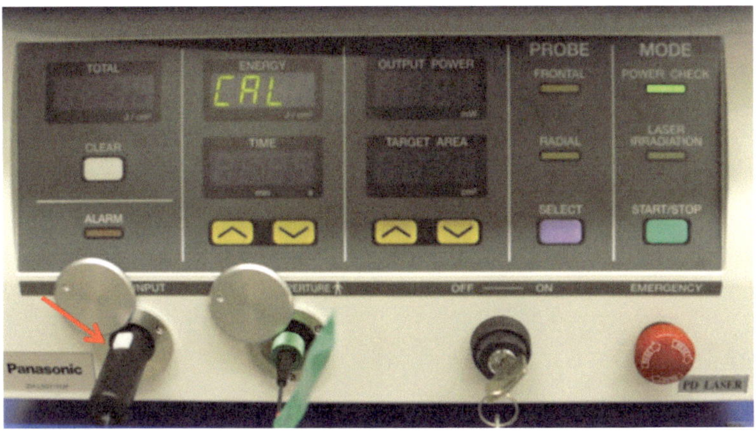

Fig. 29.7 Put the laser probe to the laser device for the output test

(f) Press the probe selection button on the laser body to select the mode appropriate for the mounted probe (Fig. 29.8).
(g) Press the START/STOP button to start the output measurement (Fig. 29.9).
(h) Make sure that the output is sufficient. If the output is low, replace the probe with a new one (Fig. 29.10).
(i) Do the output test for each probe to be used.
(j) Set the irradiation range and then complete the preparation for laser irradiation (Fig. 29.11).

6. Approach the lesion with the use of a bronchoscope that can be used in PDT. Slight increase of the dose of sedation would be needed.
7. After confirming the lesion on bronchoscopy, insert the laser probe through the multipurpose working channel and bring it close to the lesion.
8. After stabilizing the position of the laser probe relative to the lesion, start laser irradiation by pressing the START/STOP button (Fig. 29.12).
9. When bronchial secretions increase, hold the irradiation by pressing the START/STOP button then suction the secretions.
10. The assistant should clean the tip of the laser probe by wiping it gently with gauze, while the operator is doing bronchial toilette.
11. When the airway becomes clear of secretions, resume laser irradiation.
12. When the dose of irradiation has reached 100 J/cm^2, laser irradiation is terminated automatically.

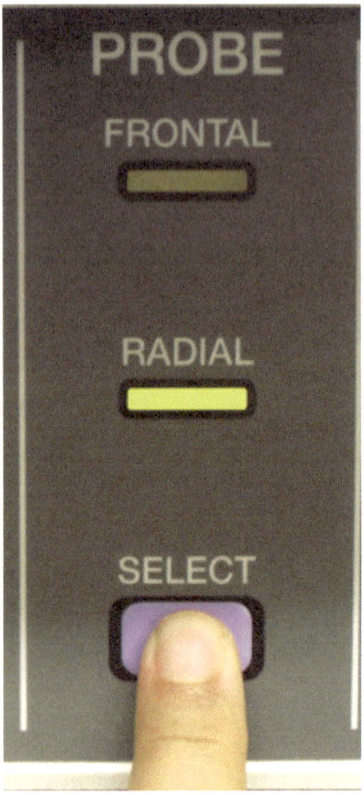

Fig. 29.8 Selection of laser probe

13. If you need to irradiate another portion of the tumor, replace the probe with an appropriate type that is needed. Repeat the output test and reset the irradiation range before performing another irradiation.
14. After irradiation is complete, turn OFF the power switch on the PD laser® body.
15. After completion of treatment, the patient should continue to limit light exposure below 500 lx for 2 weeks. The patient should also continue to wear sunglasses for 3 days, but this may be removed when sleeping or when inside a sufficiently dark place.
16. After more than 2 weeks treatment, check for sunlight hypersensitivity by outdoor sun exposure of one hand for 5 min.
17. Complete avoidance of sunlight may be stopped if there is no sensitivity detected, but instruct the patient to avoid direct sunlight until 1 month after treatment.

29.1.4 Limits and Measures

1. The timing of laser irradiation after photosensitizer administration
   The timing of drug administration before laser irradiation is important. Immediately after administration, the photosensitizer is distributed to many tissues, not only the tumor; however, the drug concentration in non-tumor tissues

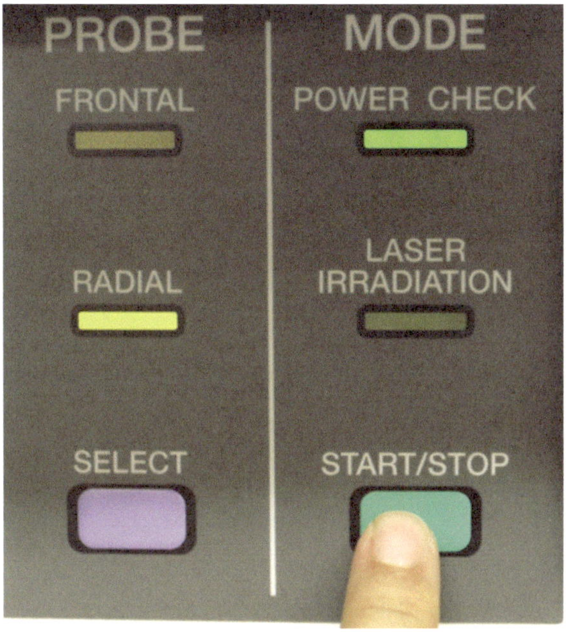

Fig. 29.9 Measurement of laser output at the tip of the probe

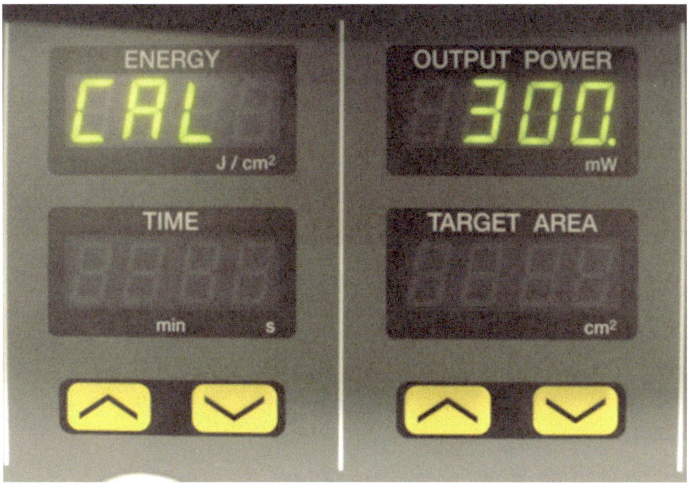

Fig. 29.10 Check the laser output

is reduced over time compared with that in the tumor. The optimal timing of PDT is 4–6 h after administration of talaporfin sodium and 48–72 h after administration of porfimer sodium. After porfimer sodium administration, it is possible to divide the irradiation sessions into 2 days; however, excretion of the drug is slow and requires strict limitation of light exposure to less than 300 lx for more than 4 weeks.

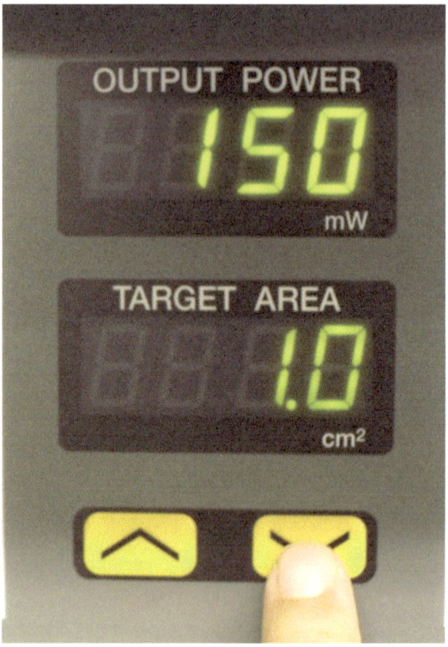

Fig. 29.11 Set the laser irradiation range (area)

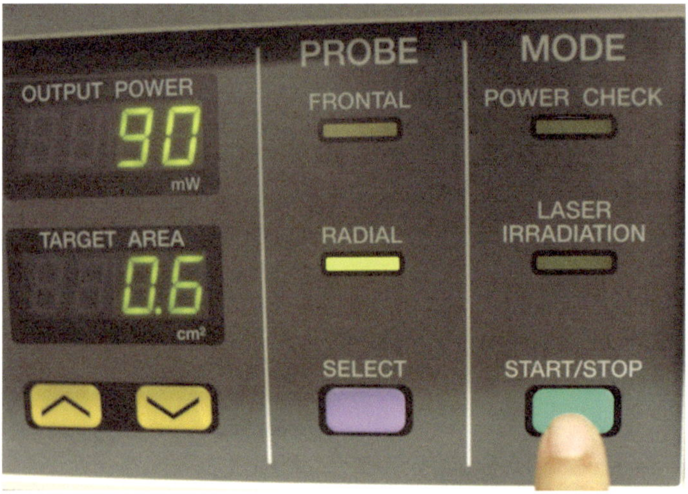

Fig. 29.12 Start laser irradiation

2. Irradiation angle of the laser
   According to the characteristics of light, laser irradiation is effective when performed at an acute angle of 60° or less to the tumor surface in order to avoid reflection of the majority. Therefore, the proper choice between a direct probe and a radial probe should be made according to the shape of the tumor (Fig. 29.2a, b).

29.2 Photodynamic Therapy for Advanced Lung Cancer

29.2.1 Indication

1. Endobronchial tumors that obstruct the main bronchus or lobar bronchus.
2. The patient has no porphyria.
3. Off-label use for treatment (in Japan).

29.2.2 Preparation

Same as photodynamic therapy (PDT) for central-type early stage lung cancer

29.2.3 Procedure

1. Administration of the drug and handling of laser equipment are same as those for PDT for central-type early stage lung cancer.
2. Dose of irradiation is 150 J/cm^2 for a radial laser probe on the peripheral side of the obstruction, 100 J/cm^2 for a radial laser probe on the middle portion of the obstruction, and 50 J/cm^2 for a direct laser probe on the central side of the obstruction. However, the optimal dose has not been established (Figs. 29.13 and 29.14).
3. Postoperative management is the same as that for PDT for central-type early stage lung cancer.

29.2.4 Limits and Measures

1. It is often difficult to observe the peripheral side endoscopically while applying irradiation to the obstructing tumor. Since the side elevation probes do not appear on X-ray fluoroscopy, use the computed tomography images to measure the irradiation position of the distal side in the insertion length of the probe from the central side.
2. It is not possible to use this method in cases wherein the lumen is completely obstructed (Fig. 29.15).
3. Since the obstruction may temporarily become more severe due to bronchial edema, it is better to administer steroids immediately after treatment in cases with almost complete obstruction (Fig. 29.16).

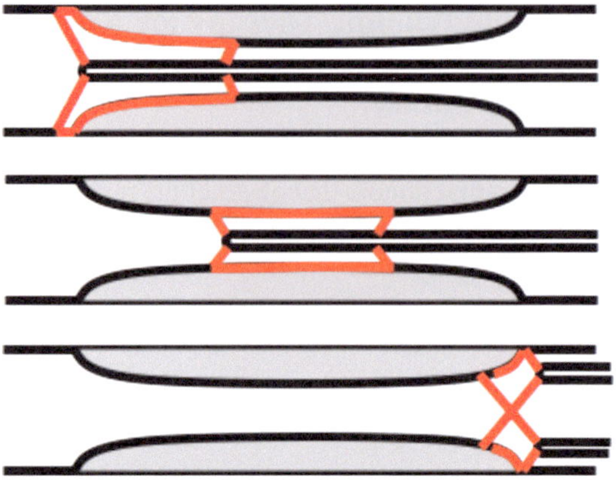

Fig. 29.13 Irradiation method and the energy density of the laser

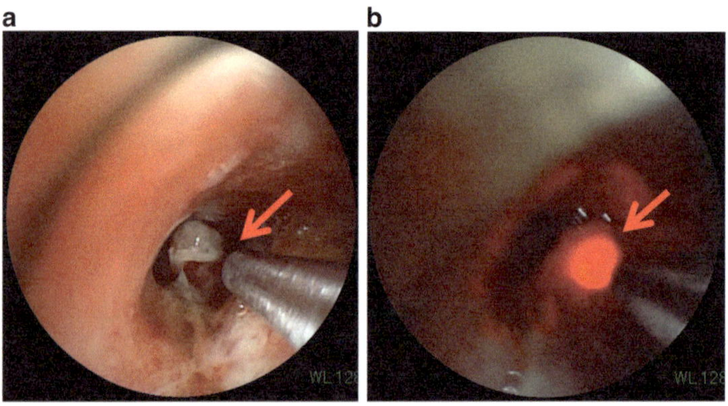

Fig. 29.14 Representative case of photodynamic therapy for advanced lung cancer. (**a**, **b**) Irradiation to a tumor obstructing the right bronchus intermedius

29.2.5 Available Literature

According to a randomized controlled trial that compared PDT with Nd-YAG laser ablation, postoperative symptom improvement was the same, but time to restenosis and median survival were longer after PDT [1].

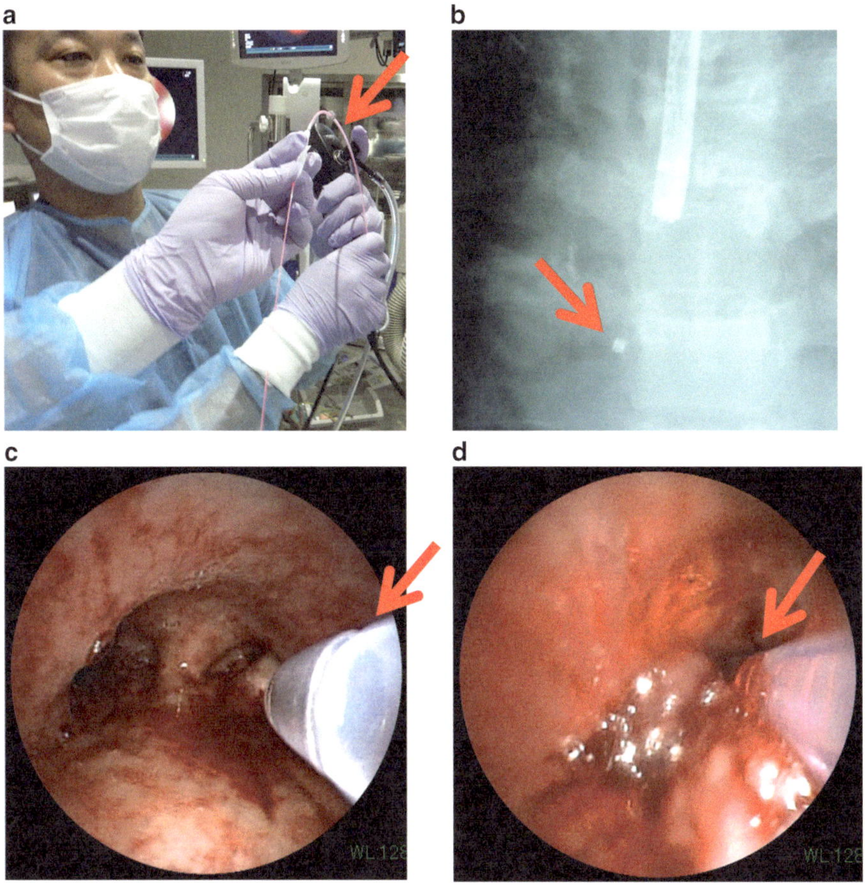

Fig. 29.15 Photodynamic therapy through a guide sheath for advanced lung cancer. (**a**) Laser irradiation through a guide sheath (SG-201C, Olympus Ltd) (*arrow*). (**b**) Check the position of the metal marker on the guide sheath tip by X-ray fluoroscopy (*arrow*). (**c**) Insert a guide sheath through the working channel of the bronchoscope (*arrow*). (**d**) Position the tip of the guide sheath more distal to the stenosis and then apply laser irradiation through the guide sheath (*arrow*)

29.3 Photodynamic Therapy for Peripheral-Type Lung Cancer

29.3.1 Indication

1. Nodular lesions within a maximum diameter of 20 mm.
2. Diagnosed as non-small cell lung cancer by transbronchial biopsy or cytology.
3. Adenocarcinoma with a solid part that is >50 % of the maximum diameter nodule diameter is excluded.
4. Inoperable cases.

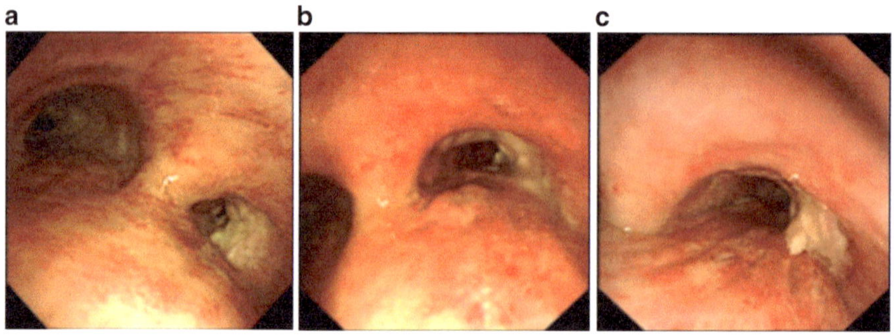

Fig. 29.16 Representative case of right main bronchus stenosis due to squamous cell carcinoma. (**a**) Before photodynamic therapy. (**b**) 7 days after photodynamic therapy. (**c**) 30 days after photodynamic therapy

5. The patient does not have porphyria.
6. To be performed under clinical trials.

29.3.2 Preparation

1. Same as photodynamic therapy (PDT) for central-type early stage lung cancer
2. Larger diameter guide sheath, radial-type endobronchial ultrasound (R-EBUS) probe, and ultrasound device (Fig. 29.17)

29.3.3 Procedure

1. Administration of the drug and handling of laser equipment are the same as those for PDT for central-type early stage lung cancer.
2. A large diameter guide sheath is guided to the lesion with the use of R-EBUS probe.
3. After placing the guide sheath into the lesion, inject 2 ml of saline through the guide sheath before inserting the laser probe. As a result, the irradiated laser will be diffused by the reflection.
4. Perform laser irradiation on the distal side of the lesion first.
5. The energy density is 50 J/cm^2 or 100 J/cm^2 of the maximum cross-sectional area of the tumor. Please note that this dose has not been established yet.
6. Postoperative management is same as that for PDT for central-type early stage lung cancer.

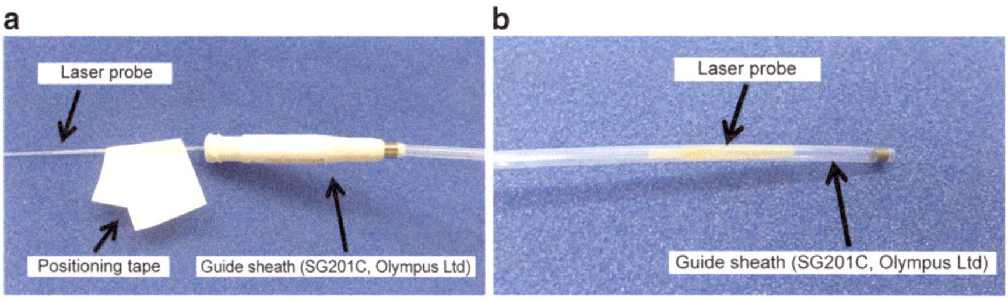

Fig. 29.17 Preparation of guide sheath and laser probe

29.3.4 Limits and Measures

1. Since the procedure should be carried out as a clinical trial, institutional ethics committee review is necessary.
2. Treatment of lesions close to the pleura may induce pleurisy; therefore, it would be advisable to apply laser irradiation as far away from the pleura as possible.
3. It is necessary to accurately guide the laser probe to the lesion. Use of a navigation system, guide sheath, and R-EBUS will provide accurate guidance to the lesion during bronchoscopy.

29.3.5 Available Literature

1. There have been no reports published on the use of bronchoscopy for PDT of peripheral-type early stage lung cancer.
2. The use of a percutaneous needle to deliver photodynamic therapy laser irradiation for peripheral lung cancer has been reported to be effective in seven of nine cases [2].

References

1. Diaz-Jimenez JP, Martinez-Ballarin JE, Llunell A, et al. Efficacy and safety of photodynamic therapy versus Nd-YAG laser resection in NSCLC with airway obstruction. Eur Respir J. 1999;14:800–15.
2. Okunaka T, Kato H, Tsutsui H, et al. Photodynamic therapy for peripheral lung cancer. Lung Cancer. 2004;43:77–82.

Part III
Edition for Nurses

Chapter 30
Actual Nursing in Respiratory Endoscopy

Akiko Kobayashi, Sugako Hirata, Mayumi Ohga, Akemi Sakatsume, Kaori Shimada, and Junko Kaneko

Abstract Collect the information necessary for bronchoscopy and share it with the medical team. Anticipate possible effects and complications of bronchoscopy for prevention and prompt management. Relieve tension of the patient by gentle talking or light touching on the shoulder. Know the needed equipment and supplies, and ensure that there are adequate stocks and no defects. The role of the nurse in the multidisciplinary collaboration during bronchoscopy is to ensure patient safety and comfort. The Safety Committee of the Japan Society of Respiratory Endoscopy recommends the standard precaution to prevent infection for respiratory endoscopy. Doctors and nurses apply standard precautions to prevent exposure to body fluids, cross infection, and spread of contamination. Except for goggles, all personal protective equipment, such as gowns, masks, and gloves, should be disposable and replaced after every procedure in patient. In addition, the members of the staff who handle and clean the equipment and scopes are mandated to follow and practice standard precautions of cleaning and environmental disinfection, as well as wearing of gowns, mask with face shield, and gloves.

Keywords Nursing care • Patient information • Prevent infection • Standard precautions • Tuberculosis • N95 mask

30.1 The Role of the Nurse in the Endoscopy Division

Respiratory endoscopy is an invasive diagnostic and therapeutic procedure for lesions of the lungs and bronchus. Before bronchoscopy, patient cooperation is needed during application of laryngeal anesthesia. Nurses should prepare every patient on what to expect, reinforce understanding of the indications of the procedure, and ensure safety. Moreover, knowledge of the underlying medical condition of the patient is mandatory in order to be prepared for possible complications, such

---

A. Kobayashi (✉) • S. Hirata • M. Ohga • A. Sakatsume • K. Shimada • J. Kaneko
Nursing Service Department, National Cancer Center Hospital,
5-1-1, Tsukiji Chou-ku, Tokyo 104-0045, Japan
e-mail: akikkoba@ncc.go.jp

T. Izumo et al. (eds.), *Respiratory Endoscopy*,
DOI 10.1007/978-981-287-916-5_30

as difficulty of breathing due to bronchoconstriction, hypoxia, and hemodynamic instability. It is likewise important for nurses to know the progress of the procedure and to take note of changes in the vital signs of the patient so that the other members of the medical team can focus smoothly on their specific tasks, such as performing bronchoscopy or doing X-ray fluoroscopy. When there is any untoward sign, all the members of the team should be made aware so that corresponding measures can be taken.

Bronchoscopy is usually an outpatient procedure. Most patients undergo the procedure for the first time and are usually anxious about pain, what to expect, etc. Nurses are the ones who receive the patients upon their arrival to the unit; therefore, it is their job to relieve the anxiety of patients by clearly explaining to them the flow from preparation to the end of the test. We should aim to communicate and give our patients a sense of security in order to make them relax, as much as possible, before bringing them to the examination room. After the procedure, it is an important role of nurses to instruct patients on what to watch out for, what to avoid, and what to do in case complications occur.

In recent years, endoscopic technology has advanced. Aside from ensuring patient safety and comfort, nurses are encouraged to learn new knowledge and to keep updated with the latest technology in order to continue self-improvement.

30.2 Nursing for Patients Undergoing Bronchoscopy

Bronchoscopy is an invasive procedure that has accompanying risks, such as bleeding. In addition, patients are also exposed to sedatives and anesthetics during the procedure. In our hospital, about 90 % of bronchoscopy procedures have been performed on an outpatient basis. Bronchoscopy with biopsy of lung cancer is usually performed for definitive diagnosis, staging, and determination of disease status after surgery, chemotherapy, or radiation therapy. In this chapter, the flow of bronchoscopy, as well as caring for a patient undergoing the procedure, will be described.

30.2.1 Actual Nursing Care

30.2.1.1 Before Bronchoscopy

Collect the information necessary for nursing care (Table 30.1).

Prevent and anticipate complications during bronchoscopy in order to prepare for therapeutic strategies that may be needed.

Table 30.1 Patient information that needs to be known in advance

Demographics (age, gender, performance status, height, weight, social background)
History of present illness before bronchoscopy
History of previous illnesses, such as drug allergies, bleeding diathesis, etc.
Subjective symptoms
Test results (electrocardiogram, pulmonary function tests, etc.)
Indications for bronchoscopy and informed consent
Previous bronchoscopy examinations

Table 30.2 Process flow of patients

(1) Preoperative checklist
Signed informed consent
Vital signs and general status
Remove from the body any metal that may obscure X-ray fluoroscopy examination
(2) Corresponding to the patient
Nurse in charge greets and introduces herself/himself to the patient
Ask the patient regarding any apprehensions or questions about the procedure
Strive to reduce anxiety

30.2.1.2 Management of Emotional Distress of Patients

Emotional distress of patients and their families are usually from both fear of undergoing the test and knowing the results. Even if a patient has undergone a previous bronchoscopy procedure, the magnitude of anxiety depends on his/her impression of the previous experience. Based on prior information collected, consider and empathize with the psychological situation of the patient in order to give a sense of security and relieve anxiety.

30.2.1.3 Preparations (Table 30.2)

1. Informed consent

Table 30.3 Complications associated with bronchoscopy

(1) Lidocaine intoxication
(2) Hypotension due to sedatives
(3) Hypoxia
(4) Pneumothorax
(5) Airway bleeding
(6) Fever, pneumonia

Before the procedure, a signed consent is secured from each patient after sufficient explanation from the doctor about the need for the procedure, as well as the possible risks and complications of treatment.

2. Vital signs and general status
   Filling out questionnaires, vital signs (blood pressure, pulse rate, body temperature) to observe the general state of the previous inspection.
3. Fasting instructions
   In order to prevent aspiration, eating and drinking should be prohibited 2 h before the procedure.

30.2.2 Nursing Management of Complications During the Examination and Treatment

At our hospital, at the start of every procedure, a "briefing" is performed among the doctors, nurses, and other members of the team in order to share information, such as patient's name, procedure, diagnosis, and the possible complications to watch out for. The possible complications associated with bronchoscopic procedures are shown in Table 30.3; a description on the nursing management of each is given.

30.2.2.1 Lidocaine Intoxication

The symptoms of lidocaine intoxication include decreased or loss of consciousness, tremors, and convulsions. Check for physical signs, such as bradycardia, cardiac arrhythmia, and the like, during pretreatment and inform the rest of the team. In addition, observe for the presence of tremors and seizures or loss of consciousness and report these to the doctor. In some circumstances, lifesaving measures may be necessary. The maximum dose of lidocaine is 8.2 mg/kg; for a body weight of 50 kg, maximum dose is 410 mg (20.5 ml of 2 % lidocaine).

30.2.2.2 Hypotension Caused by Sedatives

Sedatives are used in order to calm the patient and avoid pain, as well as to avoid unnecessary body movements that can affect the procedure. The nurse in charge reports the condition of the patient to physicians and administers additional doses of sedatives upon the instructions of the physician. Upon the time of administration of sedatives, it is necessary to pay careful attention to decreases in blood pressure and notify the physician as necessary. Derangements in vital signs on the monitor should be confirmed manually.

30.2.2.3 Hypoxia

Along with the vital signs, the value of SaO_2 should be measured continuously. Before the procedure, the doctor initiates oxygen support at 2–3 l per minute via nasal cannula; this level of support is adjusted as necessary to keep the SaO_2 value within normal. If there is a tendency for the tongue base to obstruct the airway during sedation, chin lift is effective in securing the airway.

30.2.2.4 Pneumothorax

The endoscopy room of our hospital is equipped with an X-ray fluoroscopy machine, which can be used to check the status of the lung immediately after bronchoscopic biopsy. In case a pneumothorax develops, the nurse in charge and head nurse should anticipate and quickly prepare the required materials for thoracic drainage, if deemed necessary. In addition, the patient should be monitored for hemodynamic instability, chest pain, dyspnea, and other signs of pneumothorax immediately after the procedure and at the recovery room. Changes in the vital signs or status of the patient should be reported immediately to the physician.

30.2.2.5 Airway Bleeding

Bronchoscopic biopsy may lead to bleeding, especially in patients with bleeding tendencies, such as those with low platelet count. When bleeding occurs, epinephrine diluted 5,000-fold should be prepared. This solution is applied by the doctor on the site of bleeding, along with other maneuvers, until hemostasis is achieved. During and immediately after hemostatic treatment, vital signs are checked manually and on the monitor to check for early abnormalities. At our hospital, the protocol is to observe the patient at the recovery room for at least 1 h before discharge. The unit should also be equipped with the necessary instruments to manage bleeding and hemodynamic instability.

30.2.2.6 Fever, Pneumonia

Antibiotics may be prescribed by the doctor if infection during inspection and treatment is suspected. It is necessary for the nurse to give instructions on the correct intake of medications. After discharge, patients should be advised to watch out for signs of fever, cough, sputum production, and dyspnea which may indicate pneumonia. Therefore, patients should be given instructions on how to contact the hospital in case such symptoms occur.

30.2.3 Nursing After Inspection

At our hospital, flumazenil is administered to antagonize the effect of midazolam at the end of the procedure. After administration, vital signs are taken while the patient lies on the examination table. Look for signs of recovery from sedation, such as response to name calling. Vital signs and oxygen saturation should be normal before bringing the patient to the recovery room either on a wheelchair or on a bed.

30.2.3.1 Observation in the Recovery Room

After the procedure, each patient is wheeled in to the recovery bed to rest and for observation. In the recovery room of our hospital, the SaO_2 value and the pulse rate of every patient are displayed on the central monitor. Also, in anticipation of complications, such as hypoxemia and bleeding, oxygen and suction device are available at each bedside. Equipment for calling the nurse should be made available, and curtains should not be fully closed to enable observation of the respiratory conditions and body movement of the patient. Intravenous access and fluid replacement are also maintained. Flumazenil is made available on standby, in case there is a delay in weaning off from sedative effects.

When the patient awakens, talk to the patient using relaxing words of encouragement. Describe the current status and give assurance that it is expected to have some uncomfortable feeling, such as throat discomfort, mild hemoptysis, and cough.

30.2.3.2 Recovery Room Discharge Criteria

After about 1 h of observation, confirm that the patient is fully awake and stable before sending home as outpatient. Depending on the status of the patient, the tie of observation at the recovery room may be extended. At our hospital, this assessment is performed using “recovery exit criteria” (Table 30.4).

Table 30.4 Recovery and discharge criteria

(1) There is no dyspnea
(2) There is no hemoptysis
(3) The patient can walk straight

30.3 Nursing Processes for Basic Bronchoscopy

30.3.1 Checklist

1. **Drug agents**

   - Pethidine, 1 ampule (35 mg) for analgesia
   - Midazolam, 1 ampule (10 mg) plus 20 ml saline for sedation
   - Flumazenil, 1 ampule (0.5 mg) for antagonizing the effects of midazolam
   - Two percent Xylocaine, 20 ml for additional local anesthesia during bronchoscopy

   *At National Cancer Center Japan, the dose of pethidine is usually 17.5 mg (1/2A); for patients more than 80 years old or those who weigh less than 50 kg, 8.75 mg (1/4A) of pethidine is used. The first dose of midazolam is usually 3 mg; for patients more than 80 years old or those who weigh less than 50 kg, 2 mg of midazolam is used. Additional dose of midazolam is 1 or 2 mg. The dose of flumazenil is usually 0.25 mg.

2. **Other materials**

   - Banded mouthpiece (Fig. 30.1)
   - Syringe, 10 ml for midazolam
   - Syringe, 5 ml for flumazenil
   - Syringe, 1.0 ml for pethidine
   - Syringe with Luer slip tip, 10 ml for intermittent application of Xylocaine during bronchoscopy
   - Clean gauze for blindfold for eye protection
   - Sterile petri dish as container for 2 % Xylocaine
   - Suction tube for oral suction
   - Small plastic tray or kidney basin as container for the drugs to be injected
   - Oxygen cannula

3. **Medical equipment**

   - Monitor for heart rate, electrocardiogram, blood pressure, oxygen saturation concentration
   - Suction device (for oral suction)
   - Oxygen breathing apparatus
   - Emergency cart
   - Hanger for devices (Fig. 30.2)

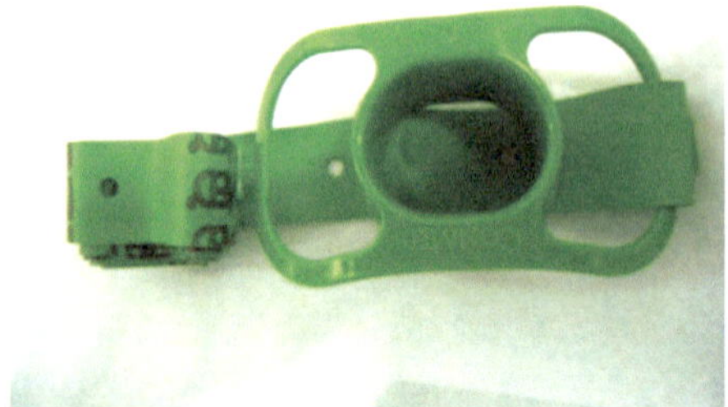

Fig. 30.1 Band with mouthpiece

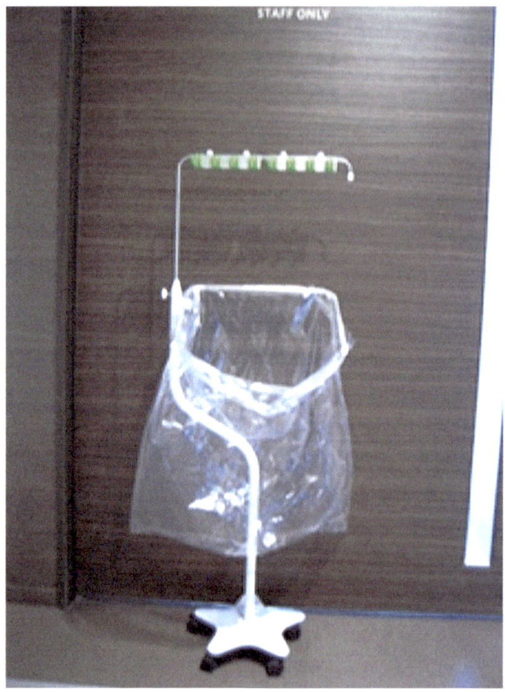

Fig. 30.2 Hanger for devices and treatments tools to be used

30.3.2 Preparation

1. **Environmental improvement of the laboratory**
   The standing positions of the operator and assistants, as well as the layout of the examination room, should enable smooth and comfortable entry of the patient (Fig. 30.3).
2. **Position of monitor**
   Place on the side of the patient's leg and arrange in such a way that the operator, assistant, and nurse can view the procedure.

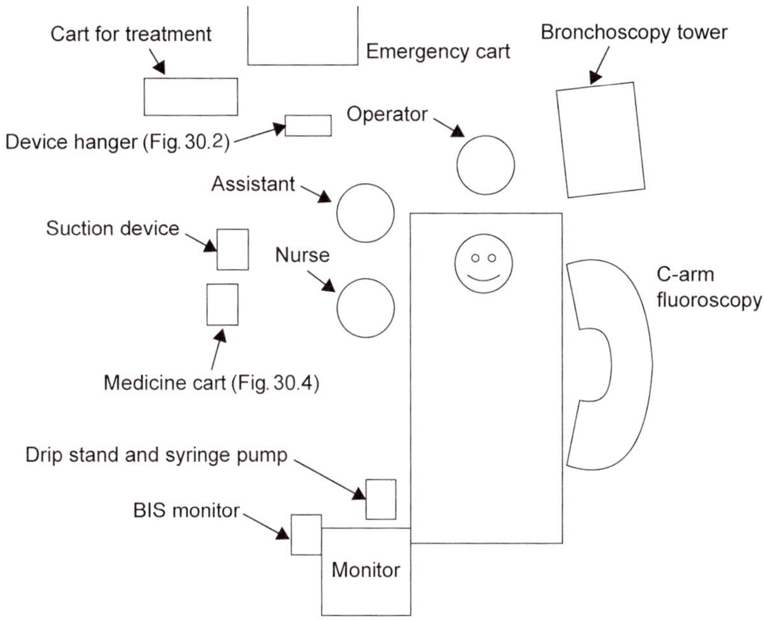

Fig. 30.3 The layout of the examination room

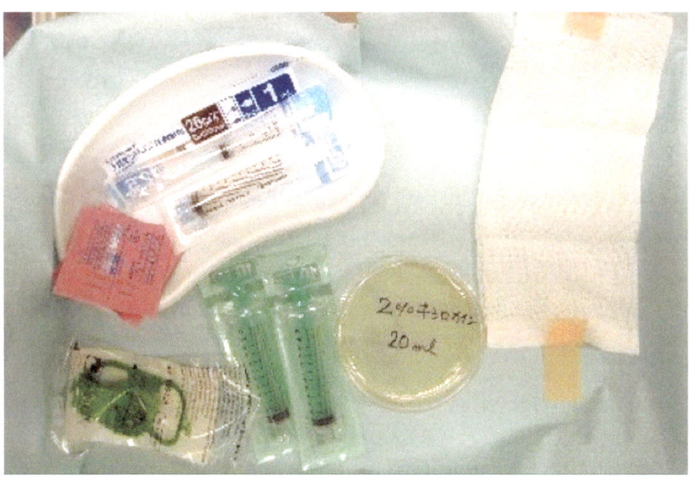

Fig. 30.4 The instruments on the nursing cart

3. **Emergency cart**
   It should be always contain the necessary medicines and equipment and be ready for use anytime. In our hospital, there is one emergency cart for every floor. As soon as an emergency cart is used, the materials are immediately replenished.

30.3.3 From Patient Entry into the Examination Room to Start of Bronchoscopy

1. **Place the patient in a supine position on the examination table**.
   - Bronchoscopy is performed with the operator standing on the head side of the patient.
   - Consider the patient's body type and physical symptoms when positioning the patient on the examination table. Anticipate the needs that will make the patient comfortable, such as placing the comfort pillows to knee, etc.
2. **Attach the monitors to the patient.**
   - While maintaining the peripheral intravenous access secure, attach the pulse oximeter to the fingertips.
   - Attach the blood pressure apparatus to the arm opposite the one with peripheral intravenous access. If this is not feasible, use the lower leg.
3. **Try to keep the patient warm.**
   - Consider the cold and heat felt by the patient. If necessary, cover the patient with a cotton blanket from the chest to the feet.
4. **Put a clean gauze over the eyes as a blindfold.**
   - This is done to prevent chemical liquids from accidentally getting into the eyes and possibly cause blindness. While covering the patient's eyes, alleviate fear by explaining that this is for eye protection.
5. **Place the mouthpiece with band.**
   - Firmly fix and tighten the band so that it does not come off during the bronchoscopy procedure.
   - In case dentures are removed, the mouthpiece will also serve to protect the gums.
   - Because the patient cannot speak during this time, instruct him/her to give you signals, such as hand movements, to which you can respond accordingly.

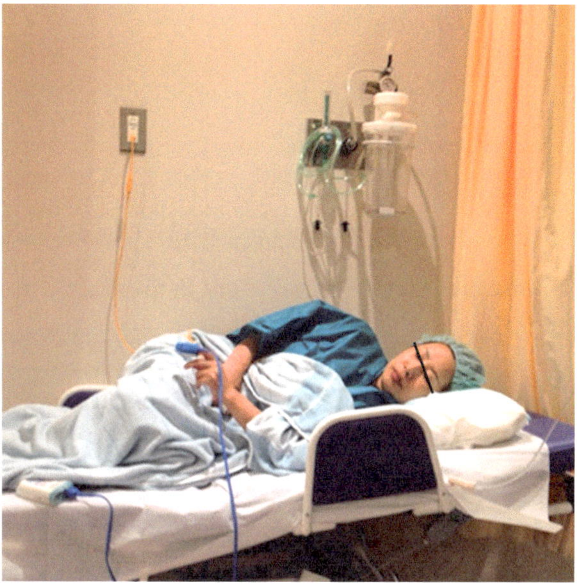

Fig. 30.5 Appearance after preparing the patient from steps 1 to 6

6. **Place the nasal oxygen cannula (2 L/min).**
7. **After preparing the patient from steps 1 to 6** (Fig. 30.5), measure the vital signs before the start of treatment.
8. **Thereafter, measure the blood pressure at 5-min intervals.** In addition, report the baseline SpO_2 value to the doctors and start oxygen administration when instructed.
9. **Start intravenous anesthesia, such as pethidine and midazolam, according to the doctor's instructions.**

   - While administering the drugs, tell the patient that he/she will become slightly sleepy. In addition, tell the patient to say if there is pain during intravenous administration in order to alleviate anxiety.
   - When the doctor gives instructions to give a medicine, confirm the name and dosage. During administration, say the name and dose of the medication that you are giving.

10. **Measure the vital signs after induction of sedation.**

    - Make sure that you are aware of the signs of the side effects of sedative use, such as respiratory depression and decreased blood pressure. Strive to detect abnormalities early.
    - Adjust the position and enlargement of the vital signs monitor so that it will also be visible to the doctors (operator and assistants) and technicians.

30.3.4 During Bronchoscopy

1. **Notes on scope insertion**

   - Oxygen saturation and blood pressure may decrease during scope insertion. It is important to anticipate and watch out for these changes, which can happen suddenly. Always be ready to respond to these changes; prepare the sedative antagonist and the emergency cart should be in the vicinity at all times.

2. **Measures for pooled secretions in the oral cavity**

   - Instruct the patient in advance to indicate by hand signal when he/she feels any sensation of aspiration. Also, anticipate for signs of pooling of secretions, such as low SpO2 value, and/or listen to instructions from the doctor. In such cases, suction the oral secretions as often as necessary.

3. **Correspondence at the time of sedation**

   - Repeat and confirm the instructions from the doctor before preparing the drug to be administered.
   - Upon administration, say out loud the drug name and dosage so that all members of the medical staff are aware. Do this when additional doses are given; give the cumulative dose given.

30.3.5 After Completion of the Bronchoscopy Procedure

1. **Check the vital signs.**

   - During and after administration of the antagonist flumazenil, upon the doctor's instructions, keep in mind that blood pressure can increase rapidly. At our hospital, we report to the doctor if systolic blood pressure exceeds 180 mmHg.

2. **Observe for signs of wakefulness.**

   - After the end of the procedure, while the patient is still on the examination table, check for eye opening in response to verbal stimulation.
   - Suction pooled oral secretions as necessary.
   - After clearing oral secretions, check the state of arousal again and remove the mouthpiece when the patient is awake.
   - Vital signs are measured again and reported to the physician.
   - Upon the physician's instructions, transfer the patient to the recovery room.
   - When transferring the patient, watch out for sudden drop in blood pressure, dizziness, and other symptoms, such as weakness. In such cases, slowly move the patient and hold in a seated position for about 2 min. After confirming the absence of subjective symptoms, proceed with the transfer.

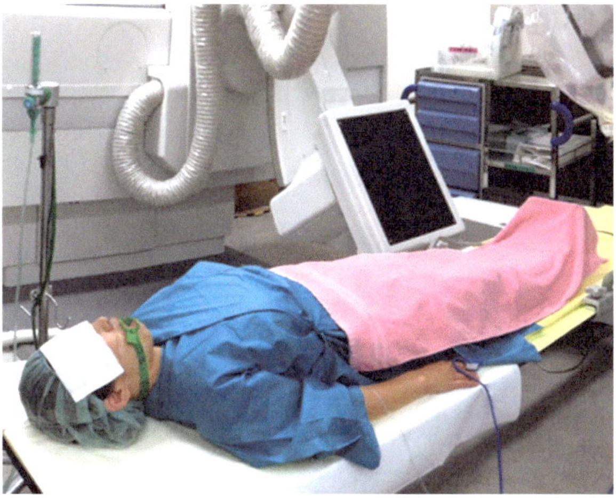

Fig. 30.6 Place a sedated patient in moderately inclined back rest

3. **Correspondence at the recovery room.**
    - Endorse the intraoperative course, latest vital signs, and drugs administered to the patient to the recovery room nurse who will take over the care of the patient.
    - Communicate with the family or companion of the patient about the end of the procedure and that recovery may take about 1 h of observation.

30.3.6 Observation After Bronchoscopy

- Usually, administration of antagonists shortens the duration of action of sedatives, and patients are already awake upon entry into the recovery room. However, delay in restoration of wakefulness is possible. In the latter case, prevent aspiration by placing the patient in a moderately inclined back rest (Fig. 30.6).
- In patients who are not yet fully awake, breathing may become shallow, SpO2 may decrease, and choking may ensue due to accumulation of oral secretions. If coughing does not improve symptoms, report immediately to the doctor.

30.3.7 Preparation of the Operator and Assistant

- In cases wherein fluoroscopy guidance is used during bronchoscopy, the examination room should be in a radiation controlled area.
- Wearing of personal protective equipment, such as lead gown, goggles, mask, gloves, and gown, is mandatory.

30.4 Improvement of Hospital Infection Prevention Measures in the Respiratory Endoscopy Examination Room

30.4.1 Actual Standard Precautions

30.4.1.1 Air-Conditioning Maintenance at the Endoscopy Center

In carrying out respiratory endoscopy, 6–12 times per hour of ventilation is required. The room is equipped with negative pressure to prevent air contamination by diseases, such as pulmonary tuberculosis. If possible, it would be ideal to always do a procedure in a room with negative pressure setting.

30.4.1.2 What to Do When Air Disinfection Is Required After a Procedure for a Suspected Tuberculosis Case

If an airborne infectious disease, such as tuberculosis, is suspected, information sharing among the staff involved is important. The doctor should immediately inform the nurse who, subsequently, will prepare for the needed disinfection protocol. This way, the next procedures can be carried out smoothly. At our hospital, if tuberculosis is suspected, the doctor informs the head nurse at the time of scheduling the procedure. The head nurse informs the nurse in charge the day before the procedure. On the day itself, this information is disseminated among the nursing staff in the morning in order to make the necessary precautions in avoiding contact with other patients. The nurse in charge wears an N95 mask before greeting a patient.

30.4.1.3 Responding to Health-Care Workers Exposed to Tuberculosis

In cases where in air precautions were not done because tuberculosis was not initially suspected, but bronchial lavage culture shows *Mycobacterium tuberculosis*, all the staff involved during the procedure are considered to have been exposed to the bacterium and should be advised close follow-up. All exposed staff should be reported to the hospital infection control office and should undergo a T-spot TB test or a chest X-ray examination.

30.4.1.4 Management of the Bronchoscope and Peripheral Equipment

After sufficient washing, the bronchoscope is placed under high-level disinfection. The peripheral equipment and the surrounding environment also require appropriate cleaning.

Bibliography

1. Asano F, Miyazawa T. Kikanshi-kyo best technique. Tokyo: Chugai Igakusha; 2012.
2. Fukuoka M, Tsuchiya R. Nihon Kokyuki Naishikyo Gakkai, editors. Kikanshi-kyo Rinshoi no Tameno Technique to Gazo Shindan. 2008:18.
3. Inoue T, editor. Bena Kango Care no Rinsho-chi Kodo-shitsutsu Kangaeru-koto. Tokyo: Igaku Shoin; 2005.
4. Miyawaki M, editor. Shin-taikei Kangogaku Zensho; Kiso Kango-gaku 4; Rinsho Kango Soron. Tokyo: Medical Friend Co. Ltd; 2012. p. 2–18.
5. Nihon Iryo Fukushi Setsubi Kyokai, editor. Byoin Setsubi Sekkei Guideline (Kucho Setsubi Hen). 2013.
6. Kyokai NK, editor. Shimpan Kangogaku no Kihonteki Sekimu (Teigi Gainen, Kihonho, Rinri). Tokyo: Nihon Kango Kyoukai Shuppannkai; 2009.
7. Nihon Kokyuki Naishikyo Gakkai, editor. Shokaki Naishikyo no Kansen Seigyo ni Kansuru Multi Society Guideline. 2012.
8. Nihon Kokyuki Naishikyo Gakkai Anzen Taisaku Iinkai, editor. Tegakisho Kokyuki Naishikyo Shinryo wo Anzen ni Okonautameni. 2013. pp. 18–21.
9. Nihon Shokaki Naishikyo Gishikai Kango Iinkai, editor. Shokaki Naishikyo Kango Gyomu Kijun; Naishikyo Kensa Chiryo ni Okeru Kango Gyomu Kijun. 2008.
10. Nomura K, Hiraide A, editors. Gan Kango Jissen Series 3 Hai-gan. Tokyo: Medical Friend Co. Ltd; 2007.
11. Omi A, et al. Kikanshi-kyo Kensa no Kango. Kokyuki Care. 2005;3(5), pp. 562–567.
12. Otsuki A, Sasada S. Kikanshi-kyo Kensa no Jumbi ya Monitoring ha Dosuruno? Kokyuki Care. 2014;12(7), pp. 109–113.
13. Tatsuta M, Wakabayashi E, Tone T, editors. Tenitoru-yoni Nagarega Tsukameru Shokaki Naishikyo Kango. Kyoto: Kimpodo; 2011.

MIX
Papier aus verantwortungsvollen Quellen
Paper from responsible sources
FSC® C105338

If you have any concerns about our products,
you can contact us on
ProductSafety@springernature.com

In case Publisher is established outside the EU,
the EU authorized representative is:
Springer Nature Customer Service Center GmbH
Europaplatz 3, 69115 Heidelberg, Germany

Printed by Libri Plureos GmbH
in Hamburg, Germany